Immune
Resilience

Immune
Resilience

The Breakthrough Plan to
Protect Your Body and Fight Disease

ROMILLY HODGES,
MS, CNS, CDN

AVERY
an imprint of Penguin Random House
New York

AVERY

an imprint of Penguin Random House LLC
penguinrandomhouse.com

Most Avery books are available at special quantity discounts for bulk purchase for sales promotions,
premiums, fund-raising, and educational needs. Special books or book excerpts also can be
created to fit specific needs. For details, write SpecialMarkets@penguinrandomhouse.com.

ISBN (hardcover) 9780593330838
ISBN (ebook) 9780593330845

Printed in the United States of America
1st Printing

Book design by Laura K. Corless

This book is dedicated to all those who lost their lives or loved ones as a result of COVID-19. And to those who still struggle with its aftereffects.

And to I, H, D, M, and K. Without you this book would not exist.

———————————

The author will donate a portion of her proceeds from Immune Resilience *to organization(s) supporting immune-related research.*

CONTENTS

||||||||||||||||||||||||||||||||||

CONTENTS

CONTENTS

Why Do You Need Immune Resilience?

wasn't always a nutritionist. In my "previous life," I was a research analyst (research has always been my happy place) at a business and technology think tank—pretty much as far away from nutrition as you can get. It was my job to gather information about current business practices, understand the complex, evolving landscape of business technology, synthesize trends, and communicate them back out to our executive members across the globe. Then at age twenty-eight, I had my first child—a wonderful bundle of joy—who struggled with digestive issues from the get-go, including reflux and abdominal pain as an infant, then head-to-toe eczema as a toddler. Everyday things caused skin irritation and hives, even the simple tasks of washing hands, walking through grass barefoot, or eating raw fruits or vegetables. A referral to an allergist helped me understand that all these issues were immune-related. Or, more specifically, driven by an immune malfunction: a riled-up immune system that was misinterpreting normally benign, everyday things as threats.

During this period, other than conventional medication recommendations such as steroid creams, the only guidance I received for my child was avoidance of those things that provoked an unwanted immune response. No expert I saw had any answers to my recurring questions: How did this come to be? How could we prevent this from getting even worse? What could we do to help restore immune tolerance? Without much to go on, I decided to turn my research skills to finding these answers. And what I found was a whole world of potential new understanding of how our immune system works, what it does for us, what keeps it in balance and strong, and what can weaken it.

Through my online sleuthing, and the assistance of a kind, functional medicine-in-training physician, I learned enough to resolve the eczema and dial down the environmental reactions. We added anti-inflammatory, kid-friendly smoothies, vitamin D, fish oil, and probiotics. We identified and removed trigger foods that were causing the eczema outbreaks, but I didn't really understand *how* these were helping. I wanted to know more about supporting immune resilience, and even perhaps ward off what's known as *atopic march*—the progression in over 50 percent of children with allergic conditions from food allergy to hay fever to asthma, and even increasingly another challenging immune disease called eosinophilic esophagitis (an inflammatory condition of the esophagus that can make it hard to swallow). Another nagging thought grew at the back of my mind: if my family was going through this, then there must be others—children, adolescents, adults—suffering with an immune system gone simultaneously haywire and vulnerable who would benefit from knowing what I was discovering.

In my early thirties, I went back to school and got a master's degree in human nutrition. I learned from expert teachers in functional medicine about systems biochemistry, which explains the underlying biological mechanisms that either improve or hinder health, i.e., what *causes* things like our immune system to either work well or not. After I graduated, I worked to complete my supervised hours for board and state certification, and I learned from experienced, groundbreaking physicians and doctorate-level practitioners who were themselves educators of physicians and other clinicians about the biochemistry of our immune system and how to work with dietary and lifestyle inputs to improve resilience. I completed certification through the Institute for Functional Medicine, which teaches practitioners how to harness evidence-based dietary and lifestyle strategies to address the root causes of health and disease. With my ongoing interest in immune health, I continued to build my knowledge of the intricacies of our elaborate defense system, how it must learn to respond appropriately to every new substance it encounters from the moment we're born (no small feat!), and how easily it can get derailed by our modern lifestyles. Then in practice, I worked (for many years) in an interdisciplinary team of physicians and nutritionists, providing comprehensive dietary and lifestyle care to hundreds of "ticked off" and struggling immune systems—my most powerful teachers of all.

I helped my child, who is still, so far, free of eczema, hay fever, asthma, and other day-to-day immune symptoms, and I hope to help all of you reading this book understand that there is so much you can do to alter how strong your immune system is and how it behaves. By helping my own child, and now helping others through my clinical practice, I have seen it's not so hard to do, as long as you know *what* to do.

And today, unexpected natural events have shown just how important it is to do it. At the very moment of writing this book, the role of immune health has been thrust fully into the spotlight by SARS-CoV-2, the virus behind the COVID-19 pandemic. SARS-CoV-2 has made its way to nearly every country, and infected hundreds of millions of people—all mothers, fathers, sisters, brothers, children. Sadly, it has taken millions of lives, too. Several times during the pandemic, COVID-19 became the leading cause of death in the United States (as measured by daily rates). It became the third leading cause of death for 2020 as a whole. This situation, never experienced before in our lifetimes, has driven home just how vulnerable our densely populated, hyper-connected society is to highly contagious new diseases.

Before COVID-19, most of us in more developed countries thought of infectious pathogens as a relatively minor inconvenience, though still one we'd rather avoid. Or at least prefer to move through relatively easily. Symptoms of an infection like congestion, vomiting, diarrhea, itching, or fever can make us feel miserable. They can keep us off work or disrupt vacation and leisure plans. They can interrupt important societal care structures if, for instance, you have small children or elderly parents that need you, or other friends and family that rely on your support. They can cause embarrassment if they are prominently displayed like skin infections. Rarely they can be life-threatening, although with COVID-19 and growing drug-resistant pathogens this rarity is unfortunately diminishing. Even before COVID-19, infectious diseases accounted for 15.5 million physician consults per year and cost an estimated $120 billion annually in US health care expenditures and lost productivity. The flu virus alone is estimated to cost around $10 billion in direct medical costs and $77 billion in indirect costs per year.

But how to combat these invisible threats? The microbes that cause infectious diseases are too small for us to see them coming. We generally have no idea when and how we're going to be exposed—on our daily commute, at school, at lunchtime, on vacation, even at (yes) hospitals and other medical care facilities. And aside from popping some vitamin C during flu season, maybe some zinc and echinacea, most of us just let our immune system get on with it and hope that medical help will rescue us if an illness gets out of hand.

The trouble is that the right kind of medical help *isn't* always there, even if you're lying in one of the best hospitals, surrounded by the best doctors in the world. SARS-CoV-2 laid clear the reality that we don't have ready and waiting medicines to prevent and treat all infections. Even the medicines we do have are being blunted by the ongoing spread of drug-resistant germs (microbes like some bacteria that are no longer defeated by today's antibiotics). Prescription guidelines that are rightly changing to reduce the use of pharmaceutical antimicrobials against minor infections, to try to reduce the risk of provoking drug resistance, mean that the use of medicines against infections will be dialed back further still. There is also an increasing recognition that, in individuals with vulnerable immune systems (of which there are a growing number), infections can persist beyond the acute phase into chronic "syndromes" that significantly impact quality of life and productivity. Several are implicated in the development of autoimmune diseases, where the immune system is triggered into misdirecting its fire toward the body's own cells.

Of course, none of us can ever completely avoid getting sick. No amount of science has shown that we can do that. However—and there is no doubt about this—if we want to give ourselves the best chance of fending off and successfully weathering infectious bugs, and reduce our need for medicines in the first place, we need to start with a strong, resilient immune system. Science shows that how we choose to eat and live can affect how well our immune system operates. By making better choices, we can support our in-built, sophisticated defenses that protect us against an attack by harmful bacteria, viruses, parasites, or fungi. And we can improve our ability to weather the "storm" of an infection when we do get sick.

SIGNS OF A WEAKENED IMMUNE SYSTEM

Perhaps you're wondering just how you'll know if you need to pay attention to your immune health. In other words, is your immune system already resilient or not? Well, the first thing to know is that it's a good idea for *all of us* to pay attention to our immune system. And even though this book mainly focuses on immune resilience against *infections,* it's important to know that through supporting immune resilience, we're supporting overall health, too, since most of today's chronic conditions involve some form of dysfunctional immune activity that can trigger and perpetuate the disease process.

Of course, there are more specific indicators that your immune system needs some help. The most obvious indication is getting frequent infections. Perhaps you're always catching colds or have chronic sinusitis or laryngitis, recurrent urinary tract infections, or other infections that are hard to shift. Perhaps you need antibiotics more than twice per year, or get two or more severe infections like bronchitis or pneumonia per year, both of which can be considered examples of above-normal rates of infection. But there are other potential indicators still. Any of the following may mean your immune system operations are being hampered:

- *You don't regularly eat "healthy" foods or a balanced diet.* Your immune system, like other systems in your body, relies on a steady input of vital nutrients to do its job. Poor food choices can also compromise immune function just as much as nutrient deficiencies.

- *You're under significant stress.* Stress tanks immune resilience. It's one of the reasons we can more readily get sick during stressful events such as exams or big work deadlines.

- *You don't exercise regularly.* Exercise is great for immune health. When you're not regularly physically active, your immune system suffers and resilience drops.

- *You're not sleeping well.* Poor sleep is another sign that your immune system may be compromised, since sleep is an important time for your immune system to be active in surveillance as well as in the clearance of potentially harmful germs.

- *You have digestive issues.* Much of your immune system is located in your digestive tract. Having recurrent diarrhea, constipation, or gas and bloating can be signs that things are not well in your gut, and that may be harming your immune defenses.

- *You have low energy or brain fog.* Energy and a healthy immune system go hand in hand. When your immune system struggles, you can often feel your energy tank as resources get diverted toward the immune system's latest fight.

- *You struggle with low mood.* Just like it affects your energy, a poorly functioning, overstressed immune system can zap your mood. Higher levels of inflammation produced by a stressed immune system have also been linked with feelings of depression and anxiety.

- *You've got eczema, allergies, an autoimmune disease, or other immune-related conditions.* A misfiring immune system that inappropriately attacks things that it should consider "safe" is a sign that it's overstressed, dysregulated, and vulnerable to other mistakes.

- *Your wounds don't heal quickly.* Your immune system is involved in repairing your body after injury. Delayed wound healing indicates your immune system isn't as responsive as it should be.

- *You have one or more chronic diseases.* Inflammation, one of the hallmarks of a poorly functioning immune system, is causatively linked with nearly all major chronic diseases including diabetes, heart disease, stroke, dementia, and cancer. Chronic diseases may also increase the risk for more severe infectious disease, as has been seen with COVID-19.

- *You're aging.* Join the club! Your immune system will decline in function as you grow older, and needs taking care of to help preserve and retain healthy levels of immunity for as long as possible.

How Our Immune System Changes with Age

Medical professionals understand that our immune system loses its effectiveness as we age. There's a scientific term for this: *immunosenescence*. As we get older, we are less able to produce as many immune cells as before, our thymus gland (one of the important immune cell "training grounds") shrinks in size, and our immune responses in general get more sluggish and even dysfunctional. This is why vaccines are less effective in older individuals, why *varicella zoster* virus often resurfaces as shingles as we age, and why 75 percent of flu-related deaths are in adults over sixty-five years of age. It's estimated that around 20 percent of us are living with some level of compromised immune status due to aging.

Older individuals do have a secret weapon, however: Time gives immune systems more experience of different bugs, so older age means more naturally built-up immunity, i.e., more stored cellular memory for dealing with harmful germs. So, if you happen to get sick while your also-exposed mother or grandmother doesn't, that's a likely reason.

YOU HAVE MORE INFLUENCE OVER YOUR IMMUNE RESILIENCE THAN YOU THINK

Have you ever really stopped to think about why infectious diseases don't affect everyone they encounter in the same way? Some people can fight off infections with just minor symptoms, while others really suffer. Not everyone who catches a serious infection dies; fatality rates from any one disease are always less than 100 percent. Even for the legendary bubonic plague in the fourteenth century, half of those who contracted it survived. This illustrates clearly that there are differences between each of our defense systems that change the course and outcome of an infection. What's tremendously exciting is that a great many of these differences are responsive to environmental cues—that is, it is within our ability to change them and to improve how our immune system functions. We can build *resilience*. We just need to know how.

As you read through this book, that is exactly what you'll discover. This isn't simply a book about classic nutrients for immune function (although those are important and are covered, too). Instead, you'll find a comprehensive view of all the natural dietary and lifestyle influencers and interventions that you can use to improve your immune defenses.

In the following chapters, you're going to learn what you need to optimize your immune resilience fully. I'm going to show you how to incorporate everyday nutrition strategies through the Immune Resilience Diet, as well as exercise, clean living, sleep, stress reduction, and nature. You'll learn about less considered aspects of immune function such as having healthy physical barriers like our skin, respiratory tract, and gut, and the roles that beneficial microbes play. You'll also read about how modifiable underlying health conditions affect immune function and can be improved with diet and lifestyle strategies. And this is all based on the latest scientific evidence and cutting-edge clinical application.

Why do we have to cover so much ground in this book? Can't I just pop some extra vitamin C and be done? Well, sure. But it's not going to get you very far on its own. If we take some vitamin C, but our immune system is compromised in other areas—say our microbiome is off, we have eczema, we're eating tons of pro-inflammatory foods, and we're only getting six hours of sleep per night—just taking the single nutrient is like plugging only one hole of many in a leaky bucket. The bucket still isn't going to be able to do its job well. Human beings are complicated! Or sophisticated, more like. We have to consider all the angles if we truly want to build immune resilience.

As you read this book, I hope you develop a profound appreciation for the vast machinery that is our immune system, like I have, and the broad spectrum of influencing factors. In addition to being evidence based, these recommendations are uncomplicated, widely accessible, and have a long, long history of safe use. Applying all this knowledge and practical guidance within these pages will set you up to master how to have your immune system working at its very best.

OTHER HAPPY SIDE EFFECTS OF TAKING CARE OF YOUR IMMUNE SYSTEM

Although this book focuses on restoring and optimizing our own natural resilience against harmful germs, there are many other benefits that come with having a solid immune system. *For one, you'll help improve your energy, mental clarity, and general feelings of well-being.* When we don't take care of our immune system, we also don't feel our best. A sluggish or upset immune system generates inflammation, and this can impact energy, cognitive function, mood, sleep, productivity, and more. *Second, you will be helping restore balance in a system that may have a tendency toward other immune conditions like allergy or autoimmunity.* More than 50 million Americans suffer from some form of an allergy, where the immune system mistakenly attacks something external that should ordinarily be benign, like a food, pollen, or animal dander. And more than 24 million Americans have one or more autoimmune diseases. *You will also be guarding yourself against one of the most fundamental mechanisms common to nearly all chronic diseases: inflammation.* Chronic inflammation—an immune response that has been strongly implicated as a driver behind the majority of chronic diseases including diabetes, metabolic syndrome, heart disease, stroke, asthma, mood disorders, and dementia—affects 6 in 10 American adults. *You will also be helping your body fight against cancer cells.* One in three of us will get cancer at some point in our lives, acknowledged to be in part driven by chronic inflammation as well as a failure of the immune system to do its job of finding and eliminating budding cancer cells. So, although this book is focused primarily on building immune resilience against infectious disease, building a strong, balanced immune system is also the right place to start counteracting these other, really important immune concerns.

HOW TO USE THIS BOOK

Use this book as a guide, a reference tool, a roadmap builder. You'll get the most out of it by reading through the arguments for why we should build immune resilience and understanding the inner workings of our immune systems enough to get just how tied in nutrition and lifestyle can be to its effectiveness. Once you have this connected knowledge, it's my hope that you'll find that the motivation to make improvements for yourself and your loved ones comes effortlessly.

The principles and resources in this book are also my go-tos for foundational health and a strong immune system. You'll find that the vast majority of the recommendations in this book are "broad spectrum," in the sense that they are supportive against many different kinds of infections. And ideal as support both before and during illness. You'll also find specific natural interventions for unique situations such as skin infections, excess mucus, oral infections, cough, stomach upset, and more. Last but not least, you'll find recipes I hope will inspire you to enjoy looking after your immune system.

Of course, this book isn't intended to be a replacement for appropriate medical care when it's needed. For moderate to severe infections, or if your immune system is compromised due to medications or other conditions, or even if you're feeling at all unsure of how serious your condition is, it's always best to seek medical guidance. It does, however, give you options that may make it less likely you'll need that medical care in the first place, and even support the effectiveness of that care if and when you do need it. Let's face it: it's not like we can tell which known and unknown pathogens we're going to be exposed to in the future; the COVID-19 pandemic surely taught us that. Working on your immune system at this level gives you the best means of improving your defenses against *any* type of harmful microbe and improving your chances of living a long and healthy life.

Ready to get resilient?

To view the references cited in this chapter, please visit www.immuneresilienceplan.com/science.

Immune
Resilience

PART 1

Germs vs. Your Immune System

CHAPTER 1

Hidden Enemies Around Us

Humans have lived with infectious microbes since our very first beginnings and they have been, for most of our history, one of humanity's biggest preoccupations. Fortunately for us, modern science has had many shining successes against infections. To understand these successes, as well as our ongoing vulnerabilities to pathogens, we need to look at where we've come from, and where we are now.

Louis Pasteur's "germ theory," which originated in the 1870s, marked the dawn of our modern-day approach to microbes by illuminating for the first time the immense landscape of microscopic infectious pathogens that were behind the most problematic diseases of the time. It was a turning point after which medics and scientists began to develop and use hygiene principles and antimicrobial agents to prevent infection. Improvements in sanitation, water treatment, and pasteurization that were subsequently adopted have saved millions of lives and are still vital today. But despite these advances, the leading causes of death in the early 1900s remained infectious diseases, especially pneumonia and tuberculosis. Smallpox, cholera, diphtheria, and polio were also widespread. Average life span was just forty to fifty years in part because childhood infections were frequently fatal, and infections we now consider minor could lead to sepsis and death.

Against this background, it's no wonder that the first licensed vaccines in 1914, and first widely distributed antibiotics in 1928, were hailed as miracles of modern medicine. The decades that followed World War II were a golden age for vaccine and antibiotic development, culminating in the complete eradication of smallpox, near-eradication of polio, and the ability for people to live their lives unencumbered by the fear of catching diseases that could cause paralysis, brain damage, blindness, and death. The control over infectious diseases was such that their cumulative mortality rates dropped from 797 to just 36 per 100,000 people per year between 1900 and 1980. This allowed scientific and medical attention to shift to what then seemed like more pressing concerns: chronic diseases such as heart disease, diabetes, and cancer.

Aside from the tremendous difference that these medical advances made, what's also remarkable about this is that it is only relatively recently in human history, and only really in industrialized countries, that infectious diseases have taken a back seat. Of course, COVID-19 thrust infections back to the forefront, highlighting the potential for new pathogens to emerge and wreak havoc across the world. Prior to that, though, it's arguably in part down to sheer luck that prior outbreaks such as SARS and Ebola never completely took hold on our shores. And these emerging diseases are not the only reason for growing concern and interest in new antimicrobial solutions. There's increasing recognition that some pathogens can contribute to chronic symptoms and the chronic diseases that we normally consider separate from infectious ones. The scientific community is also sounding alarm bells over the ever-growing incidence of antimicrobial resistance. COVID-19 dramatically changed the collective concern around infectious diseases. But the reality is that protecting ourselves against infectious disease has always been important. The current world of infectious, disease-causing microbes is still quite vast.

TODAY'S INFECTIOUS MICROBES

The primary types of infection-causing microbes are bacteria, viruses, parasites, and fungi.

BACTERIA

Bacteria are independently living, single-celled organisms that are generally large enough to be identified under a light microscope. Most bacterial infections can be successfully treated with antibiotics. Common types of bacteria that can cause human infection when they proliferate are staphylococci and streptococci. Normally, these infections are localized at a particular site in the body, such as the throat, gums, sinuses, ears, lungs, skin, urinary tract, digestive tract, or genitals, but if they infect the blood, it causes a widespread infection called *septicemia*. Rarely, bacteria can cross into the central nervous system and cause meningitis. Other types of bacteria include *Borrelia burgdorferi*, which can cause Lyme disease. Harmful bacteria are also the cause of most instances of food poisoning.

VIRUSES

Viruses are much smaller than bacteria and operate quite differently. They cannot exist independently since they don't have their own cellular structure; instead, they are tiny fragments of genetic code that must insert themselves into the living cells of humans or other organisms (including bacteria) in order to survive. They can infect any part of the body. Viruses cannot be treated with antibiotics, and there are relatively few antiviral drugs available. Common types of human-infecting viruses are flu viruses (influenzae); cold viruses (such as adenoviruses or coronaviruses); varicella zoster virus, which causes chicken pox and shingles; herpes simplex viruses; Epstein-Barr virus, which causes mononucleosis; and cytomegalovirus. New viral strains have emerged as potential, serious threats in recent years, including severe acute respiratory syndrome (SARS-CoV-1 and SARS-CoV-2, the latter virus the cause of COVID-19), Middle East respiratory syndrome (MERS), Ebola, West Nile virus, and Zika virus.

FUNGI

Fungi can exist as simple celled organisms or branching structures made up of several cells. Fungal infections can occur at any location of the body and can usually be treated with antifungal medications. Fungal infections are usually relatively mild, such as skin ringworm, athlete's foot, oral thrush, or vaginal candidiasis. However, rarely, and particularly in people whose immune systems are compromised, fungal infections can compromise essential organ functions and become life-threatening. Valley Fever, caused by *Coccidioides* fungi, is one example of this.

PARASITES

Most parasitic infections affect people living in tropical and subtropical countries, but several can also occur in Europe, North America, and other parts of the world. Parasites range in size from those visible only with a microscope to those that are visible even to the naked eye. Intestinal parasites that are relatively common in the United States include pinworm (*Enterobius vermicularis*), hookworm (*Ancylostoma duodenale* and *Necator americanus*), *Giardia lamblia,* and *Entamoeba histolytica.*

MICROBES WITH INSIDIOUS EFFECTS

In addition to the acute effects they can cause, there is another, more insidious side of infectious diseases known to occur in those who suffer later or long-term effects from infections. These can occur well beyond the first acute stage of illness in one of three ways:

Reactivation after a period of dormancy: Herpes simplex virus type 1, for example, which can cause cold sores around the mouth, can lie dormant in the facial nerves only to later reactivate and cause new outbreaks during a period when the immune system is weakened. Varicella zoster, the virus that can cause chicken pox, lies dormant in the body after the initial infection and can become active again many years later to cause shingles (herpes zoster), a painful, blistering skin rash. Reactivations usually occur when the immune system is compromised. Sometimes medications compromise our immune system. Other times, our immune system can be compromised by stress, poor diet, or aging.

Chronic infection "syndromes": Several infections can produce long-term symptoms lasting months or years after an initial infection in some (but not all) infected individuals, often baffling medical doctors and leading to clusters of symptoms described as syndromes. Symptoms can range from fatigue, brain fog, headache, sleep disturbance, and pains to digestive issues and more. Sometimes these are mild and manageable. Other times they can significantly impact quality of life and work productivity. Epstein-Barr virus (a member of the herpes virus family that by some estimates up to 90 percent of us have encountered, and that can cause mononucleosis or "mono"), human herpesvirus-6, and *Borrelia burgdorferi* and other tick-borne illnesses can all lead to persistent symptoms in some individuals. As can SARS-CoV-2: *long COVID* is the term that was quickly adopted for chronic COVID-19 symptoms lasting more than a few weeks.

Contribution to other chronic diseases: Some delayed effects of infections can relate to diseases we normally think of as noncommunicable, or "chronic" diseases. Latent *Chlamydia pneumoniae,* a major cause of bacterial pneumonia and bronchitis, for instance, is thought to be able to promote arterial plaque formation and potentially contribute to heart disease due to its ability to enter the bloodstream and settle in other sites such as the lining of blood vessels. Epstein-Barr virus is implicated in triggering some autoimmune diseases and increases the risk for certain types of cancer. Herpes simplex, the virus type that causes cold sores and genital herpes, is implicated in the later development of some instances of dementia and Alzheimer's disease. Almost all cervical cancers, as well as some genital cancers and cancers of the throat, are caused by human papillomavirus infections.

Infections and Autoimmune Disease

Several microbial infections are thought to play a role in the development of autoimmune disease in susceptible individuals. What makes someone susceptible isn't yet well defined but is understood to include a combination of genetics, environment (i.e., diet and lifestyle factors), and an immune system that is already under stress and not fully resilient. Some potential infectious triggers implicated in autoimmune diseases include:

- *Type 1 diabetes:* rotaviruses, rubella, influenza, mumps.
- *Rheumatoid arthritis:* Porphyromonas gingivalis (a common cause of oral gingivitis), *Escherichia coli,* Epstein-Barr virus.
- *Systemic lupus erythematosus (lupus):* Epstein-Barr virus, parvovirus B19, cytomegalovirus, hepatitis C virus.
- *Sjögren's syndrome:* Epstein-Barr virus, herpes simplex virus, hepatitis C virus.
- *Autoimmune thyroid disease:* Epstein-Barr virus, *Yersinia enterocolitica, Bartonella henselae,* influenza, herpes viruses, hepatitis C virus.
- *Multiple sclerosis:* Epstein-Barr virus, *Mycoplasma pneumoniae, Chlamydia pneumoniae.*

Emerging data also implicate SARS-CoV-2 in the development of autoimmune reactions.

PATHOGEN RESISTANCE TO CURRENT MEDICINES

In addition to the acute and long-term health effects of infections, one of the biggest threats to our control of harmful microbes is antimicrobial resistance. Resistance occurs when a bacteria, virus, fungi, or parasite changes in a way that makes it unharmed by the medications we normally use to kill them. This renders them much more difficult to treat, and in some cases not treatable at all—these microbes are known as "superbugs." Current examples of resistant microbes include certain species of *Staphy-*

lococcus ("staph"), *Salmonella*, tuberculosis, *Candida*, and *Clostridioides difficile* ("*C. diff*"). Our exposure to these bugs can occur through foods, plants, animals, soil, air, other people, and public places, especially (and unfortunately) health centers.

Antibiotics, for example, used to be a trusted tool against bacterial infections, but now medical professionals are seeing increasing antibiotic resistance from more and more bacterial types. More than 2.8 million people in the US become sick due to antibiotic-resistant bacteria each year, at a cost of over $55 billion annually, and the number is growing. Just one of several drug-resistant bacteria, methicillin-resistant *Staphylococcus aureus* (MRSA), kills more Americans annually than emphysema, HIV/AIDS, Parkinson's disease, and homicide combined. These bacteria can cause resistant infections of the urinary tract, intestines, lungs, and other organs.

The reasons behind this increase in resistant microbes are several, but all come down to the fact that higher medicine usage rates mean a higher chance that bugs develop resistance. Recent data from the US Centers for Disease Control and Prevention (CDC) show that we are prescribed an equivalent of 838 antibiotics per 1,000 people in the United States each year. The vast majority are prescribed by primary care physicians for respiratory infections, many of which are actually viral rather than bacterial and therefore not treatable with antibiotics. This kind of overuse in medical, and also veterinary, practice has accelerated the resistance problem. Improper use, such as dosing too low, or stopping a course of antibiotics early is also problematic, since it increases the chance that the harmful bacteria survive the treatment and develop the capability to resist the medication.

Another driver has been the widespread preventive use of antibiotics in livestock and fish farming. In fact, the total agricultural use of antibiotics *exceeds human use*. Approximately 60 percent of the antibiotics used in food production are the same antibiotics that we rely on to prevent or resolve human infections, making the risk to human health even greater.

Compounding the problem is the stark reality that the development pipeline for new antimicrobial medications is concerningly thin. While around one new human infectious disease is discovered each year, there haven't been any entirely new classes of antibiotics discovered since the 1980s. Most antibiotics used today were identified during the 1940s to 1960s. One reason for this is that it's just not that attractive a business model for private enterprises. To develop one new antibiotic, there's the high cost of development, over $1.5 billion by some estimates. Then there's the problem that new drugs have a high risk of being soon rendered ineffective due to new antimicrobial resistance. This means that new drugs either have a blunted life span or they have to be used sparingly in order to preserve their effectiveness.

Although many experts are working on trying to solve these problems, the outlook for our continued ability to control harmful bacteria with medications is still shaky. The World Bank estimates that, without new drug breakthroughs, antimicrobial resistance could cause up to 10 million deaths per year by 2050. Other estimates are similarly bleak. Scientists have called the situation "desperate," and "one of the most pressing threats to human health." The reality for us as individuals is the growing threat of catching a germ that can't be treated medically, and that the use of antimicrobial medications will have to be increasingly reserved only for the most needed situations. It's likely that milder infections will increasingly be left to run their natural courses without pharmaceutical antimicrobial treatment.

THE UNIQUE PROBLEM OF EMERGING VIRUSES

While most nonresistant bacterial infections can, for now, still be countered by antibiotics, relatively few *antiviral* drugs exist. Have you ever wondered why? The answer lies in the different way that viruses are structured and operate. Viruses, without their own complete cellular structures, rely on their ability to "break into" their host's cells, incidentally through pathways already used by essential biochemical molecules, and hijack that cell's operational machinery—machinery that includes DNA or RNA replication (a way to reproduce genetic information) so the virus can make lots of copies of itself to send out to infect other cells. This overlap between viral functions and normal cell operations means that most of the viral targets that drugs could attempt to block would simultaneously block functions critical to our own healthy cells. It's not just that killing viruses is hard. The challenge is to kill viruses *without harming our own cells*. It's not all doom and gloom, though. There have been some notable antiviral successes such as for human immunodeficiency virus (HIV), hepatitis B, and hepatitis C—but standard medical care for most viruses is to treat the symptoms only until the individual's immune system (hopefully) dispenses with the unwelcome invader.

Vaccines have been our best defense against some viruses; the measles vaccine, for instance, is 97 percent effective at preventing infection to this highly contagious disease. However, for many other viruses, it's much harder to develop effective vaccines in part because, as the virus replicates, it churns out mutated copies of itself that then form different strains of the original virus. Vaccines developed to target one strain don't automatically work against others. Influenza (flu) viruses, for example, develop new strains each year, which makes predicting vaccine targets challenging and is why flu vaccine effectiveness rates as low as 40 percent to 50 percent are still considered a success.

During the COVID-19 pandemic, the unprecedented collaboration and effort within the scientific community led to an astoundingly fast vaccine development timeline—less than one year. Prior to this, vaccine development has otherwise typically taken ten to fifteen years. Yet even with the record-breaking development time achieved for SARS-CoV-2 vaccines, the virus still had free rein to cause chaos and suffering for a good while, and it's not yet clear how the virus's ability to mutate will influence vaccine effectiveness and development need going forward. It's also not clear whether we'll be able to replicate this accelerated vaccine development for other pathogens.

Unfortunately, although the COVID-19 pandemic has been the worst the world has seen in more than one hundred years, experts warn that more pandemics are likely in the future. And that potential pandemic-causing infections are emerging at a faster rate. Urban spread and the encroachment on wildlife habitats means closer contact with wild animals, which increases the chance of infections passing from other species to humans. Population growth and frequent travel make it easy for infections to travel rapidly through communities and from country to country. Changing climate conditions due to global warming mean that disease-carrying insects like mosquitoes will naturally spread into new geographic areas. Milder winters mean fewer deer ticks dying off each year in areas where Lyme disease is endemic, leading to greater numbers come spring-time and increased risk for human transmission.

With the battle against infectious disease taking new turns, it demands our renewed attention. Even as the scientific community works to solve these challenges through vaccines and new antimicrobials, we are not com-pletely helpless: Optimizing our own immune resilience is an important, complementary endeavor. In fact, in our evolutionary struggle to survive in a world full of potentially harmful and devious germs, it's our immune sys-tem that has been our constant stalwart. And now, with the real potential of pandemics, superbugs, and the threat of losing our antimicrobial lifelines, we need it more than ever. The next step in understanding how to do that is to build a fundamental appreciation of how our incredible immune system works. It's time for a tour of our immune biology.

To view the references cited in this chapter, please visit
www.immuneresilienceplan.com/science.

CHAPTER 2

What Makes an Immune System Resilient?

There are things so precious in life that people would do anything to keep them safe. Like your family, for instance. There are lots of different ways you can choose to do that, and most likely you're going to use several of them at any one time. You can live in a well-built house with state-of-the-art locks, perhaps a fence around the yard, maybe a sensor-triggered yard light, a dog or an alarm or home monitoring system. Of course, you can't keep them locked up at home all the time if you want your kids to grow up and lead productive lives. So you train them—not to talk to strangers, not to go down dark alleys late at night, have them memorize emergency numbers, maybe take a self-defense class. You give them a phone so that they can reach out in an emergency. In addition, you observe that they learn from their experiences, and the experiences of others, like not to touch that hot pan, to keep their bike locked up, to use antivirus software on their computer, even to stand up to the schoolyard bully.

This system of multiple safety measures and learning is much like your immune system. All through your body you also have a sophisticated network of defenses that keep you safe from harmful germs. It's a combination of structures, communications networks, biochemical weapons and offense tactics, specialized cells, training camps, and even alliances that handle the billions of germs that bombard your body every single day—germs so tiny that you can't see them with the naked eye. These include up to 1 billion microbes in and on your food and between 10,000 and 1 million microbes you breathe in daily (!). Then there's what we come in contact with on everything we touch—our hands carry between 40,000 to over 4 million bacteria at any one time. If you're an average healthy person, these germs won't make you sick. And the reason for that is your always-on, silently efficient immune system. It is one of the most sophisticated and complex systems in your body.

When you first encounter an active pathogen, let's say a harmful virus or bacteria, competition begins immediately between your immune responses and the offending germ. Because the goal of the germ is to replicate and grow, and the goal of your immune system is to prevent that and eliminate the threat. Those germs we encounter can be pretty fierce. And persistent. And smart—so smart that they have adapted cunning ways to get past your barrier structures and sneak into your cells and bloodstream. Some have elaborate disguises, even occasionally using parts of your own cells to fool your immune system into thinking they are harmless. Some adopt a Trojan horse strategy, deliberately allowing themselves to be drawn into one of your own cells so that they can then travel to other places in your body without being noticed. Some can throw a monkey wrench into your immune cells' equipment, leaving them inoperative. Others can change their identity by mutating into different variations of the same bug to confuse your immune system and render any adaptive immune responses less effective. And, importantly, these bugs are masters at seizing an opportunity—after all, many harmful pathogens can actually be innocuously dormant long-term residents in our bodies, lying in wait until an opportunity to grow and proliferate presents itself.

So, as incredible as our immune system is, providing many layers of defense and being able to mount an effective response when attacked is no small task. Our immune system is dependable in many ways, but resilience is not always guaranteed. So, what makes the difference between an immune system that is resilient and one that leaves us vulnerable to disease? It is these six characteristics, all of which you're able to influence (for better or worse) through dietary and lifestyle choices:

1. IT IS SUPREMELY RESPONSIVE, ABLE TO RAMP UP AND DOWN RAPIDLY

It's not likely that you keep a team of armed guards in or around your house. That would be pretty expensive and not likely necessary unless you're a particular target of unwanted attention. But we can all call 911 for emergency assistance if and when we need it to deal with an intruder, a health emergency, or a fire. Your immune system does much the same thing. You don't need (or want) high numbers of immune cells to be active all the time, so when you are not fighting an infection, your immune system dials back the number of cells it has in circulation to just those necessary for surveillance.

But if there *is* a threat? Your immune system can't be caught short-handed. That's why, when it needs to, it has the ability to rapidly ramp up the production and deployment of millions of white blood cells, the hallmark cells of your immune system. And when this happens, you don't just get a single patrol car, ambulance, or fire truck, you get a whole army showing up at your door, ready to do battle if necessary. You get special forces cells with unique skills eager to put them to use. You get the clean-up crew, cells ready to clear away debris from any attack that takes place and mend collateral damage. You get a sophisticated management team, working to direct the whole operation and ensure that each army unit is doing what it should in coordination with the rest. As you might imagine, this requires an ultra-refined system of communication between immune components and a ready inventory of resources to draw from.

2. IT'S A GREAT COMMUNICATOR

Although your immune system may not always make itself known to you, among and within its different layers it must be able to communicate extremely well. After all, it's orchestrating a set of vastly complex operations, with many moving pieces, all of the time. However, unlike soldiers, your immune system doesn't have technological communications devices. Instead, it relies on two main types of communication—chemical messengers and cell-to-cell communication.

- *Chemical messengers:* Many "civilian" cells (what I call those not typically classified as immune cells) as well as immune cells communicate through their own language of chemical signals using a rich assemblage of molecular messengers such as cytokines, eicosanoids, kinins, and more. These act like words and phrases, telling other cells what to do. For instance, when one of your civilian cells detects incoming fire, it sends distress messengers that say, "Hey, I'm under attack over here. I need help!" These messengers disperse throughout your body and attach to the surface of immune cells at specific "receptor" sites. The receptor transmits the message into the cell, which then sets that cell's response into motion. There are hundreds of different kinds of chemical messenger types that your cells use for communication. These do everything from signaling alarm and attracting other cells to a site of injury and attack to ramping up cell production, fine-tuning immune responses, and more.

- *Cell-to-cell communication:* Cell-to-cell communication requires a temporary physical connection between two cells so that information can be transferred. This information might be a fragment of a bacteria, for instance, that one cell has picked up and that it wants to show to the part of your immune system that knows how to produce antibodies. (This is called *antigen presentation*.) Once those antibody-producing cells have "seen" the configuration of that bacterial fragment and been exposed to the corresponding chemical signals that provide the right "encouragement," they can begin making targeted antibodies.

3. IT CAN DISTINGUISH FRIEND FROM FOE

Imagine that your job was to identify an enemy, in disguise, in a crowd of hundreds of thousands of people. It would be supremely difficult, right? Well, that's just the scenario that your immune system deals with on an ongoing basis. Each day, your body encounters billions of different substances, from foods to dust particles to toxins to germs (both friendly and not so friendly kinds). And it needs to be able to survey each and every one of these particles to establish whether or not it is a threat.

How your immune system learns whether a substance is a threat or not is through an immensely important, complicated process that starts even before you are born. At that stage, your brand-new immune system is seeing everything for the first time and has to determine how to handle each substance, each different particle it finds. As we get older, there's less and less to learn, but our immune system still needs to stay on track with deciding what's safe and what's not.

As you can imagine, the process of discernment is fraught with risk. And when things go wrong, your immune system can turn from your best friend into your worst enemy. If your immune system accidentally earmarks a should-be-harmless substance like a food or pollen as a threat, you get what we know of as an allergic response. Essentially, your immune system starts attacking something it should consider harmless, even beneficial. A similar thing can happen with your own cells: if your immune system starts to think that some of your own cells are a threat, it can start mistakenly attacking those. That's what we call autoimmunity, the prefix *auto-* meaning "self." Autoimmunity is the process behind several diseases including type 1 diabetes, Hashimoto's thyroiditis, multiple sclerosis, rheumatoid arthritis, Crohn's disease, ulcerative colitis, and Sjögren's syndrome. That's why it's so important that your immune system gets this right.

While there is documentation going back thousands of years on their existence, allergies and autoimmunity have become much more prevalent in our modern era, and remarkably so in the last few decades. While it's hard to definitively prove the exact causes, it's clear that something (and science suggests likely multiple things) about the way we live our lives now can really mess with our immune systems.

4. IT NEVER FORGETS

One of the hallmarks of your immune system is its incredible ability to store all that learning as memory. One of the most well-known ways it does this is by generating targeted antibodies. These antibodies are typically unique to each germ (or other molecules such as pollen, in the case of hay fever), which is what makes them so effective. As your immune system encounters a potentially harmful new germ, it figures out (through a process of continual refinement) how to make antibodies that act specifically against that germ and then deploys them by the millions to circulate around your body. Your immune system stores copies of those antibodies in its memory—templates that can be used to form more antibodies rapidly the next time it encounters that same germ. This is what gives us near-lifelong immunity to certain diseases like measles or chickenpox, since the next time our immune system "sees" that germ, it whips out its antibodies and neutralizes it before you even start to feel sick. Scientists estimate that our immune system can generate and store antibodies to a quintillion (that's one million trillion) different germs. That's quite a library of stored memory!

Vaccines work by tapping into these same immunological memory capabilities. When you get a vaccine, you introduce a dead or weakened version of a germ (or, in the case of newer mRNA vaccines, the template for your own cells to make copies of germ fragments) into your system for your immune system to get a good look at. This prompts it to develop antibodies and to store them in your antibody memory library for future use.

5. A LITTLE BIT OF A BAD THING DOES YOUR IMMUNE SYSTEM GOOD

Here's something very important to understand about physiology and about your immune system: sometimes a little bit of something bad can be beneficial. This is a concept known as *hormesis*, where something known to be damaging at high doses is actually helpful when used in smaller quantities.

This concept at first might sound bizarre but consider this. Most likely, the way that you've grown throughout your life is through challenging yourself. Your teachers challenged you in school, your parents challenged you at home, your job may challenge you, too. I'm sure you've also challenged yourself when there's been something you really wanted to achieve. And, for the most part, out of those challenges comes personal growth. Learning. Development. Perhaps there have been times in your life when things have been *too* challenging, though, where you've been overwhelmed by the challenge and it hasn't gone well. All of this is hormesis—something that in small amounts can have a positive effect, but in large amounts can have a negative effect.

Hormesis applies to your health and your immune system, too. All kinds of things can cause hormetic biochemical responses, being helpful in the right doses, but harmful in large amounts. Exercise, stress, or fasting are a few examples. Some vaccines also operate via a hormetic-like mechanism, providing a mild stimulation of, or stress on, your immune system with something harmful in order to prompt the development of immune memory to a particular germ. Germs themselves, in your environment, can help strengthen your immunity as long as the challenge isn't too overwhelming for your defenses—as the German philosopher Friedrich Nietzsche dramatically declared, "what doesn't kill me makes me stronger." As you proceed through these chapters, I'll point out where certain similar inputs can be harnessed to create a beneficial, hormetic effect. Each can help to strengthen, train, or mature your immune system's activity toward optimal resilience.

6. IT NEITHER BURNS THE CANDLE AT BOTH ENDS NOR LETS THE FIRE GROW TOO BIG

Your immune system should be always alert, but not always in attack mode. Just as the lack of sleep from burning the candle at both ends eventually catches up with you, so it does with your immune system.

Attack mode is costly to our bodies. For two big reasons: It uses up significant amounts of nutrients and it causes collateral damage to your other cells—innocent bystanders in the vicinity of the attack. For these reasons, your immune system needs to carefully contain its attack mechanisms and allow time to restock and heal. If this doesn't happen properly, it can lead to imbalanced and unruly inflammation.

Inflammation is a very important concept in immunity. When you have a wound that swells up, turns red, and is painful, perhaps even a bit warm to the touch, that's inflammation. Your immune system uses inflammation to fight off a germ: Upon being triggered by a harmful germ, certain chemical messengers signal your blood vessels to dilate so that more blood can enter the affected area, bringing needed immune cells to the scene. That causes swelling and redness. Then, your soldier immune cells go to work trying to destroy the germ. It's quite a fight scene (at a microscopic level, of course), full of physical and chemical weapons that you'll learn more

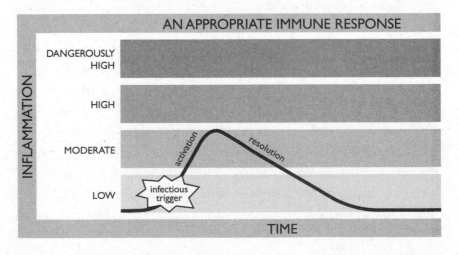

about in a few pages. Infected cells and germs get broken apart, their contents and fragments get strewn about. The goal, of course, is to direct as much of that attack activity as possible toward the target bug. However, your own nearby cells can't help but undergo some damage, too, alarming them into sending more "Help!" signals, which in turn call in more immune cell troops and so it goes on.

Once the germ is defeated, your system should wind down. The immune signals need to switch from "Help! I'm under attack," to "Folks—it's okay! We've won. It's time to clean up the mess and repair the damage." This balance between your immune system's "activation" and "resolution" responses is absolutely essential. When it works well, everything returns to its normal, steady, functional state and proceeds happily along.

However, sometimes the inflammatory response doesn't quiet down. This can create one of two scenarios. The first, and also fortunately quite rare situation, is *hyperinflammation* (such as occurs in so-called cytokine storms) where the "go-go-go" chemical messengers keep going until inflammation is so high it's out of control. Sometimes this happens when a germ is just too strong to be defeated, prompting your immune system to just keep on and on producing more inflammation to try to overcome it. The excessive inflammation can do such damage to your own organs that their function is compromised. When this happens in a critical organ or organs, or spreads throughout your bloodstream, hyperinflammation

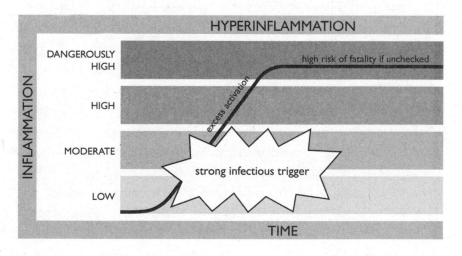

can be life-threatening and require emergency medical support. While normally rare in individuals who are not either very old or infirm, the COVID-19 pandemic has pushed hyperinflammation into the spotlight with SARS-CoV-2's ability to induce this effect in the lungs and other organs of those with severe COVID-19 infections. In fact, it's the leading cause of death in affected individuals. While rare, other viral, bacterial, and fungal pathogens, like influenza (the virus that causes the flu), can sometimes generate this effect in vulnerable people.

The second and far more common scenario is that, even when the germ is no longer a threat, the immune system does not return to a quiet baseline level. It doesn't grow and grow, like during hyperinflammation, but the fires of inflammation continue to smolder without going out. This is called *chronic inflammation*. This ongoing inflammation is not immediately life-threatening but is nevertheless problematic in different ways. Ongoing inflammation is an "alarmed" state—remember those cells that are triggered into "Help!" mode by the damage that inflammation causes? These cells continue to behave in an agitated fashion, sending distress signals around the body. With no discernible germ in sight, these signals cause confusion and spread agitation to other cells. Plus, they continue to attract the attention of your immune cells, which try to attack the "invisible" enemy, but instead end up simply causing more damage and agitation to your own cells.

There are a variety of reasons why your immune system might not know how, or be able, to effectively calm down. Typically, they include some kind of ongoing pro-inflammatory stimulus that isn't the original pathogenic germ. This might be pro-inflammatory foods found in a diet full of sugars and processed foods, chronic psychological stress, an over-sedentary lifestyle, ongoing exposures to environmental toxins, or even having the wrong kinds of microbes living in your digestive tract. Carrying too much fat on your body can also generate this nonspecific inflammation, since excess fat cells (especially those that like to hang out in our belly area) tend to be "angry cells," creating and releasing their own pro-inflammatory signals.

Infections that become chronic can lead to ongoing inflammation, too.

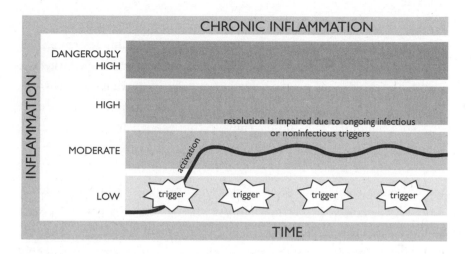

Certain germs, such as Epstein-Barr virus, the germ that causes mono or glandular fever, or *Borrelia burgdorferi,* the germ that causes Lyme disease, can do this. If your immune system can sense those pathogens are still there and tries unsuccessfully to target them, this can trigger a low-level, ongoing inflammatory response.

Another major reason why inflammation can persist in a chronic state is because your immune system isn't able to properly turn it off. Your immune system relies on specific inflammation-resolution mechanisms (a whole subsection of those chemical messengers and other molecules) to quell inflammation once it is no longer needed. These include compounds called *pro-resolving lipid mediators* that incidentally are derived from long-chain polyunsaturated fats you consume by eating good-quality fish, seafood, nuts, seeds, and antioxidants, which neutralize free radicals (and are plentiful in diets with the right kinds of foods). Another crucial mechanism your body uses to turn off inflammation is via regulatory T cells, which you'll learn more about in chapter 4.

Organ cells that are constantly bombarded by chronic inflammation can't do their jobs well. Believing there is a potential threat, they continue to repair damage caused by your equally confused immune cells. Over time this can lead to DNA damage and internal scarring of organs (*fibrosis,* to give it its scientific name), impairing their functionality.

The effects of chronic inflammation over time can be significant. The damage it causes is linked with several diseases, including heart disease, type 2 diabetes, obesity, Alzheimer's disease, and cancer. In fact, there is increasing recognition among scientists and clinicians that these chronic diseases are also diseases of *immune* dysfunction because of their direct link with inflammation—quite a thing to think about! It's also why there are many popular diets and health movements that aim to alleviate chronic inflammation. Chronic inflammation also increases the risk of your immune system learning to attack the wrong things. After all, chronic inflammation ramps up your immune system's attack cells without giving them a productive target. This is when it can start to attack foods or pollens mistakenly, triggering allergies and asthma. It can also mistakenly attack you, potentially leading to diseases of autoimmunity. Not least, when put in this situation for a long time, some parts of your immune system can eventually become tired out and less effective. Scientists call this *immune exhaustion.*

One final but significant problem with having a baseline level of chronic inflammation is that the next time you encounter a germ, your immune system is already revved up. It's already got its battle gear on and is primed for a fight. The "Attack!" chemical signals it receives are *added* to this baseline level of inflammation, creating an even greater immune response and pushing you closer and closer to that dangerous hyperinflammation level.

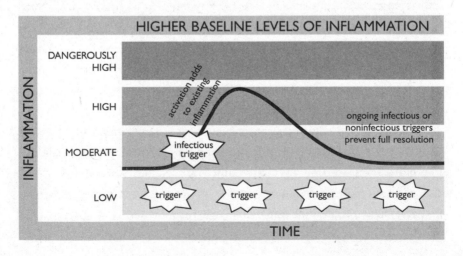

This and all the other problems associated with chronic inflammation make it important for us to be thinking about how to keep our baseline levels of immune activity in check. Not only does that allow our immune systems to operate at their best, it also helps protect us from chronic disease. You'll find that we'll come back to this concept time and time again as we look at all the different factors that affect our immune system and as you learn how to build a plan that supports optimal immune resilience.

THE THREE PILLARS OF YOUR IMMUNE SYSTEM

By now I'm sure you can start to see just how much sense it makes that your immune system has several layers of defense. And each of these has to be working well to optimize your immune resilience. It's no good locking your front door if you've left your side window wide open. It's no good having a cell phone for emergencies if you leave it at home. Shoring up each layer of defense is how you establish a foundational bedrock of strength from which your immune system can operate. Otherwise, one part can easily undermine the hard work you've achieved in another. I'm sure you're also starting to appreciate how taking just a vitamin C tablet might not be enough if you're truly looking to optimize immunity.

As you'll learn in the chapters that follow, your immune system is incredibly elaborate, and there are aspects of immunity that you may never have even realized were important—like your barrier cells, saliva, stomach acid, and the trillions of *helpful* microbes that we all have living within and on us. When you understand all these inner workings, and what either helps or hinders them, you'll see just how much you can do to keep that bucket in tip-top shape.

The layers of defense in your immune system can be grouped into three overarching pillars: (1) civilian army and fortifications, (2) immune cells, and (3) strategic allies.

1. **Your civilian army and fortification structures.** These include physical barriers and other first-line defense mechanisms that block germs from entering your body in the first place. These are the keepers of the

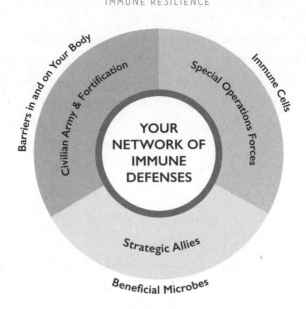

peace—essential mechanisms that help us live in harmony with the germy world around us.

2. **Your special operations forces.** These are all the immune cells that tend to come to mind first when thinking about the immune system. Germs that manage to penetrate your civilian army and fortification structures meet this amazing team of superhero cells.

3. **Your strategic allies.** Nations around the world recognize the advantages of establishing mutually beneficial alliances with other countries: with a handshake, they can share information, pool resources, and ultimately stand stronger in the face of shared adversaries. By now I'm sure you're starting to appreciate just how smart your immune system is, so it might come as no surprise that it forms alliances, too. But it may surprise you just who your immune system partners with—germs. But this time not the harmful germs that risk making us sick. Instead, it's the helpful ones, the trillions of *helpful* microbes that live at every barrier in us and on us, most abundantly in our digestive tracts. These beneficial microbes are essential allies in your fight against the daily onslaught of bad bugs, crowding out the bad guys, giving them less room to take hold and compete for available food sources.

Let's now take a deeper dive into the first of these fundamental defenses: the various but often overlooked "barriers" that are on the front lines, working constantly to block harmful bugs from getting in in the first place.

To view the references cited in this chapter, please visit
www.immuneresilienceplan.com/science.

CHAPTER 3

Fortifications and Civilian Army

Your Multitalented, Dynamic Barrier Cells and More

I n times of war, physical fortifications are important to block the entry of your enemy. Our own body's fortifications are no different. And our barrier cells excel at that. But our barrier cells are not just static fortresses, as you'll see. Instead, they are intelligent and active servicemen with numerous tricks up their sleeves to keep you safe from that invading germ. In addition, just like a civilian army, these cells have other "day jobs"—being in your military forces is not their only gig. Airway barrier cells, for instance, must also facilitate the ongoing exchange of oxygen and carbon dioxide. Barrier cells in the digestive tract must allow for the absorption of essential nutrients. Skin barrier cells regulate temperature, prevent excess water loss, and produce certain nutrients like vitamin D, which, as you'll find out later in this book, is one of our most important immune nutrients. Yet all of these barrier cells also perform vital immune functions on an ongoing basis. Let's take a tour through these roles, which fall into three main categories: structural defense, chemical arsenal, and good old-fashioned spring cleaning.

STRUCTURAL DEFENSE

Structural defense is all about your body's physical barriers—your skin being the most obvious and one that we usually take for granted. I mean, imagine if we didn't have our skin . . . it would be a free-for-all with germs gaining ready access to our internal blood system all of the time. That barrier, made up of layers of billions of tightly packed cells, provides a wall that physically stops thousands of germs in their tracks and hugely cuts down the number of germs that the rest of your immune system ends up having to deal with. And it's not a small area: the skin surface of an average-sized adult, accounting for all the openings and appendages around hair follicles and sweat ducts, is estimated at around 270 square feet (25 square meters, or roughly the size of some small studio apartments).

There are other structural defense barriers, too, like the lining of your mouth and throat, and your digestive tract (another even bigger surface area of around 350 square feet, the size of half a badminton court). Then there's the lining of your nasal passages and lungs (the biggest of all at a whopping 540 square feet!); even the urinary tract, female vagina, and the cornea (the surface of our eyeballs) have to perform similar essential barrier functions. How could the surface areas of some of these barriers be so big? It's all to do with their structure. Your digestive tract, or gut, is made with billions of tiny finger-like projections called *villi*, each around a millimeter in length. There can be up to 25,000 of these per square inch of your small intestine, which itself is over 9 feet long. These villi are why the surface area seems so impossibly large to fit into your body, and they are there by design to maximize your ability to rapidly absorb essential nutrition from the food that you eat. In your lungs, hundreds of millions of tiny airway branches and sacs called *alveoli* maximize the surface area to enable you to quickly absorb the amount of oxygen you need in every breath. The scale we're talking about is enormous when you consider that your immune system has to police these surfaces at a microscopic level.

When your barriers are damaged, such as through excess UV exposure, pollution, cigarette smoke, free radicals, injury, medications, poor diet, chemical stress, allergies, inflammation, or even the harmful bugs themselves, they are less effective at keeping pathogens out. More harmful microbes, and the toxins they produce, are able to take hold and cause infection, or even pass into our bloodstream and travel to other areas of the body.

THE GUT LINING

The lining of your gut is, perhaps surprisingly, an important *external* barrier, even as it sits out of sight within your body. Everything within the tube of your digestive tract is considered to be still outside the body, and only when it is absorbed across that barrier does it become something that is now internal to us. Anything that the body doesn't absorb is after all excreted unceremoniously at the end of its passage.

Gut health is the health topic du jour: in the last few years it has become a media darling, with dozens of published books on the topic, which gives you some indication of just how key this organ and its function are. Many of these books explain the concept of leaky gut, or *intestinal permeability*, as it's known among scientists. If you haven't heard of it, you'll get the lowdown here, including a sophisticated and nuanced understanding of how leaky gut is not an on/off switch, but rather a sliding scale that is in flux throughout the day.

Your gut lining is actually incredibly thin. Under healthy conditions, those lining cells are tightly packed and in control over what substances pass through the digestive lining and into our bodies. When this barrier breaks down, cracks or holes can appear in between barrier cells, allowing pieces of partially digested foods, inflammatory toxins, or even germs to gain access to your tissues beneath it. Scientists have written several thousand papers on intestinal permeability in the last twenty years, with ever more published each year.

Now, we all have some degree of gut "leakiness," since our gut barrier isn't designed to be completely impenetrable. Nutrients must still be able to pass through. And this leakiness can vary relatively harmlessly on a daily basis depending on what we throw its way. However, when the gut

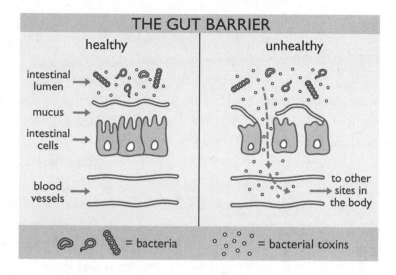

lining is strongly assaulted or continually bombarded even at a lesser intensity, it can struggle to maintain healthy levels of permeability. In rare, severe cases, problematic germs themselves can move across a leaky gut barrier and circulate in your blood, setting up localized or systemic infections. Much more common, though, is a different form of immune battering: the ongoing influx of normally excluded compounds (including bacterial toxins if you have harmful germs in residence) through the gut barrier triggers a state of alarm in your defense system. This alarmed state can cause several problems. It can increase the chance that your immune system misfires, as seen in allergies and autoimmune diseases like type 1 diabetes, multiple sclerosis, and Hashimoto's thyroiditis. It can also drive chronic inflammation. Scientists today are producing increasingly more evidence to show that leaky gut, and the inflammation that can derive from it, is linked with the development of many of our common chronic diseases.

Although some of us may have a genetic predisposition to greater gut leakiness, we can't wholly blame this phenomenon on our DNA. Many of our modern-day habits have a detrimental effect on this barrier, as you'll learn. Diets characterized by processed, low-fiber foods and full of sugar and food additives, for instance, will continually wear away at your gut integrity. Pesticides and other toxins in foods, certain medications, stress, and poor sleep also take their toll. The common pain reliever ibuprofen, for instance, can irritate and inflame the stomach and intestinal lining, increasing permeability. Antibiotics, too, induce intestinal leakiness likely because they also strip the good bugs from your intestines that are essential for maintaining gut barrier health. Bad bugs that thrive on a modern diet and lifestyle habits are known to increase permeability, too (more on both good and bad bugs when you get to chapter 5).

The good news is that it is within our power to change the trajectory of our gut barrier health, through the foods we eat—like less-processed and more nutrient-dense foods, especially colorful plant foods and sources of anti-inflammatory omega-3 fats. Fermented foods nourish our healthy microbes. Paying attention to nutrient density goes a long way, too, since several essential nutrients like vitamin A, vitamin D, and zinc are critical for barrier health. And a lifestyle that keeps stress levels in check and gives us some good zzz's. (The Immune Resilience Plan in this book will show you how.)

Even though the digestive tract and leaky gut have received much attention recently, there are other munitions your civilian army barrier cells deploy that deserve a callout, some attention, and TLC.

YOUR CHEMICAL ARSENAL

Besides being your structural defenses, your multitalented barrier cells produce secretions that combat germs in generically antimicrobial ways. These are your *chemical arsenal*: biological compounds in tears, sweat, mucus, saliva, stomach acid, even ear wax. These aren't specifically targeting any one type of bug, but rather are keeping things in check, keeping your "terrain" inhospitable to bad bugs, and making sure that they aren't allowed to gain too much of a foothold. The three kinds of chemical arsenal to know about are acidity, antimicrobial molecules, and mucus.

ACIDITY

Your body creates acidic environments at several of your barriers—your skin, for instance is moderately acidic, as is vaginal fluid. But nothing quite compares to stomach acid. Your stomach cells produce around 1.5 liters of stomach acid per day which can kill many harmful germs that you might happen to swallow. We normally just think of stomach acid as part of our digestive process, but it is also a formidable weapon when it comes to annihilating pathogens.

Consider then, the implications of the huge market for antacids, designed to suppress stomach acid production, valued at $10 billion in annual sales globally and growing year on year. Sixty million people suffer regular episodes of gastroesophageal reflux disease (GERD, or *reflux* for short) in the United States, where acid suppressants are among the top ten prescribed medications. Could this have a detrimental effect on susceptibility to infectious disease and immune dysfunction? The research strongly suggests so.

A scientific paper in the *Journal of the American Medical Association* (*JAMA*) recently concluded that medications used to suppress stomach acid are significantly linked to having multi-drug-resistant germs living in your digestive tract, and to having recurrent symptomatic episodes of a particularly nasty intestinal bug, aptly named *Clostridioides difficile*. Not only that, a previous *JAMA* research study of more than 350,000 individuals found a connection between the use of proton-pump inhibitors (PPIs, a class of acid suppressant medications including omeprazole and esomeprazole) and pneumonia; those on these medications were more than four times more likely to catch pneumonia, indicating that it's not just gut infections that acid suppression can leave you more vulnerable to. Other studies have found associations between long-term use of acid suppressants and gastroenteritis, small intestine bacterial overgrowth (SIBO, a condition where even the normal, beneficial bacteria grow out of control), as well as nutrient deficiencies of calcium, magnesium, iron, and vitamin B_{12}. Even heart attacks may be connected: one study of a large patient population of 2.9 million individuals found the risk for heart attack increased

1.2 times, and the risk for cardiac mortality doubled, in individuals taking long-term PPIs.

Having GERD is problematic because it is a risk factor for erosion of the esophageal lining, Barrett's esophagus, and potentially even esophageal cancer. However, GERD is another disease primarily driven by our modern lifestyles, including poor diets, sedentary behavior, and stress. The fact that antacids are also available over the counter, and that acid suppressants are so often prescribed in the United States, makes it seem as if they are pretty harmless. However, as the research clearly shows, they are not without risk. If you have GERD, in part 3 I'll show you how to reduce its symptoms naturally, which can help you reduce dependence on antacid medications.

ANTIMICROBIAL MOLECULES

Antimicrobial molecules, produced by your barrier cells, are the closest your body has to its own homemade, all-purpose antimicrobial ointment. Like bacitracin, but for all sorts of bugs, not just bacteria. And of course, since your body doesn't like to take any chances, these exist in several different variations to increase the chance that there will be at least one that will do the trick when a bad bug comes along.

Scientists call these compounds *antimicrobial peptides*, or AMPs. Thousands of different naturally occurring AMPs have so far been identified and more are discovered by scientists each year. AMPs work in several fascinating ways. First, they are attracted to pathogenic bacteria through their inbuilt electrochemical charges. AMPs have outer sections that are strongly positively charged, whereas microbial membranes are negatively charged. These opposites attract and help AMPs find their microbial targets. Human cells carry a neutral charge—an important feature that allows AMPs to do their work without harming normal cells. The positive charge of the AMPs induces electrical disturbance in the microbe's cell membrane that causes damage and even holes. The inner materials of that microbe then start to leak out while other AMPs gain access to the inner workings of that microbial cell and cause further destruction, including of DNA. The microbe doesn't last long once it's in these death throes and rarely has the chance to develop resistance mechanisms, which is why AMPs don't carry the same degree of resistance risk as pharmaceutical antibiotics. In fact, AMPs have continued to be effective against infections for millions of years, seemingly in part due to their huge diversity and their variety of modes of action.

Pharmaceutical antibiotics, on the other hand, often work by interfering with a narrow set of biochemical reactions that bacteria use to function. These might be reactions that help the bacteria build structural components or DNA, or reactions that are part of that bacteria's normal metabolism. The effect can be very potent—as I'm sure you've experienced when you start to quickly feel better after just a dose or two into your course of antibiotics. However, the effect is also super specific to just a part of a bacteria's function. It's thought that this narrow range of activity is what makes antibiotics more likely to provoke resistance. Bacteria are known to develop strategies to render an antibiotic ineffective such as blocking its route of entry to the bacterial cell, pumping it out of the cell just as fast as it may enter, or simply inactivating it. These work-arounds can then become encoded into the bacteria's DNA, passed onto its progeny when it replicates, and even shared among its bacterial buddies through DNA gene transfer. And then—presto!—you have drug resistance.

Scientists looking for the next antibiotic to develop are understandably interested in potentially harnessing synthetic versions of our own AMPs. However, early lab studies that tried to do this found that microbes can more easily develop resistance to AMPs, too, when they are used singularly and out of their usual balance. Something about the broad variety of natural AMPs found within us is less vulnerable to provoking resistance. It seems it's not just safety in numbers, but safety in diversity.

So, while we support our scientists in their ongoing search for much-needed lifesaving new antibiotics, it makes sense that you would also want to optimize what you already have—including your AMPs. And it turns out you can. Vitamin D, for example is one nutrient that is essential for AMP production. In fact, it *controls* the production of AMPs. You'll learn more about that and other strategies to support your AMPs in this book.

MUCUS

Mucus is another type of chemical weapon that your barrier cells produce and is secreted onto several barrier surfaces including your mouth, airways, and digestive tract. Although mucus conjures rather unappealing mental images of slime monsters and gruesome boogers, it's not just there to provide entertainment to kids and to horrify adults. It has much utility that, once you see just how it works, may rouse surprising appreciation for this lowly substance.

Mucus immediately acts as an extension to the physical barricade of cells at the barrier's surface, enforcing a distance between microbes and your own cells. "Not so fast" it says to that bug, dust particle, or food—"stand back a minute and let me get a good look at you." By suspending particles, including potentially problematic germs, in this kind of "holding gel," it gives the immune system a chance to scope them out and determine what action, if any, may be needed. You'll find out just how immune cells do that in the next chapter, "Special Operations Forces." Too little mucus means there's no order and due process to the sorting and assessment of microbes, and it sends our immune system a little haywire. Without enough mucus, you'll get excessive defense responses and increase the potential for chronic inflammation.

Mucus, unsurprisingly, is also an effective lubricant that helps the mobile components of our barriers, which you'll learn about next, move germs along and out of our bodies. It also provides a more fluid medium in which our AMPs can get to work on their targets. Without mucus, those AMPs would be rendered immobile and unable to do their job.

Mucus (along with other secretions such as tears, saliva, and breast milk) also contains several proteins with antimicrobial properties, like lysozyme and lactoferrin, and important, broad-spectrum antibodies called secretory IgA (more on those in the next chapter). Last but not least, mucus contains carbohydrate molecules called *glycans*, which are one source of nourishment to your beneficial bacteria that you'll learn about in chapter 5. This keeps our helpful bugs going in between feedings of fiber from the food you eat.

SPRING CLEANING

I wonder if, like me, you dread spring cleaning—after all, it takes up so much time that feels like it could be more productively directed elsewhere. Either way, the good news is that your body is *continually* doing its own spring cleaning of germs without you having to think about or direct it in any way, or even remotely stop what you're working on to help it. For your immune system, spring cleaning is a lot about liquid and motion—sweeping here or flushing out there—and, just like when you clean your home, it's the combination that often does the trick.

Let's think about this for just a minute, and how important it is in keeping ecosystems healthy. A stream, for example, that is running well stays clear and healthy. But water that sits and stagnates becomes a breeding ground for all manner of organisms. Obvious ways that your body uses liquid and motion against germs when it gets sick are responses like coughing, sneezing, vomiting, or even diarrhea, which are all about getting that germ *out*. But your body also uses liquid and movement continuously to keep your inner environments healthy.

Saliva flow, for instance, kick-starts your digestive process, and it helps keep your mouth clean. One milliliter of human saliva from a healthy individual actually contains about 100 million bacterial cells, washed from the surfaces of our gums and teeth. Yucky, right? But an essential way to clear out some of those germs. When we don't have enough saliva we're more prone to oral infections as well as non-oral infections like sinus and chest infections. Low saliva is actually quite a pervasive problem and can lead to dry mouth symptoms (medically termed *xerostomia*). By conservative estimates, around 20 percent of us in the United States have decreased saliva production. It is, after all, a common side effect of several diseases, radiation therapy, medications, and of simply getting older. This number goes up to around 30 percent in females and around 50 percent in older adults.

Motion is also used by some of your barrier cells, like those that line your airways. These cells have miniature hairlike projections called *cilia* that trap dust, toxins, and germs, and then move in coordinated wave-like patterns to carry those unwanted particles out of your sinuses and lungs. The liquid mucus your barrier cells produce helps this process function well. Barrier cells in your digestive tract take part in another kind of movement called *peristalsis*, which, again along with the lubricating mucus, is what moves food along our intestines. Peristalsis also performs a sweep of intestinal microbial populations, culling as it goes to prevent overgrowth and to limit the ability of a bad germ to hang around and cause trouble. Peristalsis can be easily affected by medications (the ones that tend to cause constipation like opioid pain relievers, tricyclic antidepressants, and antihistamines), and also by stress, and conditions like hypothyroidism and diabetes.

The Effect of Cigarette Smoke on Lung Cilia

Cilia are tiny hairlike projections that protect your airways by sweeping trapped pathogens, toxins, debris, and mucus up and out of your lungs. As stated by the CDC, tobacco smoke paralyzes cilia, rendering them ineffective at fulfilling this important role. With repeated smoke exposure, cilia can eventually die. Keeping your cilia healthy is another compelling reason to keep away from tobacco smoke.

Another kind of spring cleaning your immune system does is to continually replace its barrier cells. And I mean *continually*. Barriers have a huge cell turnover. That skin you can see when you look down at your arm will be completely replaced by next month. Your digestive tract cells are even shorter lived—the entire lining of your small intestine will be brand new by this time next week. That's the highest turnover of any organ in your body and hugely nutrient-demanding. This carefully controlled (by which I mean without creating gut leakiness), constant change is by design: The intestinal lining is just the thickness of a single cell layer and is under constant assault from the food and microbes you throw at it; ongoing regeneration maintains its strength and integrity. Plus, it's much harder for pathogens to form attachments to an always-shedding wall.

———————

Did you ever think there would be so many layers of defense involved in your immune system before we even get to talk about a white blood cell? All these active barrier mechanisms—your fortifications and civilian army—work on keeping the peace, and most important, keeping you safe before those white blood cells even need to get involved. That bad germ that finally encounters an immune cell will have had to navigate a blockade of militarized barrier cells, layers of chemical assault, and a constantly moving terrain—quite a feat! And if it does so, what happens next is no less impressive.

———————————————

To view the references cited in this chapter, please visit
www.immuneresilienceplan.com/science.

CHAPTER 4

Special Operations Forces

Highly Trained Immune Cells with Formidable Superpowers

At this point, we turn to what many of us think of first when we talk about our immune system: those white blood cells that counterattack any germ that manages to penetrate our barrier defenses. White blood cells are *the* cells of your immune system. Even as you read this, they are being produced in your bone marrow, just like your red blood cells, and circulating throughout your body, including your blood and your lymphatic system (a large network of major and minor circulatory vessels as well as nodes and organs such as your thymus and spleen). There are several different types of white blood cells, all with different roles in fighting germs.

When you're not fighting an infection, white blood cells (or *leukocytes*) make up just 1 percent of your blood. Even so, they perform critical surveillance duties and can rapidly respond and multiply when called to action. I'm sure you've experienced at some point—perhaps when a cut or scrape gets infected, or even when you get a pimple—how the area becomes red, usually a little hot, swollen, and tender. You'll also have seen the collections of spent white blood cells and the dead germs they've been fighting that can collect in the form of pus. These are the results of your white blood cells fighting an infection.

As you'll see in this chapter, white blood cells protect you against illness and disease by using a litany of impressive combat skills and capabilities to destroy harmful germs and cancer cells that try their luck at invading your body.

THE "INNATE" AND "ADAPTIVE" BRANCHES OF YOUR IMMUNE SYSTEM

Before we go much further, it's important to understand a little about how scientists have long divided up our immune system into two buckets: innate and adaptive immunity. It's worth understanding the fundamentals of each branch since, later on, I'll explain how nutrition and lifestyle can impact how well they function.

INNATE IMMUNITY

Your innate immune system is the defense system you've had in place since you were born. What you read about in the preceding chapter actually all falls under the umbrella of innate immunity: physical, chemical, and mobility factors that form a first line of defense. In addition to that, innate immunity includes several types of white blood cells that are supremely proactive and the quickest cells to respond to any emerging threat they perceive. Our innate immune cells are also *generalists*, meaning that they work well enough against any kind of invader. Very handy since you don't always know what kind of threat is coming your way.

Innate immune cells have names like *neutrophils, eosinophils, basophils, mast cells, macrophages, dendritic cells*, and *natural killer cells* (yes, "natural killer cells" is their given scientific name!). These cells all have special sensors that can identify when germs are present, sensors that are very good at "reading" the patterns on particular bad bugs or on the trail of toxins those bad bugs emit. Once they've sensed a germ, all these cells quickly adopt their incredible, somewhat sci-fi-esque, superpowers that turn them into formidable killing and clearing machines. And they need to be—after all, those harmful germs they come up against have already proven they are tough enough to get past your layers of frontline defense, and many of them have evolved sophisticated ways of mounting their own attacks.

Here are some of those superpowers to know about. The first is the dramatically named *cell death activation*, a favorite of natural killer cells. These cells have two different ways they can activate this power. One way is by triggering something aptly called the death receptor on their target cell—perhaps one of your own cells that has become infected with a virus or perhaps a cancer cell. This is essentially akin to a fingerprint ID–controlled self-destruct button that initiates a cell's own self-destruction mechanisms (called *apoptosis*). Not all immune cells have the right "fingerprint" to make this work, but natural killer cells do.

Natural killer cells can also produce bubble-like structures that contain chemical weapons. This is a capability they share with other immune cells such as neutrophils, eosinophils, and mast cells. They can then fuse these bubbles onto the outer membranes of their target cells (virus-infected cells or tumor cells) and release their contents in a kind of chemical attack. Some of these chemical agents (ones called *perforins*) can poke holes in the membranes of the target cell, damaging the cell's essential barriers and facilitating the entry of other types of chemicals. Other chemicals are enzymes (these ones are called *granzymes*) that also activate cell death.

Incidentally, natural killer cells are best known for their antitumor and antiviral activities. We know, for instance, that humans with impaired natural killer cell numbers or function are more susceptible to cancer formation and viral infections including herpes simplex virus, cytomegalovirus, chicken pox, and human papilloma virus.

Dendritic cells, our immune sentinel cells, have an intriguing superpower: the ability to "see" through walls and around corners, and sense what's out there. The clue to how their superpower works is in their name, since these cells are named for their probing projections that look like long arms or branches (from the ancient Greek word *dendrite*, meaning "tree-like"). Positioning themselves just inside the safe zone—tucked up behind the wall of barrier cells—they then extend one of their arms in between those tightly packed cells (without disrupting the integrity of the barrier) and out to the outside world, whether that be on the skin, into the contents of the digestive tract, or at another one of our barriers. From there they "sample" what's out beyond the barrier, pick up any useful fragments to study, and report to other immune cells if they sense danger. These could be new foods they are encountering for the first time, helpful microbes living on the surface of our barrier, and of course any threatening germs that are lurking out there that need dealing with.

The next superpower to know about is a shapeshifting ability called *phagocytosis* (pronounced "fa-go-sai-*tow*-suhs"), in which an immune cell engulfs something such as a bacterial cell, one of our own cells that has become infected, fungal spores, or simply virus particles or broken cell pieces. It's a bit like having a sea of Pac-Man creatures (remember that arcade game?), working on your side, whose role is to gobble up nasty bugs and to clear debris from the battlefield when your immune system goes into action. Neutrophils, macrophages, and dendritic cells have this ability and are therefore called *phagocytes*. To do this, they first attach to the offender in question through specialized receptors, then extend the shape of

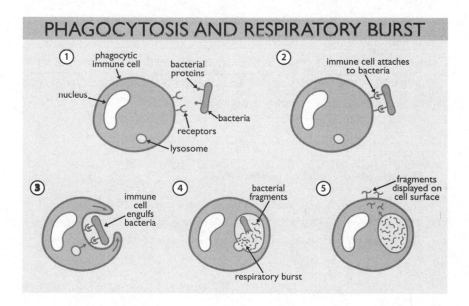

their own external membrane to smother their target from both sides, gradually drawing it inside. Like a giant, smothering hug, and quite deadly. Once inside, they unleash the next superpower: a blast of chemical compounds from lysosome capsules inside the cell that destroys the engulfed offender, scientifically termed a *respiratory burst*. These compounds are potent free radicals derived from oxygen and nitrogen, as well as strong acids, that can destroy the captured target. This process is very demanding of the body's resources and energy; oxygen consumption, for instance, can increase by ten to twenty times in cells during the respiratory burst process. And your phagocyte cells don't stop there: the fragments that remain from the destroyed germ are then displayed on the surface of the cell as a means of educating other immune cells about the invader.

But that's not all. In addition to their capabilities described above, neutrophils and other immune cells can also activate a kamikaze superpower in response to viral, bacterial, or fungal triggers. This power is an elaborate form of suicide in which the immune cell releases long strands of its own DNA, coated with destructive enzymes and antimicrobial proteins, that trap and neutralize invading germs. Pretty intense!

The next time you start to feel sick—like if you get the flu—you might now have a visual in your mind of some of what is going on inside you. All this inflammatory immune activity can make you feel pretty lousy, causing fever, aches, and pains. What's often unappreciated is that much of what actually makes you *feel* sick during an infection is the activity of your own immune system in combat with the germ.

The Role of Fevers in Immune Function

The average body temperature is generally accepted as ranging from 97 to 99 degrees Fahrenheit. A temperature of over 100.4 degrees Fahrenheit is considered to be a fever, which may occur while the body is trying to kill a virus or bacteria. This temperature elevation is usually related to the stimulation of your immune system by that germ, as it tries to fight it off. Fevers also have a functional role in immunity and are not usually harmful if they stay within controlled temperature levels and do not become excessive. Fevers are known to stimulate immune activity, promote white blood cell circulation, and enhance the cells' antimicrobial activity. The higher temperature of a fever also makes it harder for some harmful bugs, especially pathogenic bacteria, to survive. Although the strength of a fever can't always distinguish between bacterial and viral causes, a high fever is more often associated with bacterial infections.

All the innate white blood cells patrolling the vast microscopic world inside you, as well as all your civilian army cells, can call for backup when they encounter a harmful bug. The biochemical signaling molecules they send out attract other innate white blood cells to the scene. Neutrophils are among the first to respond, within just a few hours, and while working to attack the bad bugs they simultaneously amplify the alarm signals. Eosinophils, basophils, and mast cells may be present, too. Natural killer cells arrive within a few days to try to destroy infected cells before a virus replicates too far.

The activity of your innate immune system is sometimes enough to knock out the invader completely, but your immune system doesn't take any chances. That's why you also have your adaptive immune system, which has been preparing its attack even as your innate immune cells have been busy with a germ.

ADAPTIVE IMMUNITY

Your adaptive immune system is what develops over time as your body is exposed to germs. Even while innate white blood cells are getting into the fight, more signaling mechanisms set the wheels in motion for this most powerful and sophisticated response of all. Your adaptive immune system mounts a defense strategy that is *specific just to that germ*. This is great because its precision makes it a much more effective weapon against invaders. It also leaves behind less collateral damage to your own cells. Yet that precision requirement means it takes a little longer to pull together (around four to seven days on average for newly encountered pathogens) and so it relies on all your other lines of defense to hold the fort while it prepares its attack.

What triggers your adaptive immune system into action are those fragments of destroyed bugs that innate immune cells like dendritic and other phagocytic cells display like battle trophies on their surfaces. These fragments are unique to that pathogen, making them a highly informative report to share up the chain of command. Innate immune cells displaying these trophies travel to your immune system's lymphatic base camps, such as your spleen, lymph nodes, adenoids, and tonsils. There they meet T cells and B cells, your two key adaptive immune cell types, semirelaxed and milling around yet always "on call" and ready to respond. They present these fragments to those T and B cells by locking into them using one of the thousands of surface receptors displayed on these adaptive immune cells.

Your T cells and B cells read this information, along with other signaling molecules from the innate immune system's alarm bells, and are spurred into action, shedding their everyday plain clothes and emerging in their own superhero gear. T cells can evolve into *cytotoxic* T cells, warrior cells that can attack specific infected cells or tumor cells with their own array of chemical weapons. These weapons can poke holes in or chop off essential components of their pathogen targets, and even jam the machinery that viruses use to replicate. Other options in your T cell evolutionary repertoire include regulatory T cells and helper T cells. These types of T cells step into the critical roles of wise choreographer (the regulatory T cells) and assistant choreographer (the helper T cells). Regulatory T cells are like the Yodas of your immune system—full of wisdom and direction about when to act and when not to. They help channel the behavior of your cytotoxic T cell warriors, take over direction of your innate immune cells, and crucially provide the right checks and balances to ensure things don't get out of control and that immune activity winds down again after a germ has been neutralized. As you can imagine, you want your immune system to have enough regulatory T cells.

One of the signaling molecules produced by T cells (as well as barrier cells, macrophages, and natural killer cells) is a type of cytokine called *interferon gamma*. This molecule is important to know about because it can be influenced by good or bad changes in your diet, nutrient status, lifestyle choices, and toxin exposures. Interferon gamma helps your defenses in some very useful ways: It improves the antimicrobial actions of many innate and adaptive immune cells (for instance, it promotes natural killer cell activity, antigen presentation, and B cell activity). It also plays a role in balancing immune activity, keeping inflammation within appropriate levels. It is perhaps best known for its generalized antiviral effects, since that's what led to its discovery. Interferon gamma interferes with virus activity in many different ways, including how the virus tries to enter cells, how it replicates, how it transmits to other nearby cells, and even how it can reactivate after being dormant.

B cells are your antibody-producing cells. Or at least they are when they are activated into plasma B cells. The antibodies they produce travel freely around the body like an intergalactic X-wing squadron (although actually, antibodies are Y-shaped molecules). They locate patterns on the microbes' surfaces that they have been preprogrammed to identify. Once they find a match, they attach to it at the specific site they recognize just like a key fits into a lock. Sticking out like a tag, they start calling in the troops who can much more easily find and neutralize these now "labeled" bugs.

Antibodies have several other tricks up their sleeves, too. Antibodies can make those tiny, elusive virus particles clump together by forming cross-links with other attached antibodies on adjacent particles so that the virus particles can't function properly and can be more readily identified and destroyed by other immune cells. They can render a pathogen less able to get a foothold on your own cells, they can interfere with its mobility or replication, or they can even directly cripple that harmful bug, rendering it no longer infectious. If all goes well, the target succumbs and is destroyed. Job done.

Adaptive immunity also has one more important benefit: its memory. Adaptive immune cells keep a record of the germs they've seen and a blueprint of the antibodies they can use against them, ready to ramp up and deploy again (this time much more rapidly) the next time that germ comes along.

I don't know about you, but I find all these examples of immune cells and their capabilities simultaneously surreal and fascinating—and reassuring, in a way, in just how sophisticated, earnest, and intense they can be. We're nowhere near understanding it all; science is still studying our immune system, finding out more and more about how it works.

And what we'll look at next is no less intriguing (maybe even mind-blowing!): the third-party *microbial allies* that play a surprisingly extensive role in shaping and honing our own immune defenses.

———————————

To view the references cited in this chapter, please visit
www.immuneresilienceplan.com/science.

CHAPTER 5

Strategic Allies

Indispensable, Beneficial Microbes
That Broaden and Fine-Tune Your Defenses

D id you know that your body is not, well . . . all you? It may be hard to fathom, but in addition to any nasty germs it may be carrying, your body harbors a vast population of (normally) harmless and actually beneficial microbes that have been our constant and evolutionary companions since our great ape days. These microbes—bacteria, viruses, fungi, and even parasites—descended from ancient life forms on our planet long before the human lineage appeared. And their numbers are staggering: There are about 38 trillion live-in/live-on bacteria in your body right now—that's more than the approximately 30 trillion human cells you have. That's right: you may be less human, more bacterial! And these have evolved to be symbiotic—mutually beneficial and even *indispensable*—allies essential for your health.

These symbiotic microbes are found predominantly at your defense barriers together with all the opportunistic pathogens—new harmful bugs that we've just encountered that day, as well as long-term residents that lie dormant within us waiting for an opportune moment to grow. Each species, good and bad, vies to establish themselves in the challenging environment that you now know characterizes these barriers: constantly shedding cells, sanitizing antimicrobial peptides (AMPs), liquids like saliva, urine, or even shower water (in the case of your skin barrier) rushing past. The truth is that the fight for living space within and on you plays out as a turbulent and fragile balance between good and bad. Amazing, isn't it? All this happening while you can't feel a thing? As long as we're taking care of them and giving them the right tools to thrive (like the right foods and lifestyle choices), the good microbes keep the upper hand. And they even help us keep the bad ones under control—hence their status as indispensable allies. When we provide the wrong inputs, we can give the bad guys a leg up, even a podium to stand on.

YOUR MOST RECENTLY DISCOVERED "ORGAN": YOUR MICROBIOTA

Microbiota refers to the collective of microbial organisms, good and bad, that you carry within you and on you. You may also hear the term *microbiome* used in the media and other publications, which describes the collection of *genes* that exist within all of those microbial organisms. That collective gene pool, by the way, contains up to a whopping 100 times the number of human genes. What we know about our microbiota, while discovered back in the seventeenth century, has only really been uncovered in the last two decades, due to advances that have been made in clinical testing and the launch of the National Institutes of Health–funded Human Microbiome Project in 2008. In just these few short years, there has been a growing realization that there are hugely important connections between these live-in guest microbes, your physiology, and your state of health, including in your neurological, metabolic, cardiovascular, hormonal, and immune systems. More and more connections are being uncovered every day, adding to our ever-growing appreciation of just how complex our relationship with microbes actually is.

Within and on your body, there are different micro-environments—habitats, if you will—that support microbial life. Some are dry, others moist. Some are light and well oxygenated, others dark and oxygen deprived. These characteristics affect the types of microbes that can thrive there. The gut microbiota is the most extensively studied of your different microbial habitats to date. It is predominantly found in your colon, which happens to be one of the most densely populated microbial regions on earth. It is also the largest of your body's microbial populations by volume and weight—up to 3 percent of your body weight (or 4.5 pounds for a 150-pound adult) according to the NIH's Human Microbiome Project. That's heavier than the average person's brain (3 pounds)! While the gut microbiota may be the most substantial by headcount and weight, the reality is that there isn't a crevice, fold, nook, or cranny inside or outside of our body that isn't inhabited by a nonhuman species that is doing something to either help or harm our immunity and overall health. Even the womb, the last anatomical locale to be considered sterile has been found to contain microbes. Science is really only in the very earliest stages of exploring all of these ecosystems, and we have much to uncover, but what we do know so far tells us that keeping our beneficial microbes as healthy and balanced as possible is critical for our immune resilience and overall health.

WHERE DOES YOUR MICROBIOTA COME FROM?

The period during your earliest development, especially within the first six months of life, is a critical time window for your microbiota—much change takes place. In utero and during birth, you acquire microbes from your mother. A large contributor to that early microbial transfer is how you're born: The gut microbiota of babies who are born vaginally tends to reflect the microbial composition of the mother's birth canal and be more diverse. Diversity of beneficial species in your microbiota is considered a good thing—just like in other ecosystems, diversity allows your microbiota to better cope with disturbance and stress, making it less vulnerable to harmful influences. Just as your immune system works best with many different layers of defense, so too does a healthy microbiota. In fact, science tells us that increased species diversity in our microbiota is associated with better resistance to infections and even chronic diseases. Babies born by cesarean section have a gut microbiota that tends to reflect the mother's skin composition and is less diverse. After you're born, your microbiota continues to be heavily influenced by the world around you—what's in your home, in your yard, whether you have pets, what food you're fed (and whether you're breast-fed), and what medications you may be given. From the time you are two to three years old, your microbiota stabilizes, as long as the inputs remain relatively constant. However, it can be altered—for better or for worse—depending on any insults or reparations it receives. At the other end of the spectrum, aging influences your microbiota, too. Since your own immune system is also responsible for keeping your microbiota in good shape, and since aging is associated with a decline in immune effectiveness, microbial populations start to get a bit unruly as our body reaches its later years. The good news is that many of these influences are modifiable, putting you in the driving seat when it comes to the health of your microbiota.

WHEN IT COMES TO MICROBES, THINGS CAN BE GOOD, BAD, OR REALLY UGLY

The relationship you have with your live-in microbes has many different levels, and they can be good or bad, depending on the type of microbes you're harboring. Numerous scientific studies have shown that when it's working well, the relationship you have with your live-in microbes can really pay off. Your lung microbiota, when robust and healthy, can help protect you from respiratory infections. Your bladder microbiota, from urinary tract infections. Your eye and ear microbiota can help avoid ophthalmic and auricular infections. And, if you're female, your vaginal microbiota, from fungal and bacterial vaginoses. You get the idea. A happy relationship with our microbes, as you'll see in this chapter, starts with keeping bad bugs at bay, but also goes much further. These seemingly insignificant organisms can shape, tone, and balance your entire immune system.

But that's not all. In addition to directly improving your immune defenses, good bacteria in your gut are also a source of essential vitamins that we humans cannot make ourselves. In fact, your friendly gut bugs are capable of providing you with significant portions of some of your daily nutrient needs—especially for B vitamins, biotin, and vitamin K. They also produce active neurotransmitters that can alter your mood and sense of well-being. They produce about 95 percent of your body's supply of serotonin, a neurotransmitter that can help you feel happier and more balanced. They can also neutralize some of the harmful environmental toxins you encounter, help your metabolism, balance your hormones, and improve your bone health. (I told you their health effects were far reaching!)

But when your beneficial microbiota is depleted, imbalanced, or overrun with more harmful species, also known as a *dysbiotic* microbiota, the opposite happens: all those health benefits dwindle away and your immune barriers, surveillance, and responses are weaker. Inflammation spreads and grows. If left unchecked, things can get really ugly. You can end up more vulnerable to infections as well as to all kinds of chronic diseases. Heart disease, diabetes, Alzheimer's, mood disorders, osteoporosis, cancer are just some of the major conditions now known to be influenced by (and even oftentimes caused by) a detrimental imbalance of our resident microbes.

YOU ARE THE GUARDIAN OF YOUR MICROBIOTA

All kinds of things that are pervasive in our modern lives can derail the balance of good vs. bad within your microbiota. This includes food, new microbes that come along, and anything that tries to kill certain species off.

By "food," I mean predominantly the food that you eat—beneficial species tend to prefer higher-fiber plant foods, whereas more harmful species tend to do well with poor dietary choices like sugar and refined carbohydrates. Monotonous diets (those with very little variety) are also bad news, since diversity of healthy plant foods is what creates a diversity of healthy microbial species and consequently a more resilient microbiota. Another kind of food for microbes is the mucus your body produces. Mucus provides alternative nourishment for microbes, sustaining them in between your meals. New microbes that come along can include harmful infectious

Meet Andrea, Who Got Her Immune Resilience Back by Shoring Up Her Microbiota

Andrea is one such individual who had gotten into a negative cycle of poor microbes and vulnerable immunity. Andrea was in her late twenties, working as a software developer. She had a history of recurrent sinus infections since childhood, especially during pollen allergy season when her asthma also flared. She regularly experienced mild to moderate flares of athlete's foot (a fungal infection of the feet and especially between the toes) and had had two recent episodes of impetigo (a common, highly contagious skin infection). Over the years Andrea had been prescribed several rounds of antibiotics and steroids for the infections and her asthma symptoms, but she grew frustrated that these problems kept coming back and wondered if there was anything else she could be doing to help keep them at bay.

Andrea's immune system was clearly under some stress, demonstrated by her history of allergy-driven asthma and recurrent infections. It was likely that her microbiota was out of balance, too, given her history of antibiotics, which indiscriminately target good as well as bad bacteria. Additional testing revealed that Andrea did indeed have an imbalance of microbes in her gut: low levels of beneficial bacteria and some elevated numbers of potentially problematic bacteria.

The challenge for Andrea was that she was stuck in a cycle: the recurrent infections leading to medication use that further weakened her microbiota and immune function, which then led to more infections, more medication use, and on and on.

Andrea's dietary and sedentary lifestyle habits didn't help. She got little aerobic exercise: she commuted to work by car and sat for seven hours in front of her work computer, after which she sat in her car to drive home, followed by more sitting in front of the TV most evenings. While on weekends she went to the gym to work out in the weights room, this wasn't enough to keep her microbiota healthy and balanced. Her meals were often highly processed and full of refined carbohydrates and the wrong balance of fats, picked up from drive-through restaurants to and from work. We also discovered that her insulin was high, a sign that her system was struggling to keep up with the amount of carbohydrate it had to process and putting her at risk for insulin resistance down the line.

Andrea and I had an honest discussion about what she felt was feasible for her. She didn't feel like she was any good at cooking, nor did she feel like trying to cook anything after a day's work in the office. So instead of new recipes, we looked at alternative store-bought foods and restaurant-food options along her daily commute. Instead of a breakfast pastry, we went for a vegetable omelet or sugar-free granola with fresh berries and plain live yogurt. For dinners, we switched to a bun-less burger with salad instead of fries, or to pairing two differently colored vegetable sides (e.g., one green, one orange) with a meat entrée. For lunches, to eat with her salad, Andrea started to add a tablespoon of live sauerkraut. We also added thirty minutes of swimming three times per week, to increase circulation and enhance immune function, which Andrea said she preferred to other forms of aerobic exercise. On days that she didn't swim, Andrea agreed to take just a fifteen-minute walk before and after work.

Two months later, Andrea came back to see me. She was amazed that these simple changes had had such a profound effect. She reported that her athlete's foot was gone for the first time in a decade, her seasonal allergies had been much milder this year, and she had hardly needed to use her inhaler. She also had experienced no sinus infections so hadn't been prescribed any antibiotics. The last of her previous bout of impetigo had disappeared and hadn't returned. Most important, Andrea felt empowered by the experience, realizing that it was within her control to change what was happening with her body and feel unburdened from these troublesome infections. I reminded her, too, that what she was doing was also going to keep her metabolic health on track, potentially warding off diabetic tendencies that could otherwise materialize later on.

germs you may encounter the next time you touch a door handle or accidentally eat undercooked poultry. They also include beneficial microbes you may ingest through live, fermented foods. Killing agents that affect the microbiome include, most obviously, antibiotics. But could also include other medications as well as pesticide residues in your food.

When we *don't* give our helpful microbiota what they need to thrive, more of the harmful microbes grow, and our immune system grows weaker and more vulnerable. In turn, it is less able to keep all the microbes under control. Dysbiosis occurs, and the situation can get progressively worse. Many individuals I've worked with have become trapped in this scenario of dysbiosis and vulnerable immunity, though by following the principles laid out in this book, they were able to break the cycle and move back into a better relationship with their microbes and improve their immune resilience.

WHAT MAKES GOOD BUGS SO HELPFUL FOR YOUR IMMUNITY?

Your helpful bugs prove their worth as the third pillar of your immune defenses in several ways. They inhibit the growth of bad germs; they help ensure your own barrier cells stay strong and healthy; and they are intimately involved in training and "toning" your immune system. Let's look a little closer at each of these areas.

1. PATHOGEN RESISTANCE

When your surfaces are well populated with good bacteria, there's just no room at the inn for bad bugs. The bad bugs get much less space to form attachments to your barrier surfaces and achieve a stable foothold from which to grow. Good bugs also use up some nutrients needed by less desirable species, and often more efficiently. This leaves less food available for the bad bugs, and less nutrition means less growth. The net effect is that good bugs, when tended to properly, can outcompete bad ones for limited food and physical space.

Another tool the good bugs have to help resist the bad ones are *short-chain fatty acids*, or SCFAs. These SCFAs have names like acetate, propionate, and butyrate. Don't be alarmed by the term *acids*; the human body is full of acids and bases, working in balance to enable all biochemical functions to occur. Beneficial bacteria produce SCFAs when they consume the soluble fiber you eat in your diet (more about that in part 2) and these SCFAs can reduce the virulence of pathogenic bacteria, rendering them less harmful.

Your symbiotic bacteria also have other chemical "weapons" that make things inhospitable to harmful bugs. Scientists call them *bacteriocins*. Similarly to the AMPs you've read about, bacteriocins act as natural sanitizers. They can degrade the external membranes of harmful bacterial cells, creating holes through which internal contents then leak out. Others stick themselves into the replication machinery that other bacteria rely on to multiply, causing them to die out.

Bacteriocins have an especially smart trick, though. Bacteriocins produced by one species kill only *other* kinds of bacteria, sometimes other species in the same bacterial family, sometimes species in an entirely different bacterial family, but not a bacteria's exact own kind. Let's see how this can help us keep problematic bugs under control: *Escherichia coli* (known more commonly as *E. coli*) is a species best known for its ability to cause serious food poisoning. Some sub-strains of *E. coli*, however, are not harmful and can actually be very helpful. *E. coli* strain Nissle 1917 is one beneficial type of *E. coli* that produces bacteriocins that targets and destroys its nasty, pathogenic cousins. And while it's at it, *E. coli* Nissle 1917 is also known to help stamp out other harmful gut infections like the "-ellas": *Klebsiella*, *Morganella*, *Shigella*, and *Salmonella*. Researchers who have studied highly infectious diarrheal outbreaks have found that individuals who don't get the disease tend to harbor this kind of helpful *E. coli* in their digestive tracts. A similar effect can be observed on your skin, where good and bad types of *Staphylococcus* bacteria fight it out for dominance. *Staphylococcus epidermis*, one of the best-known beneficial skin bacteria, produces bacteriocins that kill the pathogenic black sheep of the family, *Staphylococcus aureus*.

The activity of bacteriocins is why, once dysbiosis starts, it's harder for your microbiota and immune system to regain balance without you changing something that resets the cycle. Think about it: each bacterial strain thrives only in its own community, a "bubble" or "clump" of the same strain of bacteria that are unharmed by the bacteriocins they produce but are collectively inhospitable to other kinds of bacteria. If a harmful bug manages to get a better foothold, it produces its own bacteriocins that keep other types of bacteria, good or bad, at bay. There's very little respect for "workplace diversity" in your microbiota. Instead, your microbes harbor more of a primitive smash-and-grab mentality, where each looks out only for its own kind.

This has important implications. When our microbiota undergoes a period of stress, such as when you take an antibiotic, or even when you are simply not sticking to a "healthy" diet or lifestyle, your microbiota is potentially vulnerable to harmful shifts. I don't know about you, but one of the most challenging times for many of my clients (and for myself) is during the holidays, when we're surrounded by sugary temptations, maybe consume more alcohol than we normally would, perhaps are partying a little harder and sleeping a little less, forgoing that trip to the gym to get some holiday shopping done. What this does for our microbiota is shift its inputs, weakening our helpful bacteria and providing an opportunity for the bad bugs to grow. When you take an antibiotic, the effects can be even more drastic: antibiotics don't discriminate between good and bad bacteria, so a significant portion of your microbial slate is wiped clean. Then the race begins to see who can repopulate first—the good guys or the bad? Whoever claims their territory first will be able to keep other species out because of compounds like bacteriocins and because they've won the competition for space and food. It's a major reason why antibiotic use is followed by pathogen-induced diarrhea in one out of every ten individuals.

All this means that it's really essential to keep nourishing the good guys so that they can continue being able to resist the bad bugs. Think of it like tending a garden: if you don't keep feeding what you've planted, the weeds will take over before you know it. And then it's much harder to reestablish balance.

2. SUPPORT FOR YOUR BARRIER CELLS

Beneficial microbes help maintain the strength and integrity of your barrier cells. One major way they do this is through those same SCFAs you read about earlier. The SCFA butyrate is a very easily accessible fuel for your intestinal cells, which can use it to perform their daily functions, maintenance, and to stay healthy. In fact, intestinal cells can use butyrate to produce up to 70 percent of their daily energy needs. And remember those B vitamins that your friendly gut microbes produce? Well, B vitamins are needed to make those energy production cycles run smoothly and quickly. Even though you also consume B vitamins in your diet, most of those are absorbed in your small intestine, leaving little for your large intestine (your colon) to use directly. Your friendly colonic bacteria make sure that you always have enough for your intestinal cell's energy production right there where and when they're also needed. Handy, huh?

SCFAs play another very important role in the function of your barrier cells. They regulate the assembly of "tight junctions" between barrier cells. This means that not only are your barrier cells healthier with the energy they derive from SCFAs, they are also better *connected* to each other in the presence of SCFAs. Better bricks and better mortar build a better wall.

Only your friendly bacteria have the internal machinery necessary to produce these SCFAs. Your own cells can't produce them, and neither can the bad bugs. You can consume them in some kinds of foods like butter, but the most important source of SCFAs is your gut microbiota because, when it's healthy, it produces a far greater quantity than you could consume through food. Microbes need the right type of foods to produce SCFAs, though, and they love complex, fermentable fibers. These kinds of fibers, as you'll learn more about in part 2, aren't an ingredient that our own digestive enzymes can act on. As such, they remain intact all the way to our colon, where beneficial bacteria, which possess the right kinds of enzymes, can turn them into SCFAs.

3. TRAINING AND "TONIFYING" YOUR IMMUNE SYSTEM

As you now know from chapter 2, one of the most important processes your immune system goes through is that of "maturing": developing a robust yet balanced immune defense network and learning about the world you live in—how to discern what is safe, what is a threat. And one of the most fascinating recent discoveries is that our beneficial bacteria are essential to the success of this process. In human research, the relationship between dysbiosis and dysfunctional immune development, resulting in potential allergies, autoimmunity, and infectious disease, is now well established. Studies of germ-free mice, or mice treated with antibiotics at birth, provide the clearest evidence of just what that dysfunctional development can look like: smaller immune organs such as the thymus and spleen, less active T cells and natural killer cells, and B cell activity that is skewed out of balance and toward the production of allergy-related IgE antibodies. That all-important "Yoda-like" regulatory T cell development in the lungs, gut, and on the skin is impaired, leading to increased risk for food allergy, allergic asthma, and allergic dermatitis.

The process of immune learning and discernment is highly complex and involves multiple levels of interaction between you and your beneficial microbes. But it's easier to visualize if we take a look at a couple of examples of how this can occur: First, lactic acid that is produced by helpful bacteria (of the *Lactobacillus* kind), as well as other microbiota-derived compounds in the intestines, are what trigger dendritic cells to extend their long arms into the contents of the intestines where they scout around to capture, learn about, and respond to what's out there. That part is immune learning. When a dendritic cell finds contents related to beneficial bacteria it potently promotes our immune system's development of regulatory T cells that support immune balance and appropriate tolerance to things that should be benign, like foods. That part is immune discernment. Second, when absorbed, short-chain fatty acids and other molecules produced by beneficial bacteria can directly alter the expression of genes in your immune cells that promote yet more important regulatory T cells. Once again, supporting immune discernment.

So the good bugs in your microbiota turn out to be indispensable allies in the very development and calibration of your immune system. They teach your immune cells how to be educated, mature, responsible, and effective adults, rather than impulsive, inappropriately behaved adolescents who don't quite get it right all the time (nothing against adolescents—just referring to my own experience here). I know which I'd rather have manning my defenses.

In addition to supporting learning and discernment, beneficial microbes create "tone" in your immune system, conditioning it to be alert to any infectious challenge that might come along. "Check me out, check me out," hears your immune system when friendly microbes are around. And your immune system does just that. After all, a mutually beneficial relationship isn't one of implicit trust—your immune system must continually verify and even control those friendly microbes, too.

Beneficial bacteria prompt your barrier cells, who can't be sure when they first sense microbial activities whether it's a friend or foe out there, to produce more AMPs, as a precautionary measure. Other cells, like macrophages and neutrophils, also respond to friendly bacterial activity by increasing their readiness to respond to infections. Even adaptive immune cells, such as your B cells, jump to attention when friendly microbes are around. Let's take a look at how they do this.

When they sense friendly bacteria, activated B cells working in partnership with barrier cells start producing a generically protective antibody called *secretory immunoglobulin A* (secretory IgA or sIgA). This is an important antibody that works on the surface of your barriers and makes up part of your first line of defense. sIgA can keep microbes out of the inner mucus layer closest to your barrier cells, control the motility and fitness of different bacteria, and neutralize many of the toxins they produce. Part of sIgA's role is to keep the levels of symbiotic microbes under control, as well as to hunt for pathogens. All good so far? sIgA is also "sticky" and able to attach to the outer coating of microbes. Now let's see what happens to patrolling B cells after sIgA has been released and stuck onto a microbe— even a friendly microbe. All of a sudden, B cells get their binoculars out and start studying what's out there on the surface of that barrier. They're interested and alert now. The next time an unfriendly bug comes along, those B cells see it earlier, then respond with a faster, stronger hammer of germ-specific antibodies.

This dance at arm's length, between your beneficial microbes and your immune system, prevents your immune system from sleeping on the job. Instead, it is kept on its toes, prompted to keep figuring out what's out there and how to respond. This of course improves the chances of discovering a bad bug quickly, if indeed there's one out there, and triggering an immune response against it.

CROSS-TALK BETWEEN GUT MICROBES AND OTHER SITES IN YOUR BODY

Conceptually it is easier for us to understand that our microbiota has effects on immune cells that are hanging around in the same neighborhood. After all, they are within shouting distance, or at least we'd expect them to bump into each other at some point as they roam around the same streets. With this thinking, and from what you know about how our microbiota helps keep us safe from harmful contagious germs, it's perhaps not surprising that oral probiotics and fermented foods that directly target the gut microbiome have been shown to improve your resistance to infections in the *digestive tract,* like diarrheal infections, and shorten how long you're affected by that stomach bug.

More recently, however, it's become apparent that microbiota in one location can influence immune responses over on the other side of town, likely through the signaling molecules they emit as well as their immune training and toning effects. Even one or two towns over. In other words, the characteristics of and changes in our microbiota at one site can alter immunity and inflammation at other, more distant sites in the body.

Multiple research studies have shown this. Oral probiotic supplements, for example, can boost the levels of sIgA in your saliva (according to some scientific reports). This despite the fact that the capsule form (as used in this particular research) won't release its contents until far away from your mouth. Other research studies report that oral probiotics may cut the risk of bacterial vaginosis and reduce levels of inflammatory compounds in the blood of arthritis patients. These locales aren't even part of the digestive system! Several other studies have proven that taking oral probiotics or consuming fermented foods improves resistance against lung infections, too: One of the toughest scientific evidence review organizations, Cochrane, reports that multiple human trials show taking oral probiotics can cut the risk of contracting a respiratory infection, such as a cold, flu, or pneumonia, by about half. And reduce the use of antibiotics by 35 percent. That's incredibly impressive! These robust scientific data collectively illustrate just how much of an effect our microbiota has on our immune resilience and how supporting a healthy *gut* microbiota can support whole-body immunity.

AN OVERLOOKED MICROBIAL HUB: YOUR ORAL MICROBIOTA

Perhaps to the chagrin of your dentist, your mouth is really an overlooked part of your body, even though there is so much evidence showing how it is connected to your overall health and immune resilience. Oral infections and microbial imbalances, such as gingivitis, gum disease, and tooth decay, are now known to have wide-reaching impacts. The reason is thought to be due to inflammation that begins locally but then travels as pro-inflammatory compounds in the blood to other parts of your body. The bottom line is that these oral problems have now been associated with conditions that might not immediately spring to mind when we're talking about our mouths: cardiovascular disease, for instance, is strongly associated with periodontitis. Individuals who have periodontal disease are two to three times more likely to have a heart attack, stroke, or other serious cardiovascular incident. Microbial imbalances in the mouth have also been linked with rheumatoid arthritis, as well as esophageal, pancreatic, and colorectal cancer, and adverse pregnancy outcomes.

Another good reason for taking care of your mouth microbiota is that microbes are constantly immigrating and emigrating between the mouth and the lungs, and from the mouth to the digestive tract. *Porphyromonas gingivalis,* that keystone pathogen for periodontal disease, as well as other oral pathogens, are also able to induce dysbiosis, impaired barrier function, reduce sIgA production, and promote chronic inflammation in the digestive tract once swallowed. Inflammatory chemicals produced by harmful bacteria in the mouth can also be aspirated into the lungs.

Taking care of your oral microbiota is therefore highly relevant.

HOW ROBUST IS YOUR MICROBIOTA?

Given what you now know about the importance of your microbiota on immune and overall health, it's a good time to take a little pulse check. Use this quiz to find out whether your microbiota is likely healthy or whether it needs some extra TLC.

Likely indicators of an imbalanced microbiota	
Have you taken antibiotics within the last 6 months?	Yes ❑ No ❑
Have you taken 5 or more antibiotics in your lifetime?	Yes ❑ No ❑
Do you have any frequent digestive symptoms such as reflux, gas, bloating, diarrhea, or constipation?	Yes ❑ No ❑
Do you have any metabolic conditions such as overweight, obesity, insulin resistance, or diabetes?	Yes ❑ No ❑
Do you have any allergic or autoimmune conditions?	Yes ❑ No ❑
Do you eat less than five servings of fruits and vegetables per day?	Yes ❑ No ❑
Possible indicators of an imbalanced microbiota	
Are you sedentary for 6 or more hours per day?	Yes ❑ No ❑
Do you live in a built-up area?	Yes ❑ No ❑
Do you spend time in nature less than twice per week?	Yes ❑ No ❑
Do you suffer from depression, anxiety, or other mental health problems?	Yes ❑ No ❑
Do you have any skin conditions?	Yes ❑ No ❑
Do you have trouble sleeping?	Yes ❑ No ❑
Do you have frequent infections such as stomach bugs, colds, chest infections, urinary tract infections, vaginitis?	Yes ❑ No ❑
Do you eat more refined grains than whole grains?	Yes ❑ No ❑
Do you eat legumes or beans less than twice per week?	Yes ❑ No ❑
Do you eat nuts or seeds less than twice per week?	Yes ❑ No ❑
Does your diet lack daily fermented foods?	Yes ❑ No ❑
Do you eat processed (packaged) foods on a daily basis?	Yes ❑ No ❑

INTERPRETATION

If you answered yes to any of the likely signs or three or more of the possible signs, you likely have some disturbance of your microbiota. Don't panic: there are strategies you will learn from this book that can help bring your microbiota back to health.

The environment that you provide for these bugs to live in—especially through what you eat, drink, and how you live—determines who will gain the advantage: helpful bugs or harmful assailants. While the factions fight it out, what you habitually choose to consume directly influences which species thrive and which ones don't. Your choices impact the *diversity* of species as well. Remember: diversity is good for immune resilience. If you feed your microbial allies the right things, you will bolster your immune resilience.

To view the references cited in this chapter, please visit
www.immuneresilienceplan.com/science.

PART 2

Are You Helping or Hindering Your Immune System?

CHAPTER 6

Eating for an Army

Foods to Eat (and Not to Eat) to Fortify Your Immune System

Every bite we take, every meal we eat spurs a wondrously complex chain of events in our body. From that very first taste, that food (let's say it's a piece of broccoli if we are being good) travels from the mouth down our esophagus to our stomach, then through the small and large intestines. Along the way, the food is broken down enough to be absorbed into our blood, which then circulates nutrients along 100,000 miles of blood vessels to finally reach trillions of cells that need the nutrients to perform their everyday functions. That you know already. What you may not know is that foods don't just provide the building blocks for the body to get things done, they also provide the very *information* to cells about what to do. That seemingly innocuous, branchy piece of broccoli has nutrients and phyto-nutrients that give the cells marching orders on what to do, how to behave, and whether to be good . . . or bad.

It does this by getting right in there with our DNA and altering how our cells read and apply our genetic code. It involves a complex process of biochemical reactions (the study of which is called *nutrigenomics*). We can see how this works by looking at one example: a phytonutrient we derive from broccoli called *sulforaphane*. Sulforaphane is particularly effective at dialing down unruly pro-inflammatory genes in certain immune cells, meaning that genes go from a state of being actively "read" to more "silent" and inactive. This helps our immune soldier cells maintain a healthier low baseline level of inflammation and a levelheaded response (rather than a reckless, overreactive response) while dealing with a harmful invader. Nutrigenomics is a relatively new science, so we are only just beginning to unpack the myriad connections between diet and gene expression, but it is important because we now have a newfound understanding that food components not only feed our cells' ability to function, but they also signal the cells to tell them *how* to function. Good or bad, depending on what kind of food you eat. All this puts incredible power at the end of your fork.

Although foods are usually more subtle in their effects than the pharmaceuticals, they do exert persistent influence—after all, food interacts with our body and our immune system several times per day *for a lifetime*. And through that persistence comes tremendous power. Plus, foods are *pleiotropic*, meaning they have dozens, hundreds, if not thousands of different kinds of effects in our body simultaneously. Just as tiny water droplets carve great valleys, so does food create powerful sea changes inside us.

To understand what we need to alter about what we eat, we have to have a hard, honest look at our current dietary habits, specifically massproduced foods, our addiction to sugar, and their pitfalls. I'll then offer food-based steps you can take to optimize immune resilience. Through finding the right balance of food types, you'll be able to set a solid foundation for a healthy, robust immune system, from nutrient density, to nourishing your microbiome, to optimizing your immune system's genetic expression. Even though it sounds like it could require huge, complicated changes in your diet, you might be surprised to find out that it boils down to just "Two Rules of Two": two food groups to avoid, and two you should get more of. But before I get ahead of myself, let's understand where we are, collectively, with food, and why.

THE UNINTENDED CONSEQUENCES OF MASS FOOD PRODUCTION

Let's discuss what us health professionals call the standard American diet for a minute. After all, it's what so derails our immune resilience. Large-scale food industrialization combined with high-stakes commercial interests have changed the way we eat over the past century. Originally, delivering cheaper commodity foods that could be widely distributed literally saved millions of people from starvation during and after the Great Depression. But there were unforeseen consequences to our overall health *and* immune health that were to unfold as such mass food production continued.

By the 1950s we were fully entrenched in the industrialized food wave, and even preferred it: "modern" food was cheap, reliable, and no longer reminded us of more difficult days. Instead it bore little resemblance to the whole foods it came from and was either tamed tidily into packages like cans, frozen TV dinners, or boxes, or delivered fast and with pizzazz from the first Kentucky Fried Chicken, Burger King, and Pizza Hut restaurants. Soft drinks, candy, snacks, convenience foods, and other nutrient-poor, high-sugar products loaded with poor-quality fats that were advertised with catchy commercial jingles made greater profits for food manufacturers than most fruits and vegetables, which in turn the food industry had little incentive to promote. And so it continued.

Over the last few decades, it has become evident that our new food choices, combined with factors such as more sedentary lifestyles that have us attached to our computers, glued to our TVs and iPads, and sitting in our cars, have created huge new problems: rates of obesity, heart disease, and diabetes have skyrocketed. The signs of immune stress are also apparent in the unprecedented rates of allergies and autoimmunity. And now, more recently, in our collective vulnerability to global infections like COVID-19. After all, obesity, high blood pressure, and type 2 diabetes, diseases that are directly promoted by our Western diet and lifestyle, are known risk factors for more severe COVID-19 infections and higher mortality rates. This chapter will help explain why.

Believe me, before I became a nutritionist, I too had been the classic food industry target. In my twenties, I worked long hours in New York City, surviving on way-too-carby bagels that I picked up on my morning commute, quick sandwiches or pasta lunches from the neighborhood deli, and frequent, indulgent work dinners at restaurants—almost always with dessert. Those long days, and meals high in refined carbohydrates from the bread, pasta, and dessert, would also see my energy crash, usually around 3:00 p.m., when I would reach for my favorite caffeine-y, sugary treat—a store-bought chai tea latte. It was only much later I discovered it had the equivalent of 10 teaspoons of sugar, eeek! And then there was the frequent work travel—more hotel, airport, and restaurant food loaded with more sugars, other refined grains, poor-quality fats, and low in nutrient density, fiber, and phytonutrients.

My younger self carried me through this period without any outward visible signs (I was one of the lucky ones). Yet, although I couldn't see it, at a biochemical level I was absolutely setting myself up for potential metabolic disease to develop and for my immune system to take a hit. Even though my fasting blood sugar was within normal range, my doctor, who fortunately favored ordering predictive tests, found out that my hemoglobin A1C, an indication of average blood sugar, had climbed from 4.8, to 5.0, to 5.4 percent, over the course of two years, inching its way up toward prediabetic levels of 5.7+. My levels of insulin, the hormone the body produces in response to dietary carbohydrate and which critically enables cells to take up glucose from the blood, were probably through the roof trying to keep up with the poor-quality foods I was throwing at it. Insulin is something I look at frequently in the clinic now; it can help predict type 2 diabetes five to ten years before fasting glucose or hemoglobin A1C can.

What do I know now that I didn't know then? Well, a lot. As I reached my thirties, I found myself the mother of an immune-compromised child and made it my business to learn more about the long-term impacts foods and other environmental factors can have on our entire immune system— the good, the bad, and the ugly. For instance, conditions caused by dietary sugars, like insulin resistance and type 2 diabetes, have a lot to do with our immune resilience. Diabetics are well known to be more susceptible to infections and fare worse when they do catch one. (See more about how diabetes impacts immunity and what to do about it in chapter 14.)

Even without diabetes, the reality is that damaging effects of high blood sugar start long before we end up in a state severe enough to warrant a medical diagnosis. Every time we pound our immune system with sugars and other wrong kinds of foods we chip away at its essential protective capabilities. We're also feeding the bad bugs that hang out in our digestive tract and other areas of our body—the bugs that thrive on those foods can turn into problematic infections themselves. Those undesirable bugs also use our poor food choices to produce inflammatory compounds that then send our immune cells into a hyperalert, reckless state, primed to overrespond to harmful bugs (or even to benign things that they mistake for harmful bugs, like foods, pollens, and our own cells). As those bad bugs grow in numbers, they also crowd out our microbial allies.

Ready to turn away from this dangerous path to chronic immune fragility and disease? This understanding certainly made me want to.

TWO FOOD CATEGORIES TO REDUCE OR AVOID

Now to the first set of my Two Rules of Two. I like to keep things simple. While there are only two categories I tell every client to stay away from if they want to build their immunity, each covers a large range of foods. These are:

- Simple carbohydrates, especially added sugar
- Processed foods, especially "ultra-processed" foods

Let's take a closer look at each of these to find out why.

PROBLEM 1: SIMPLE CARBOHYDRATES, ESPECIALLY ADDED SUGARS

Simple carbohydrates (carbs) come in two main forms: added sugars such as table sugar, high fructose corn syrup, and agave nectar, and refined grains like white rice and white flour, which have had their nutritious outer parts removed. I call these "naked" carbs because they come stripped of important vitamins, minerals, fiber, and phytonutrients. I also count a third type—skinless, starchy potatoes (as used in French fries, potato chips, and mashed potatoes)—as naked carbs.

Most added sugars are a disaccharide, that is, a "double sugar," two simple sugar molecules that form a compound. Table sugar is about half glucose and half fructose. Other kinds of sugars contain mostly varying combinations and amounts of fructose, glucose, and galactose. Simple carbohydrates in refined grains and starchy potatoes (think white flour pizza and pasta, white rice, bagels, bread, potato chips, and French fries) contain chains of easily accessible glucose molecules and are treated very similarly in your body to plain sugar.

Even though we now have a much better understanding of the scourge that sugar is in our society, we're still consuming huge amounts of it—global sugar consumption continues to trend upward and sits at over 171.5 million metric tons per year. Per capita consumption in the US averages a whopping 124.4 pounds per year (that's the equivalent weight of a small adult!). Sugary drinks account for nearly half that intake, and it's not hard to see how: there can be up to 16 teaspoons of sugar in a can of cola and 15 teaspoons in a fast-food milkshake. A store-bought iced, blended coffee drink can have up to 21 teaspoons! This is so much more than the American Heart Association's recommendations of a limit of 6 teaspoons of sugar per day for women and 9 teaspoons for men, which I'd argue is still much higher than optimal (you'll find my specific sugar recommendations in part 3).

No surprise, sugar and other simple carbs are not friends to our immune system. Here's why.

SIMPLE CARBS SIDE WITH THE BAD MICROBES
AT THE EXPENSE OF THE GOOD

Simple carbs provide an easy food source that allows harmful, sweet-toothed microbes to grow, strengthen, and proliferate. Scientists have also seen how these poor carbohydrates improve these bad guys' mobility and ability to outwit our immune system. One of the most obvious places we encounter this is right where simple carbs make their first contact: in our mouths. Dentists (and moms!), after all, are the ones who remind us most frequently about how sugary foods promote the growth of harmful bacteria and fungi right there in our mouths, which can lead to infection and tooth decay. *Streptococcus mucans* is one such sugar-loving bacteria that feeds on simple carbs, producing acidic compounds that then draw the minerals out of teeth and gradually degrade tooth enamel, leaving those pearly whites not so white anymore.

This feeding of bad bugs when we eat simple carbs occurs in other parts of the body, too. After all, eating simple carbs raises the levels of sugar in our blood, and this reaches every nook and cranny—skin, eyes, urinary tract, vagina, between the toes, you name it. Bacteria and fungi, like *Candida*, thrive in this higher sugar environment, and especially so when our immune system is compromised by that same circulating sugar. The *British Medical Journal* has noted *Candida* grows more rapidly and attaches itself to our cell surfaces more readily when sugar is present, making it much more likely to cause infection. Candidal vaginitis or bacterial vaginosis infections, common and troublesome for many women that I've worked with, are very sensitive to dietary sugars. Often, we can completely reverse vaginal infections simply by dialing down sugars and those other naked carbs.

Aaliyah, a high-school teacher in her thirties, came to me with exactly this problem. Her gynecologist had diagnosed her with bacterial vaginosis, and she had been prescribed several rounds of antibiotic creams to try to treat it. The problem was that, while the creams helped for a while, her symptoms would come back not long after she finished each course. As we reviewed her diet history, it became clear that sugars and simple carbohydrates (in the form of sweet treats and sugary drinks) were most likely exacerbating the problem.

To Aaliyah's delight, simply swapping out those foods for complex, high-fiber carbohydrates such as legumes, whole grains, and vegetables made a huge difference to her symptoms. And when she combined that with probiotic and natural antimicrobial suppositories (see page 313), she was able to completely eliminate her symptoms and deal with any subsequent flareups (usually when she deviated in her food choices or experienced a period of significant stress).

At the same time they enable bad bugs, simple carbs deprive us of the good microbes we need to help us in our immune battles. We know from chapter 5 just how important a healthy microbiota is to our overall immune resilience. When we consume higher amounts of simple carbs, the bloom of harmful microbes crowds out the beneficial ones, causing dysbiosis and decreased diversity of beneficial species, that other important immune resilience measure. Recent research also suggests that eating too much sugar stalls the production of important proteins that encourage the growth of beneficial bacteria. So it's not just a question of crowding out the good microbes with sugar-loving bad ones—there are additional signaling mechanisms that simple carbs initiate that further undermine the growth of beneficial bugs.

COVID-19 and Blood Sugar

Even in the early stages of the COVID-19 pandemic it became evident that certain chronic illnesses were associated with more severe SARS-CoV-2 infections and worse outcomes. Type 2 diabetes in particular, a disease of insulin resistance and blood sugar dysregulation, has been associated with more than three times the risk for a mild infection to progress to a severe, life-threatening form.

While it's still too early to understand all the reasons why this is the case, a significant contributor to this unfortunate situation is likely to be the substantial hinderance to the immune system of higher circulating blood sugar. In fact, scientists at EPFL, a world-renowned university in

Switzerland, conducted a deep review of published COVID-19 data in 2021 concluding that high blood sugar likely facilitates the progress of the infection at every stage. They pointed to evidence that high blood sugar helps the virus evade and weaken innate immune cells in your lungs, gain entry into your cells, accelerate its replication and dissemination to other cells, and induce a potentially dangerous avalanche of inflammation.

SIMPLE CARBS DIRECTLY IMPAIR IMMUNE FUNCTION

At the same time as feeding the bad guys, simple carbs take aim at our immune defenses, impairing important activities, derailing nutrient utilization, and damaging barriers.

Remember back to chapter 2 where we reviewed some of the important characteristics of our immune system? Science has shown that high levels of blood sugar impede our immune system's ability to recognize pathogens, to produce signaling molecules, to recruit other immune cells to assist at infection sites, and to produce antiviral interferon gamma and other important antimicrobial substances. High blood sugar also has damaging effects on our tiny and more fragile peripheral blood vessels, weakening the nutrient supply to our immune barriers such as our skin and gut lining, and impairing saliva production (recall that other first-line immune defense mechanism). Not least, all kinds of things start to go wrong with our immune cells, from sluggish phagocytosis to weaker production of granzyme (a cell-killing enzyme), leading to a decrease of productivity and fending off harmful germs.

We have evidence now that diets high in simple carbs also damage our gut lining. Researchers have observed that when a sugar solution is applied to human intestinal cells, the tight junctions between cell become more pliable and lose their integrity. Mucus thickness is reduced, too, providing more space for harmful microbes to attach to our cells, and less nourishment for beneficial microbes. Skin cells have also been observed to lose their organized, tight structure in the presence of higher glucose concentrations, and are less able to replace dead, sloughed-off cells with new healthy cells to keep the skin barrier intact.

SIMPLE CARBS DRIVE UP INFLAMMATION

Simple carbs promote inflammation in three ways:

1. *Via the gut microbiota:* Dietary simple carbs cause a shift in the types of bacteria that reside in our digestive tract. Overall species diversity is reduced and the balance shifts from anti-inflammatory kinds of bacteria to pro-inflammatory kinds. These pro-inflammatory bacteria are particularly adept at producing something called *lipopolysaccharides* (LPS). These are nasty toxins that damage the lining of our intestines by weakening tight junctions and degrading healthy mucus. They then gain entry to our bloodstream across that damaged barrier and travel around our body wreaking havoc. LPS specifically attach to receptors on our immune cells called *toll-like receptors* and signal the alarm to that cell that there is a harmful invader trying to make us sick. The immune cell then goes into a state of attack and releases inflammatory compounds even though there may not be any invader present. The inflammatory compounds damage surrounding cells and perpetuate the alarm response in other cells, sending the immune system into an ongoing state of high alert. The net result? You're inflamed.

2. *By generating more AGEs:* AGE is short for "advanced glycation end product," which refers to any kind of molecular glycation throughout the body, just like the glycation of hemoglobin (which is measured as hemoglobin A1C). The problem with AGEs in general is that they are *AGE-ing* to all cells, including those responsible for immune defense. AGEs create free radicals that damage anything that they happen to come across—other cells, blood vessels, and important proteins, for instance. The damage from AGEs is called *oxidative stress* and your body perceives it as an injury. What happens next is the body's standard response to injury: inflammation. Several immune cells also carry surface receptors that are activated by AGEs and turn up their inflammatory activity.

We do have several natural means to counter AGEs. One involves antioxidants (when we have enough of them), which can neutralize those free radicals. In addition, macrophage immune cells are able to phagocytose AGEs to protect your body, but they can also be overwhelmed if there are too many AGEs. And in doing so they are "killed" by the AGE (so AGEs can stress our macrophage reserves).

3. *By cornering the body into producing a particular type of saturated fat:* Palmitic acid is a specific type of long-chain saturated fat that the body produces when it has more sugar than it can immediately use for energy or keep in short-term storage. The sugar-turned-into-fat connection might seem surprising, but it is one of the key mechanisms by which excess sugar intake promotes fat storage and weight gain. Palmitic acid, in higher-than-normal amounts and in an already pro-inflammatory environment created by sugar, does two very harmful things. First, it switches macrophages in fat tissue from an anti-inflammatory type to a pro-inflammatory, "angry" type. These macrophages start producing lots of inflammatory signaling molecules. Second, it amplifies the effects of pro-inflammatory LPS on those toll-like receptors, making them even greater activators of our inflammatory response.

> It doesn't take much sugar to get into an inflammatory state. Research shows that just one 600 ml (20 ounces) sweetened beverage per day can be enough to drive up high-sensitivity C-reactive protein, a commonly used measure of inflammation, into recognized inflammation territory.

Now, it's true that one bit of cake, cookie, or ice cream isn't immediately going to leave you ravaged by the next harmful bug that comes along. What I'm really talking about here is a long-term pattern of eating that continually puts pressure on our immune system and its trusty sidekick, the microbiota, and gradually wears them down.

Julia is the perfect example of how a long-term sugar and simple carbo-hydrate habit so undermines our immune resilience. She came to see me, seeking help for a series of skin problems that had been plaguing her for the last five years. The longest-running issue was recurrent cellulitis (a bacterial skin infection) on her lower legs and forearms, which, in addition to being potentially serious, made her feel self-conscious. Julia was prone to getting an infection whenever she broke the skin: a minor bump on her knee or a scratch on her arm from her daily gardening work would quickly become raised, pustulous lesions. "I always wear long sleeves and pants, never a dress or shorts, even in the summer," she confided to me. "Swimming is out, too. I just don't want others to see." No one, not least someone in their youthful mid-thirties, should have to feel that way about their body.

She had been under the regular care of her primary care physician and had been treated with several rounds of antibiotics over the years. Re-cently, though, these had stopped being effective, and her doctor told her that his tests revealed she now had a drug-resistant form of *Staphylococcus aureus* on her skin. "I'm worried now that there isn't a good way to control this and that it could get worse at any point," she explained. "I've tried diluted tea tree oil which helps a bit, but it's not enough to make it go away. Help!"

Julia was carrying around thirty extra pounds (being overweight is a risk factor for cellulitis), but she explained that while she tried to eat healthy meals, she was plagued by sugar cravings and regularly gave in to the office candy tin and pastries that her colleagues brought in to share. Add to that her regular morning iced chocolate mocha drink (we calcu-lated it had over 30 grams of sugar per serving) and, as we reviewed her food intake together, Julia could see that she was eating way more sugar and simple carbohydrates than she really wanted to. This eating pattern, combined with the history of frequent antibiotics, meant that it was highly likely Julia's microbiome and immune system were suffering significantly and having a knock-on impact on her ability to fend off this harmful super-bug. It was the biggest hole in Julia's immune resilience bucket.

Unsurprisingly, dialing down her sugar intake was a central compo-nent of the nutrition plan that Julia and I put together for her. Since there is invariably more than one hole we need to plug, we also worked on several others (you'll see what those were when we circle back to Julia in chapter 11), and together these helped bring about dramatic improvements in her condition and restored her confidence in her own abilities to fight off this invisible invader.

PROBLEM 2: PROCESSED FOODS, ESPECIALLY "ULTRA-PROCESSED" FOODS

While sugars deserve a spotlight all of their own, it's not the only food habit that is harming us and our immune systems. Industrially processed foods are the second large food category that can similarly undermine our defenses.

Ultra-processed foods is a term derived from the NOVA food classification system, the most robust system to date created to classify foods based on their degree of processing. NOVA classifies foods into four groups: unprocessed or minimally processed foods, processed culinary ingredients, processed foods, and ultra-processed foods. The most problematic category are those ultra-processed foods, and those are the ones we want to make the most effort to avoid.

Because, really, ultra-processed foods are not even real food, even though food manufacturers sell them to us as such. Just look at what they're made of: according to NOVA's definition, they are "industrial formulations typically with 5 or more and usually many ingredients. Besides salt, sugar, oils, and fats, ingredients include additives that typically imitate sensorial qualities of more 'natural' foods or to disguise undesirable qualities of the final product." These ingredients include varieties of chemically modified sugars, modified oils such as hydrogenated or interesterified oils (a process that chemically turns liquid oils into solid fats), unnatural protein substances such as hydrolyzed proteins and protein isolates, as well as artificial flavors, flavor enhancers, colors, sweeteners, emulsifiers, thickeners, humectants, sequestrants, firming, anti-caking, anti-foaming agents, foaming agents, bulking agents, gelling and glazing agents. I don't know about you, but this doesn't sound appetizing to me.

Like sugar and refined carbs, ultra-processed foods have been found to have potentially very harmful effects. One of the largest studies ever completed on the effects of food processing on health and mortality was conducted on nearly 20,000 Spanish university graduates with an average age of thirty-seven years. It found that consuming more than four servings per day of ultra-processed foods was associated with a 62 percent increased mortality rate during just the two-year follow-up period, compared with consuming less than two servings per day. Similar research has been conducted in the US using NHANES III data from just under 12,000 individuals identifying a 31 percent higher risk of death during the follow-up period in individuals who had the highest level of intake of ultra-processed foods. In short, the more ultra-processed foods we eat, the worse it is for our health and longevity. And they are also bad for our immune resilience. . . .

ULTRA-PROCESSED FOODS IMPAIR IMMUNE RESILIENCE

There are several problematic components of ultra-processed foods that make them bad for our immune resilience. First, they are typically the source of most added sugars and simple carbohydrates that we now know are so damaging to our immune system. That alone is enough to flag them as problematic.

Then they are also typically high in poor-quality saturated fats or vegetable oils *together* with simple carbs, which have a harmful effect of an even greater order of magnitude on our immune system. This combination worsens gut permeability, allowing an even greater flood of LPS to enter our blood, activate our toll-like receptors on immune cells, and unleash a stronger inflammatory response. And it's why you often see news headlines warning about the dangers of high-fat diets according to the latest research study; most of the time, the diets used in those studies are this exact combination of poor-quality high fat *and* high simple-carb foods. Industrially produced ice cream, pizza, French fries, and potato chips are examples of poor-quality fat-plus-naked-carb combos that create this one-two punch. The more ultra-processed foods we eat, the more harmful bacteria we grow in our gut (like harmful *E. coli* strains, according to one study), reinforcing the cycle.

What these foods *lack,* of course, is also a large part of the problem: they are largely devoid of essential vitamins, minerals, fiber, and phytonutrients, and they displace helpful, nutrient-dense foods in our diet. Filling ourselves up on hyperpalatable ultra-processed foods leaves us with little appetite for healthier, nutrient-dense foods. In the United States, ultra-processed foods make up an average of 58 percent of calorie intake. This means that in addition to all the immune-harming foods we're eating, an awful lot of healthful, nutrient-dense, immune-supportive foods also don't get eaten.

ULTRA-PROCESSED FOODS LOCK US INTO EATING MORE

Ultra-processed foods are high in calories but less satiating. This confuses our body and hinders our ability to regulate our weight and food intake. When comparing unprocessed to ultra-processed diets whose main meals are the same calorie-wise, scientific research tells us that those eating the ultra-processed meals eat more snacks between meals and gain weight. It has even been shown that your subconscious brain can better remember where you last saw that packet of potato chips than that apple (which is why I recommend just keeping junk food out of the house as much as possible). The jury is out as to exactly why, but the ultra-processed foods clearly make it difficult to self-regulate appetite and make healthy food choices.

This addictiveness of ultra-processed foods is one reason, as a population, we have such a hard time giving them up. On the one hand, we want to eat healthier—surveys of consumer food trends show that one of our biggest collective eating priorities is for foods without the artificial ingredients and preservatives that are characteristic of ultra-processed foods, and that nearly two-thirds of us report trying to eat "healthy" most, if not all, of the time. On the other hand, in North America we buy ultra-processed foods at an average rate of nearly 240 pounds per person per year, a number that hasn't changed much over the past twenty years. Clearly, despite best intentions, we are still locked into eating these highly processed, immune-damaging foods.

TWO FOOD CATEGORIES TO EAT INSTEAD

The best thing you can do for yourself and your own immune resilience is to take charge of your own food consumption. We all need to be educated consumers to navigate the deliberately confusing world of food manufacturing and marketing. Identifying and reducing added sugars and limiting ultra-processed foods is an excellent start. Part 3 will show you how. Avoidance 80 percent of the time or more is even better! As you do this, you're going to naturally reduce your intake of immune-harming food components—not only simple carbs, but also artificial food ingredients and preservatives, as well as "stripped" calories that lack that all-important nutrient density, fiber, and phytonutrients. You'll be eating more whole foods, too, as a natural side effect of choosing less processed foods.

As you make these shifts, there are two more important food habits to incorporate that will specifically help your immune system:

- The right kinds of plants
- The right kinds of fats

Let's take a look at why. . . .

SOLUTION 1: THE RIGHT KINDS OF PLANTS

We know that consuming higher amounts of unrefined plant foods improves overall health and lowers the risk for many chronic diseases, but eating this way also provides substantial immune benefits. Several research studies show that the right kinds of plant foods—varied, colorful, fiber-rich ones in minimally processed forms—improve our immune barriers and cellular functions, feed the beneficial microbial species in our microbiota, and keep baseline levels of inflammation in check. Plus, eating abundant plant foods turns back the aging "clock," keeping our immune system rejuvenated and robust. Arguably the most studied high-plant food diet—the Mediterranean Diet—is now also widely accepted as protective against conditions that derail our immune defenses, like insulin resistance and diabetes.

One particularly interesting study conducted in Spain shows just how much of an impact eating more plant foods can have on our ability to ward off infections. Families in this yearlong study had their diets tailored to traditional Mediterranean Diet principles, i.e., more fruits, vegetables, and nuts, and virtually eliminating fast food, baked goods, and candy. Amazingly, participants had fewer episodes of cold- and flu-like symptoms, and when they did occur, they were milder. Antibiotic use fell by a huge 75 percent. Many other studies have found similarly impressive effects in improving immunity. So what is the takeaway? Those of us eating more plant foods (and fewer processed foods) are significantly better protected against common infectious diseases.

What is it in unrefined plants that makes them so super beneficial for our immune system? Two big components: fiber and phytonutrients.

FANTASTIC FIBER

Dietary fiber is found only in plants and is a type of nondigestible carbohydrate. This means it can't be broken down into digestible sugar molecules and absorbed through the gut lining. Instead, it passes through the digestive tract relatively intact. Despite this, it has huge impacts on our overall health and immune system: Researchers who have specifically looked at fiber intake report that those who consume the highest levels reduce their risk of major diseases, including infectious diseases, by *over half*. Scientific evidence shows that consuming more microbe-friendly fiber is a useful strategy to improve our resistance against acute and chronic infections by stabilizing the microbiota and bolstering intestinal and overall immunity. It also helps to dial down inflammation and support the health of the gut lining, in large part through its effects on those same microbial mediators.

Fiber can be either soluble or insoluble. Soluble fiber dissolves in water, whereas insoluble doesn't. Foods such as oat bran, barley, nuts, seeds, lentils, peas, apples, strawberries, and pears contain soluble fiber, which acts as both a primary source of food for our microbiota and an excellent regulator of blood sugar, since it slows the absorption of dietary carbohydrate into the blood. And in helping our all-important microbiota, fiber's immune effects become even more powerful: it's soluble fiber, after all, that is the prebiotic food that feeds beneficial bacteria and enables them to produce those short-chain fatty acids like butyrate that you learned about in chapter 5. Certain types of soluble fiber stand out as having particularly far-reaching effects on immune health:

1. *Beta-glucans:* Found in mushrooms (especially in medicinal varieties), oats, barley, yeast, seaweed, and algae, beta-glucans are known to attach directly to specialized receptors on the surface of immune cells, including macrophages, dendritic cells, and natural killer cells. These selectively activate immune responses, including cytokine-signaling molecules and antibody production: beta-glucans have been shown to increase the levels of protective antibodies (like sIgA) in our saliva.

2. *Arabinogalactans:* Arabinogalactans have been a part of the human diet for millennia as they are found in common plant foods like carrots, radishes, pears, maize, wheat, and tomato. In human studies, they have demonstrated an ability to decrease the incidence of cold episodes by 23 percent! That's an impressive improvement using just one humble intervention—fiber. Scientists have also observed they can improve function in natural killer cells and macrophage cells, as well as increase antibody production and immune communications. Medicinal herbs such as echinacea and spices such as turmeric also contain arabinogalactan fibers.

3. *Inulin:* Inulin is a common type of soluble fiber that is especially high in chicory root. Other good sources are onions, leeks, garlic, and asparagus. A recent animal study found that when mice were given inulin, they were much better protected from the flu virus than the mice who didn't have added inulin in their diets. They noticed, too, that bone marrow in inulin-fed mice actually produced more patrolling

white blood cells, that these were better able to mount an immune response, and that they were also better able to regulate that response to avoid excess lung damage when infection did occur. What does this mean to you? Soluble fiber helps set an "immune equilibrium," balancing innate and adaptive immunity in a way that provides increased protection against infection and also helps the body get over the flu more quickly without excess damage to its own cells.

Although insoluble fiber isn't as well recognized for its immune-enhancing properties as soluble fiber, it still plays an important role. Most plant foods have a combination of both insoluble and soluble fiber, just in varying amounts, so you're usually getting some of both. Insoluble fiber is most often concentrated in the skins and outer parts of grains, seeds, vegetables, and fruits. Insoluble fiber doesn't dissolve in water, but it can absorb it, allowing it to bulk up stool to keep things moving through our digestive tract more easily. This is helpful, too, as anyone with a tendency toward constipation will attest to! Along the way, it also supports your "spring cleaning" defense mechanism, providing a sweep through the intestines and carrying out bacteria and their toxins that we don't want hanging around in there.

Unfortunately, fiber intake in the United States and other economically developed countries falls short of official recommendations: by some reports, only 5 percent of us living in developed countries consume the US Institute of Medicine's recommended 25 (adult women) or 38 (adult men) grams of fiber that we should all be getting each day, and 90 percent of us consume only around *half* that amount. On the bright side—there's plenty of room for improvement!

PLENTIFUL PHYTONUTRIENTS

In addition to fiber, plant foods contain an amazing abundance of diverse phytonutrients, also known as phytochemicals. *Phyto* derives from the Greek for "plant." These are chemical components that don't get reported in the Nutrition Facts labels you see on the back of food packaging. In fact, phytonutrients are sometimes even classed as "non-nutrients." But they shouldn't be so sidelined, and luckily, they are now increasingly recognized as having very active roles in our physiology. They aren't absolutely essential for life in the same way that vitamins and minerals are, but they do have a significant impact on disease prevention and healthy aging. They keep our body working well and so help keep us healthier and alive for longer. And there are thousands of them! More than 25,000 have so far been identified, and more continue to be discovered. Some of the big ones you may have already heard of: epigallocatechin gallate (EGCG) from green tea; curcumin from turmeric; carotenoids from deeply hued yellow, orange, and green plant foods; resveratrol from grapes and wine; and sulforaphane from cruciferous vegetables such as broccoli and cauliflower, to name just a few.

Let's take garlic as an example of a plant food with many different phytonutrients. According to classical nutrition analysis, garlic contains 67 nutritional components: vitamins, minerals, and subcategories of macronutrients. That's already pretty impressive. But can you believe there are 2,200-plus more phytonutrient compounds that are active in this tiny bulb?! Now, science doesn't yet know what all of these compounds do. But we are learning more and more. Allicin, the most studied active phytochemical in garlic, is known to change the levels of immune messenger and signaling molecules, enhance the development of new immune cells, and support immune cell phagocytosis. It is quite potently antioxidant, antiinflammatory, and antimicrobial against harmful species in its own right, just like many other plant phytonutrients are. And, like many others, it can turn on your own internal antioxidant systems, including several enzymes that are involved with neutralizing oxidative stress and toxins, protecting your cells from damage. (Antioxidants aren't just for the beauty industry; they play a critical role in protecting your bystander cells from the inevitable damage caused by an immune response as well as the wear and tear of daily living.)

Allicin and other phytonutrients are powerful influencers within that recently understood scientific concept, nutrigenomics. This important new understanding of how your genetic code is used in the body is still being teased out, but we already know several very crucial takeaways.

The first is that your genes alone are not your destiny; you have the ability, through altering your environmental inputs like diet and lifestyle, to change which genes are active, or "turned on," and which ones are silent, or "turned off." This is a huge shift from previous scientific thinking that your genetic "lottery" is what determines your health outcomes (if you're encountering this for the first time, take a moment to let that sink in). This means that, although you inherit your genes from your parents, many genes only become active when the biochemical regulatory stars align and allow them to be read by your cellular gene transcription machinery.

Second, we also know that phytonutrients are one of the most important nutrigenomic influencers. These "gene whisperers" are smart about how they selectively alter gene expression and can turn on certain beneficial genes and turn off other harmful ones. Let's revisit broccoli for a moment. That sulforaphane it gives us is now understood to be able to exert its anti-inflammatory, regulatory properties at a genetic level. So when it encounters an LPS-activated immune cell that has gone haywire, sulforaphane is able to go into the cell nucleus, alter the reading of pro-inflammatory genes, and dial them down. Now you can see how far beyond merely supplying nutrients we've come. The phytonutrients you ate for your last meal are right now circulating to the far reaches of your body, providing these kinds of instructions to your cells about how to behave.

Third, it turns out that our biological aging has a lot to do with a specific nutrigenomic pathway called *epigenetics* (*epi*, meaning "over" or "upon," since this mechanism of nutrigenomics involves planted biochemical marks on your genes that regulate their on/off status). In fact, several eminent scientists have discovered patterns hidden within the epigenetic marks on our genome that are able to closely predict chronological age and that can tell whether, at a cellular level, you are aging faster or slower than your chronological age suggests. What is even more exciting is the potential for epigenetic regulators like sulforaphane to alter those aging-related imprints and turn back the biological aging clock, restoring some of the resilience and healthfulness of youth to your immune system and more. I am fortunate to be involved in designing some of the emerging human clinical research in this area and the early results are very promising.

PLANTS AND MICROBES ARE COMPLEMENTARY IN THEIR EFFECTS ON IMMUNE FUNCTION

One final note on plant foods (for now) I want to make is how phytonutrients, fiber, and our gut microbiota have intricately intertwined roles.

First, gut microbes are essential for harnessing many of the immune benefits of many (and perhaps most!) phytonutrients because several dietary phytonutrients are still in forms that either are poorly absorbed from our digestive tracts or are in the precursor (not yet activated) form. Healthy microbes help us solve these problems by metabolizing many phytonutrients into more absorbable, active forms. Phytonutrients also act like prebiotics by enhancing the growth of beneficial bacteria and increasing their production of SCFAs. And finally, each of the groups of phytonutrients, fiber, and microbiota have their own direct benefits for healthy immune resilience, as you can see in this depiction:

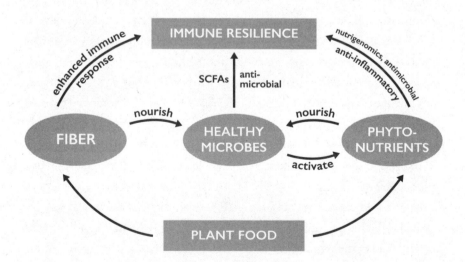

One foolproof way to get phytonutrients into your diet is to look for brightly colored plant foods, since it's those very phytonutrients that give them their strong pigmentation. (In part 3 and in the recipe section, you'll find lots more guidance and recommendations for increasing your plant food intake, like my Phytonutrient-Loaded Salad recipe (page 332).

SOLUTION 2: THE RIGHT KINDS OF FATS

So many dramatic news headlines have circulated around fats that most people are understandably just plumb confused. Are all saturated fats bad? Are all omega-6 fats bad? Are all fats bad altogether? Do fats make me fat (after all, the word is the *same!*)? Here's a sneak preview—the answers are no, no, no, and . . . no. But there's more nuance to understand.

Yes, those stripped, refined carbohydrate-plus-fats foods might reliably cause problems, but we shouldn't conclude that all fats are bad in every circumstance. Fats are a vital component of human diets and are essential for immune health. Healthy diets, such as the Mediterranean Diet, contain fats in the form of nuts, seeds, olive oil, and fish. And we know that certain saturated fats like the SCFA butyrate produced by beneficial gut microbes and found in some foods like butter and ghee are unquestionably helpful to our immune system and digestive tract. In addition, there is a growing recognition that other components of our diet, such as fiber and phytonutrients, influence how our bodies respond to fats. These nuances have yet to be fully teased out by scientists but likely play a significant role in how fat affects us (and they are a big reason why scientists still disagree so much over fats).

One of the unfortunate outcomes of the oversimplified reporting on fats is that fats tend to be labeled "good" or "bad." Most fats, and especially saturated fats, have been vilified as a group since the late 1970s. There was the "fat-makes-you-fat" movement, which ushered in a wave of low-fat products, usually high in sugar, which did nothing but continue to worsen the rising rates of obesity and diabetes. And there was also the argument that saturated fats increase the risk for heart disease by raising LDL cholesterol, based on early data that has since been questioned by scientists from the most prestigious research institutions of the world. More recent analyses have differentiated these saturated fats by their molecular chain length and suggest that it's really only likely to be some types of *long-chain saturated fats,* such as those found in greater quantities in conventionally reared animal foods, that may be the ones to be sure to keep in check. As you'll see in part 3, while animal foods are included in the Immune Resilience Diet, their quantities are limited, and higher quality grass-fed options (which actually have better fat profiles, including more unsaturated fats) are emphasized.

We shouldn't fear fats. In fact, the only kind of fats we should really try to avoid are those we've covered already in this chapter—industrially produced fats mostly found in processed foods. Aside from that, it's a question of learning how to achieve a balance of fat in your diet alongside other immune-supportive and healthy foods. Balancing the different kinds of fats: saturated, monounsaturated, and polyunsaturated. And choosing good-quality sources.

SOME FATS ARE ABSOLUTELY ESSENTIAL, INCLUDING FOR YOUR IMMUNE SYSTEM

The first thing to know is that two types of fats are considered essential in our diets since they perform vital functions and cannot be made in the body. These are the long-chain polyunsaturated omega-3 alpha-linolenic acid and omega-6 linoleic acid. Yes—that much maligned omega-6 fat is actually absolutely necessary for our survival. Deficiencies of these fats causes deterioration in cell membranes that is most visible on the skin as a dry scaly rash, decreased growth rates in infants and children, poor wound healing, vision deterioration, and increased susceptibility to infection. Signs can start to appear in as little as seven to ten days of total avoidance.

These fats are used by our cells to form other fats within the omega-3 and omega-6 families:

Linoleic acid, found in high amounts in nuts and seeds and their oils (as well as vegetable oils, but I don't recommend those as a healthy source), can be used to form another kind of omega-6 fat called *arachidonic acid* (AA). We also consume some arachidonic acid directly when we eat animal foods. AA is used during an innate immune attack to generate pro-oxidant molecules that attack harmful bugs, and it's this action that earns AA the reputation of being a pro-inflammatory fat. However, AA is also used to regulate the development of innate immune cells and improve the function of our gut barrier. It can also be used to form some specialized anti-inflammatory molecules, which means that AA can have both pro-inflammatory and anti-inflammatory roles. Other types of omega-6 fats can be formed from linoleic acid, including *gamma linolenic acid* (GLA), which has anti-inflammatory properties. GLA can also be found in small amounts in green leafy vegetables and nuts. It is found in concentrated amounts in evening primrose and borage oils, which are commonly used dietary supplements. Infants can get a significant amount of GLA from breast milk.

Alpha-linolenic acid is used to form the additional omega-3 fats *eicosa-pentaenoic acid* (EPA) and *docosahexaenoic acid* (DHA). EPA and DHA are in turn used to form various anti-inflammatory compounds that can "mop up" excess inflammation after an immune attack. Omega-3 fats also regulate the pro-inflammatory signaling mechanisms including those of AA, making sure they don't go overboard. They do this by inducing the production of regulatory T cells and dialing down the activation of toll-like receptors by those harmful LPS. Like AA, they support barrier integrity and enhance mucus production during and after infections.

Both kinds of omega fats are essential—so why all the fuss about omega-6 fats? The problem is that the average Western diet has too many omega-6 fats relative to omega-3 because of our higher consumption of industrialized vegetable oils (like soybean, corn, cottonseed, sunflower, and safflower oils in processed foods) and from our higher collective meat intake. At the same time, we tend to under-consume omega-3 fats from oily fish and seafood, flaxseeds, chia seeds, and walnuts, creating a relative deficiency of omega-3s. This imbalance of polyunsaturated fatty acids raises levels of omega-6 AA relative to omega-3s, which, against a background of pro-inflammatory stimuli like poor diet and dysbiosis, means a greater production of pro-oxidant signaling molecules that generate inflammation, without the necessary anti-inflammatory fats to balance them.

This is the reason why we often hear that omega-6 fats are "bad," and omega-3 fats are "good." But as you can now see, it isn't that black-and-white. The goal should not simply be to avoid omega-6 fats, since they have essential roles in immune resilience. Diets that have sufficient amounts of *both* of these types of fats, within appropriate ratios, have been shown to be protective against infections.

The solution is to increase our intake of omega-3 fats, and to switch our intake of omega-6 fats to healthy sources, aiming for a ratio of between 3:1 and 5:1 omega-6 to omega-3 fats (rather than the 16:1 or more that easily occurs in a standard American diet). Part 3 will show you how.

IMMUNE CELL MEMBRANES NEED A BALANCE OF FATS

You know now about phagocytosis, the ability of some immune cells to use their own outer cell wall to engulf and destroy many pathogens. This ability relies on that wall being stable, yet malleable. Think about it—if, as a cell, one of your main jobs is to completely change shape and use your outer cell wall to literally swallow something else (which is what phagocytosis is), it makes sense that you need some flexibility to be able to do that. But cell walls are made of fats—two layers of fats to be exact. And the balance of fat in those walls affects how well your immune cells can do this: Saturated fats lend rigidity, stability. Unsaturated fats bring flexibility and malleability. And this makes a difference to phagocytosis. When put to the test in a scientific lab, researchers found that cells whose membranes were deliberately enriched with additional long-chain saturated fats lost up to 28 percent of their ability to perform phagocytosis. When enriched with unsaturated fats (especially polyunsaturated fats like the omega-3s and 6s), their ability to carry out phagocytosis increased by over 50 percent. So we can say that too many of the wrong kinds of saturated fats hinders phagocytosis and that we need a good amount of unsaturated fats to support it.

Is it possible to have too many *un*saturated fats? The answer is also likely yes. After all, saturated fats bring stability and thereby support integrity as well. And having too many unsaturated fats in our cell walls makes them more vulnerable to oxidative stress, since those types of fats are prone to damage from free radicals. Unsaturated fats need antioxidants (the fat-soluble ones such as vitamin E and plant phytonutrients) to protect them against free radicals and oxidative stress. As you might imagine, having high levels of unsaturated fats, without enough antioxidants, isn't ideal either. Oxidized fats don't perform their jobs well, and can pass on that damaging oxidative stress to other cellular components. Once again, it comes back to *balance*.

The good news is that the composition of fats in our cell walls reflects how we eat. The more omega-3s, for instance, that we eat, the more get into our cell walls. This puts us in the driver's seat when it comes to making a difference in the makeup and functions of our cell membranes.

WE CAN HARNESS THE ANTIMICROBIAL ACTIVITY OF FATS

There are yet more reasons why we want to include a balance of healthy fats in our diet. Scientific studies have reported some eye-opening facts about their antimicrobial activities, including those of *caprylic acid* and *lauric acid*, types of medium-chain saturated fats found in coconut oil, oleic acid, a monounsaturated fat found in olive oil, and the polyunsaturated omega-3 and omega-6 fats. Staphylococci, streptococci (including pneumococci), mycobacteria, and helicobacters, as well as Epstein-Barr, measles, Zika, influenza, herpes simplex, and SARS-CoV-1 viruses have been inhibited to varying degrees in lab studies using these fats. Caprylic acid from coconut oil is also especially good at inhibiting fungi. In fact, it is regularly used in supplement form by natural health practitioners to combat *Candida*. It is thought that these effects are due to the ability of fats to weaken the outer membranes of bacteria, certain viruses, and fungi.

WHAT ABOUT PROTEIN?

Protein is an essential dietary component that provides a vital resource for building and repairing structural components in your body, offers an alternative fuel source, and yes, helps build a strong immune system. In particular, *L-glutamine*, a type of protein building block, is an essential fuel for your gut barrier cells and immune cells. Some athletes, fitness gurus, and self-proclaimed health experts think that protein is the be-all and end-all. But, of course, the reality is more nuanced. While it has been clearly shown

Is Being Vegan Good for Our Immune System?

This is a question that comes up a great deal. Vegan eating is surging in popularity among individuals seeking healthier ways of eating and a lighter planetary footprint. My response is always this: first, if you're following a vegan diet for ethical reasons, I absolutely respect that. I also agree that making more ecological and sustainable food choices is essential for personal and planetary health (more on the connections between environment and healthy immune resilience in chapter 9). And yes, eating more plant-based proteins supports immune resilience. After all, prestigious journals such as the *Journal of the American Medical Association* (*JAMA*) have published on the fact that eating more of your protein sources from plants reduces your risk of dying from an infectious disease.

However, I do have a few caveats:

Sugar is vegan. So are fruit juices, refined grains, fried potatoes, potato chips, and candy. Vegan diets that are high in sugars and processed foods are not going to do your immune system any favors. If the plant foods you're eating are still industrially processed and stripped of nutrients, phytonutrients, and fibers, then it isn't really better than a processed omnivore diet. And, to complicate things, there are more and more industrially processed vegan foods hitting the market, like vegan burgers, bacon alternatives, and vegan sausages, catering to the growing vegan movement. These are particularly tempting for those switching over from an omnivore diet to a vegan one, yet their ingredients usually aren't the beneficial ones we're looking for.

Getting adequate nutrition on a vegan diet requires more careful planning. While meats, fish, and eggs have the whole suite of essential amino acids (the building blocks of protein) that we need in every bite, vegan sources of protein most often contain only some of those amino acids. It's for this reason that vegans have to find complementary sources of protein to make up the full set of amino acids that they need. Rice and beans, as well as other grain-plus-legume combinations fit the bill here, much better than the meatless meats mentioned above do. As do nuts and seeds in combination with legumes.

Micronutrients also need dedicated attention. First, vitamin B_{12} is found only in animal foods, so vegans need to source their B_{12} by consuming fortified foods or taking supplemental B_{12}. Too little vitamin B_{12} can lead to anemia and irreversible nervous system damage, as well as other conditions like infertility and heart disease. In my experience, vegan diets also tend to be low in zinc and iron (I check this in clinic both through analyzing client diet journals for their nutrient content as well as through lab testing). Vegans need to check they're getting the recommended daily allowances of these important minerals, all of which help our immune system run as it should. Another important mineral is harder to find on vegan diets: calcium. Vegans need to pay attention to finding nondairy calcium sources such as fortified nondairy milks, green, leafy vegetables (except spinach, whose calcium is in large part bound to oxalates, which prevents its utilization), almonds, and sesame seeds. Since we often don't convert sufficient amounts of alpha-linolenic acid (the plant-based omega-3 fat) into EPA and DHA, vegans can be deficient in these important fats. DHA from algae oil is one way to help make up that shortfall, some of which your body can also retro-convert to EPA.

I'm not saying it's impossible to be vegan and healthy, but it does require some extra care. The Immune Resilience Diet in part 3 is designed to be mostly plant-based, with a small amount of animal protein. However, if you want to stick to the vegan foods in the diet instead, just take note of the guidance above, and keep tabs on how you feel. Symptoms such as poor wound healing, frequent infections, fatigue, anxiety, depression, mood swings, pale skin, headaches, dry or damaged skin, a sore or swollen tongue, or unusual cravings can be signs your body isn't doing as well on that diet.

in research studies that having an overall protein *deficiency* suppresses immune function and renders us more susceptible to infection, *too much protein,* especially animal protein, is associated with increased gut permeability and impaired barrier function, which as you know, is detrimental to your immune system. Some research also suggests too much protein accelerates aging, which will of course also affect the immune system. The reality is that our protein needs change, depending on several things—age for sure, but other factors can come into play dictating the amount we need, such as regular intense exercise or being pregnant (both situations need more protein).

So what's the right amount to eat? The answer is, of course, that it's about balance, and about understanding that protein needs are specific to each individual and even vary for that individual under certain circumstances. In general, a good amount of protein for us adults to aim for is the Dietary Reference Intake set by the Institute of Medicine: 0.8 g/kg of our body weight. Higher amounts, up to 1.2 g/kg or more are needed for athletes, those doing heavy physical work, pregnant women, children, those post-infection or with wound healing, and in older individuals. We use up more protein during an infection because we use those essential protein building blocks to generate many more immune cells and immunoglobulins. As a result, researchers have observed that we tend to crave higher protein foods following an infection, presumably to replenish lost stores. (Isn't the body cool?)

QUIZ: HOW WELL DO YOUR DIETARY PATTERNS SUPPORT IMMUNE RESILIENCE?

Take this quiz to find out how good your diet is in supporting a robust and healthy immune system:

1. How often do you eat candy, cakes, cookies, sweetened drinks (including sodas or coffees), or other foods with added sugars?

   A. Rarely or never / B. Once a week / C. 2 to 4 times a week / D. Every day

2. How often do you eat industrially produced bread or savory baked goods?

   A. Rarely or never / B. Once a week / C. 2 to 4 times a week / D. Every day

3. How often do you eat refined grains, fries, or potato chips?

   A. Rarely or never / B. Once a week / C. 2 to 4 times a week / D. Every day

4. How often do you eat industrially produced sauces, pre-prepared meals, and packaged snacks?

   A. Rarely or never / B. Once a week / C. 2 to 4 times a week / D. Every day

5. How often do you read labels to know how much sugar or industrially produced ingredients are in your food?

   A. Always or almost always / B. Sometimes / C. Rarely / D. Never

6. How confident are you that you could recognize ultra-processed foods?

   A. Very confident / B. Somewhat confident / C. I'm unsure if I could identify ultra-processed foods / D. I don't think I can identify ultra-processed foods

7. How often do you eat out in fast-food restaurants?

   A. Rarely or never / B. Once a week / C. 2 to 4 times a week / D. Every day

8. What proportion of your grocery store shopping cart contains minimally processed foods including fruits, vegetables, whole grains, legumes, nuts, seeds, meats, or fish?

   A. 75 to 100 percent / B. 50 to 75 percent / C. 25 to 50 percent / D. 0 to 25 percent

9. How often do you include two or more different-colored plant foods in your meals and snacks?

   A. Always or almost always / B. Sometimes / C. Rarely / D. Never

10. How often do you include sources of omega-3 fats in your diet from walnuts, flaxseeds, chia seeds, leafy green vegetables, fish, and seafood?

    A. Every day or almost every day / B. A few times per week / C. Once per week / D. Rarely or never

HOW TO INTERPRET YOUR ANSWERS

If you scored mostly As: Congratulations! You're doing a fantastic job at keeping your diet dialed in to support your immune resilience. Keep it up!

If you scored mostly Bs: Not bad at all! I can tell you're making a substantial effort to dial in your eating habits and your immune system will be benefiting from that.

If you scored mostly Cs: I'm sure, as you've already guessed, there's room for improvement. Don't worry, though—it's just time for a cupboard cleanout and some adjustments to your shopping and eating habits. You can do it—let the knowledge you've gained in this chapter and what's still to come in this book empower you to start to make new choices in the grocery store, in restaurants, and at home.

If you scored mostly Ds: Don't despair. First of all, you're not alone, and we can't beat ourselves up over what we've already eaten. Knowledge is power, so use it to turn things around! Not only will this support a stronger immune system, but your body will benefit from it in so many other ways. You have the biggest opportunity ahead of you!

Eating plants high in fiber and phytonutrients, together with good-quality and balanced fats and proteins, is the foundation of a healthy immune resilience diet. Now let's take a look at how to build on that healthy foundation.

To view the references cited in this chapter, please visit
www.immuneresilienceplan.com/science.

CHAPTER 7

Your Workhorses

Vitamins and Minerals You Can't Do Without

t was a PhD chemist, working over a century ago, who first coined the term *vital amine*. Dr. Casimir Funk, Polish by origin, educated in Switzerland, and working at the Pasteur Institute in Paris, wrote his seminal book *Die Vitamine* in 1912. Within the next several decades, other eminent scientists continued his work as they discovered the long list of essential vitamins and minerals our bodies need. These nutrients are considered imperative to source regularly in your diet since your body cannot make them itself.

Your immune system, just like every other body system, is completely reliant on these essential nutrients and the food sources that contain them. (They are called "essential" for a reason.) Yet many of us fall short of recommended intakes. Reports have shown that, depending on the nutrient, around 25 percent to 75 percent of people in the US and other developed nations have a dietary intake that is less than what is recommended by the official guidelines. This means that your body is most likely not getting what it needs to function optimally, as well as to fight against intruders.

Here are just some of the ways in which vitamins and minerals support a healthy immune response.

- *They support physical defense barriers such as the skin and intestinal tract.* Cells that line physical barriers are in a constant state of turnover. Older cells that rise to the surface of that barrier are brushed off, and new cells must replace those that are lost. Nutrient demands are therefore high at these barriers to begin with, even before immune function is layered on.

- *They help in the production of all chemical barriers.* This includes natural antimicrobial substances, mucus, and secretory IgA antibodies. Some essential nutrients even have their own intrinsic antimicrobial properties (like vitamin C, copper, and zinc).

- *They aid essential immune activities such as the respiratory burst, phagocytosis, signaling, and antibody production.* Levels of essential nutrients in your body alter the potency of your immune system's activity. When you are deficient in certain nutrients, the capacity of your immune system to perform these functions goes down.

- *They enable your immune system to quickly ramp up cell production when needed.* Here is another intensely nutrient-demanding immune activity, since the quick proliferation of millions of innate and adaptive immune cells to fight a germ draws on every single one of our essential nutrients.

- *They protect your cells from damage while the immune system attacks a pathogen.* Many essential nutrients are also either antioxidants in their own right or support other major antioxidant systems in your body.

- *They help control the immune response to prevent excess inflammation.* Several essential nutrients are involved in overseeing the balance between your immune system's "attack" and "refrain" modes, ensuring that inflammation stays within manageable levels during an immune response and returns to a healthy baseline when the threat is over.

THE RISKS OF MARGINAL NUTRIENT DEFICIENCIES

These days, nutrient deficiency diseases such as scurvy, rickets, and pellagra are rare in more developed countries. Now nutrition scientists are in the process of better understanding *marginal* nutrient deficiencies/insufficiencies—the sliding scale of everything that exists between optimal nutrient levels and outright deficiency. Marginal nutrient deficiencies don't always manifest in obvious ways, yet they can still be detrimental to our health and immune system, especially over the long term.

Science has shown us that having inadequate essential nutrient levels can lead to a decline in function of both your innate and adaptive immune systems. Even though they don't always manifest in obvious ways, these insufficiencies can weaken your immunity, increase the risk for infection, and make it harder to fight off harmful bugs. Depending on the nutrient, marginal deficits can affect your barrier function, reduce antimicrobial secretions, reduce immune cell counts, reduce the ability of immune cells to proliferate during infection, impair phagocytosis, respiratory bursts, and perforin attacks, impair the production of signaling molecules, and dampen the antibody response. So simply put, it is crucial if we want to optimize immune resilience to make sure we are getting enough of these essential nutrients. This is especially true for the biggies like vitamin C and zinc, but other nutrients are just as important, as you will learn in this chapter.

WHAT IS OPTIMAL?

The quantity of essential nutrients we need varies from micrograms per day for, say, vitamin B_{12}, an amount that would fit easily on a pinhead, to around a gram per day for a large nutrient like calcium. Since 1941, the Food and Nutrition Board of the US Institute of Medicine has set guidelines for nutrient intake, which can help clarify how much of each nutrient we should be getting, on average, per day. Although the earliest guidelines focused solely on avoiding severe deficiency disease, since the 1990s the guidelines have sought to incorporate new research, as it emerges, on the links between marginal nutrient deficiencies and chronic disease. It was an important shift in scope, and one that is still evolving today. This new directive for the guidelines also introduced defined "Tolerable Upper Intake Levels" as recognition grew that *too much* of a nutrient can be damaging, too; more is not always better when it comes to nutrients. They are another "Goldilocks factor": we need them in amounts that are "just right."

Here are the basics to know about the Institute of Medicine's nutrient guidelines:

- Dietary Reference Intakes (DRIs), the collective term for all the different guidelines, can be found at the National Institutes of Health Office of Dietary Supplements website: ods.od.nih.gov.

- Within the DRIs you'll find Recommended Daily Allowances (RDAs), which are average daily intake levels that *should* meet the needs of up to 98 percent of otherwise healthy individuals. Where there is insufficient evidence available for an RDA, the DRIs will instead provide what's called an Adequate Intake (AI) level, which is an amount assumed to ensure basic nutritional adequacy.

- Tolerable Upper Intake Levels are also included in the DRIs and provide guidance as to the maximum daily intake levels that are unlikely to cause adverse health effects.

Even with the Institute of Medicine's guidelines, though, determining optimal nutrient intake levels can be challenging. Optimal nutrient intake levels vary—your nutrient needs are different from the next person's, and even your own needs change depending on what you're asking your body to do, what it's dealing with, where your starting nutrient levels are. For instance, when you are stressed, have trouble sleeping, or aren't exercising as much as you should, this increases oxidative stress and the need for antioxidants such as vitamins C and E. The simple act of sweating—whether it is on a sweltering day or from intense, aerobic exercise—increases the need for minerals such as iron, potassium, magnesium, and zinc due to the loss of these compounds through your skin. Anyone with a chronic condition such as diabetes, obesity, or any impairment of digestive function (such as irritable bowel syndrome, Crohn's disease, colitis, or short bowel syndrome) can experience an increased need for dietary micronutrients simply because they absorb less of them than the next person. Most medications, including antibiotics, can deplete one or more nutrients as well, especially over the long term. Wound healing and postsurgical recovery are both nutrient-demanding healing processes, in particular requiring more protein, but also greater quantities of vitamins and minerals like vitamin A, vitamin C, vitamin K, and zinc. And when someone is identified as deficient in a particular nutrient, nutritionists and other health providers may sometimes use doses higher than RDA amounts (under close monitoring) to restore repletion (the opposite of depletion), where nutrients are brought back to optimal levels.

As a clinician trained and working in the field of personalized nutrition, I am faced with evaluating these influencing factors and more in each client whom I work with. I use a combination of dietary intake analysis, a detailed dietary and health history, laboratory findings, physical signs of nutrient deficiency, and more to identify where the daily intake of each nutrient may need to be adjusted from the general reference guidelines. After all, the general guidelines are just that—averages that in reality don't always apply to the unique individual sitting in your office.

Not long ago I worked with an active, health-conscious thirty-something named Steve. He loved to hike and camp backcountry trails with a group of his friends all over the US and around the world. They would go on multiday expeditions and, although they were drinking stream water, they filtered and sterilized it appropriately. The trouble for Steve was that, while the rest of his crew experienced no problem at all, Steve would nearly always get sick with a stomach bug, lasting usually for a week or two. And this had been going on for years! Steve wanted to know if he could do something to reduce his susceptibility.

I started Steve on a multi-strain probiotic as well as a prebiotic supplement, but we also identified nutrient gaps that were major holes in Steve's immune resilience bucket: Since his vitamin D levels were well below ideal, and he had few sources of omega-3 fats in his diet, we added supplemental D and omega-3 fats into Steve's routine, as well as omega-3 foods, and made sure, through testing, that this was bringing his levels into a healthy range. I also gave Steve an antimicrobial combination herbal supplement to use during his next trip. The next two hikes—both weekends away on the Appalachian Trail—went well, with no symptoms. Then Steve's resilience was really put to the test nine months later by a one-week expedition up Mount Kilimanjaro in Tanzania. Success—Steve didn't get sick! A big part of what we'd done together was give his immune system the nutrient building blocks it needed to more effectively keep bugs at bay.

OPTIMIZE NUTRIENTS *BEFORE* GETTING SICK

Nutrient repletion, as this story illustrates and as you might well imagine, is best optimized *in advance* of an infection. Once illness hits, it's not that easy to stay replete, let alone correct a deficiency, especially if your appetite drops off. Not only that, infections themselves rapidly use up several nutrients: Vitamin C, for instance, is very quickly used up during an infection and it can take gram-level dosing to restore the body's levels to what it was before. Glutamine, a protein building block, is incidentally also used rapidly during infections. Many infections can also pillage your nutrient levels by impairing absorption, increasing excretion, interfering with utilization, or simply increasing your metabolic demand for those nutrients. By ensuring you are getting your nutrients *before* an infection, you not only help stave off sickness in the first place, but you also improve your ability to "weather the storm" and recover afterward. In short, you become more *resilient*.

NUTRIENTS FROM FOOD VS. SUPPLEMENTS

The absolutely best way to source the essential nutrients your body and immune system need is through food. Food-based nutrients are safe and effective, and when we prioritize eating a nutrient-dense, balanced diet (like the Immune Resilience Diet I detail in part 3) we naturally include healthier foods with beneficial phytonutrients and fiber and shun the less healthy ones laden with chemical additives and poor-quality ingredients. Modern, processed foods are often very nutrient poor and eating those gets in the way of choosing a food that would otherwise add to your daily nutrient tallies. In my experience, you can't out-supplement a poor diet, one of the likely reasons why it's been challenging to get clear evidence of benefit from simply adding a supplemental multivitamin to a poor diet.

That said, staying fully nutritionally replete through diet alone is challenging. My years of clinical nutrition have shown that it takes dedicated intention and little wavering to fully meet all your nutritional needs through food. There's also the challenge of waning average nutrient levels in mass-farmed fruits and vegetables. One study of nutrient levels in twelve fresh produce items found that between 1975 and 1997, average vitamin A levels dropped 21 percent, vitamin C levels dropped 30 percent, and iron levels dropped 37 percent. Several other studies have found similar declines across many nutrients, and we can only assume that most produce today continues to have less nutrient density than it did before the modern farming era. Scientists don't have definitive answers as to why, though they acknowledge that something about modern farming practices— whether it be breeding for improved traits such as size and growth rate, nutrient-depleted soils due to over-farming, longer transport and storage times, or a combination—is the likely culprit. Nutrient levels may still be better retained in older cultivars rather than the newer breeds of fresh produce, and in varieties that are grown in richer small-farm soils. But good data on these differences are unfortunately lacking.

For these reasons I also recommend taking a good-quality multivitamin and mineral supplement (hereafter referred to as *multivitamin*) as an insurance policy against nutrient deficits, even as you pay close attention to diet. As we look at the most important immune-related nutrients over the rest of this chapter, you'll see my guidelines for the amounts to look for in your multivitamin as well as specific circumstances where you'll want to either avoid a nutrient (for example, iron is not something everyone should have in their multivitamin) or where you may need to add a supplement to your maintenance-level multivitamin. There are situations where it can be a sound strategy to go above the RDA level; there is good rationale, for instance, for choosing a higher level of vitamin D supplementation during winter months in northern latitudes.

Another complication is that finding good-quality supplemental nutrients is not that simple. There are many to select from and not all carry the nutrients that you need. There is also very little regulation of the dietary supplement industry in the US—quality standards are very basic and approval by the FDA is not required before products are introduced to market. There's a great deal of variation in the quality of nutrient ingredients used in supplements and often undesirable filler ingredients that are added, too, like artificial dyes, anticaking agents, and titanium dioxide (a possible human carcinogen). Inadvertent contaminants such as lead, mercury, or polychlorinated biphenyls (PCBs) can sneak in if proper testing of ingredients and the final product isn't conducted. As a practitioner, I use and recommend only products whose manufacturers I have performed due diligence on and am satisfied that they have the right quality processes in place to ensure the nutrients will be effective and there isn't anything harmful lurking. I have listed the top companies I recommend and which you can feel sure of getting a good-quality product from in the Resources section of this book.

One important last point before we dive into the vitamins and minerals you need to know for immune health is that we must avoid excessive nutrient intake at levels that may be unsafe. We are most at risk from this when we are taking more than one supplement providing the same nutrient and also consuming fortified and natural food sources. It's important to check the cumulative intake levels of nutrients across *all* your supplemental and non-supplemental intake sources to ensure they stay within Tolerable Upper Intake Levels.

VITAMINS AND MINERALS TO KNOW FOR IMMUNE HEALTH

VITAMIN A (RETINOL)

Vitamin A is one of the most researched nutrients for immune health. And for good reason, since it is involved in most aspects of your defense systems. Retinol (preformed vitamin A) is essential for keeping your body's barriers armed and intact—it is needed for the physical integrity of your barriers, for mucin production, as well as for AMP (remember—your natural antimicrobial proteins?) and secretory IgA production. It contributes to the phagocytic and respiratory burst functions of innate immune cells (both of which are impaired when vitamin A is deficient) and, in its carotenoid form (a form that can be converted to retinol in your body), protects bystander cells from oxidative damage. Retinol also has a regulatory role that helps build up and calibrate your immune response: it helps shape the development and maturation of immune cells, ensuring that they can successfully proliferate in response to any pathogen invasion, and it balances helper T cell and regulatory T cell formation. Retinol is essential for the proper production of antibodies and is known to improve your body's response to vaccines.

Its wide range of influence is likely why a vitamin A deficiency is associated with an increased risk for morbidity and mortality from all types of infections. Even a mild vitamin A insufficiency is associated with increased risk for respiratory and gastrointestinal infections, especially in children, and with worse outcomes in those children who end up hospitalized. In certain areas of the US, especially low-income areas where more nutrient-poor foods and insufficient nutrient-rich foods are consumed, up to half of the population can be deficient or insufficient in vitamin A.

WHERE TO FIND VITAMIN A

Vitamin A as preformed retinol is found in animal foods such as liver, egg, butter, and milk. Carotenoids, sometimes known as pro-vitamin A (beta-carotene is the primary one), are found in yellow, orange, red, and green brightly colored plant foods such as sweet potato, pumpkin, butternut squash, carrots, cantaloupe melon, tomato, spinach, and other green leafy vegetables. Carotenoids can be converted to retinol in the body, but simultaneous fat intake (carotenoids are fat soluble), healthy iron levels, and good thyroid function are necessary for this to occur well. In addition, the enzyme that converts carotenoids to retinol in our body runs slower for some of us than others (something you *can* blame on your genes). The net result is there are some potential (and often hidden) challenges with relying on plant-only sources for your vitamin A.

SHOULD I SUPPLEMENT WITH VITAMIN A FOR IMMUNE HEALTH?

Yes, as part of your daily multivitamin at an amount that provides at least 50 percent of your RDA level. In general, adults should choose a multivitamin with a mix of retinol (usually as retinyl acetate or retinyl palmitate) and natural forms of pro-vitamin A carotenoids (usually beta-carotene). Retinol content should be 2,500–5,000 IU (750–1,500 mcg RAE—see box below) per day. Vegans and those with low thyroid function should lean toward the higher side of that range.

Decoding Vitamin A Units

Vitamin A unit measures are somewhat complicated by the fact that there has been a transition from using International Units (IU) to micrograms of retinol activity equivalents (RAE). The reason for using RAE is that it accounts for the variable potency of the different forms of vitamin A (retinol vs. carotenoids) in your body. For instance, 1 IU of retinol is equal to 0.3 mcg RAE. However, 1 IU beta-carotene is much less potent, equating to just 0.05 mcg RAE.

CAUTIONS

If you are a smoker or former smoker, be cautious with excess pro-vitamin A intake since several large trials have found that taking 20 mg synthetic beta-carotene or more per day may increase the risk for lung cancer (this doesn't apply to natural sources of supplemental carotenoids, which are usually listed on supplement labels with the food source they are derived from).

AM I AT RISK FOR VITAMIN A INSUFFICIENCY?

Complete this questionnaire to find out if you may have insufficient levels of vitamin A.

Likely factors/signs	
Deterioration of night vision (often a first sign)	Yes ❑ No ❑
Bitot's spots (foamy patches) in your eye(s)	Yes ❑ No ❑
Possible factors/signs	
Dry eyes	Yes ❑ No ❑
Dry hair	Yes ❑ No ❑
Dry mouth	Yes ❑ No ❑
Dry/itchy/bumpy skin	Yes ❑ No ❑
Bumpy skin on the back of upper arms	Yes ❑ No ❑
Thin, brittle, or soft nails	Yes ❑ No ❑
Tooth decay	Yes ❑ No ❑
More frequent infections	Yes ❑ No ❑
Reduced tear production	Yes ❑ No ❑
Poor wound healing	Yes ❑ No ❑

If you answered yes to either of the first two likely signs, start adding vitamin A foods to your diet (including those from animal sources if possible), begin supplementation according to the guidelines above, *and seek professional advice about the cause of your symptoms and the potential need for vitamin A repletion through additional supplementation.* If you answered yes to three or more of the possible signs, add more vitamin A foods to your diet and follow the supplement guidelines above.

VITAMIN C

Vitamin C is another nutrient that hits so many aspects of our broad immune system. Starting with our defense barriers, vitamin C is used to make collagen, a key building block for barriers that helps them stay supple and strong. It is essential for healing from physical trauma or surgery; being deficient in vitamin C has been shown to impair wound healing. Vitamin C also has its own intrinsic antimicrobial properties, thought to be due to its acidity: research that has looked at the topical application of vitamin C to cold sores, for example, showed that it could shorten the duration of the cold sore and reduce the shedding of viral particles, making it less contagious.

Innate immune cells have much higher concentrations of vitamin C than other cells, likely because vitamin C is useful for so many of their activities. It stimulates their mobility, antiviral interferon production, bacteria-killing activities, and phagocytosis. It works on both ends of the respiratory burst process: Vitamin C used in concentrated amounts during a respiratory burst is a pro-oxidant, meaning that it can damage and destroy microbes. But vitamin C in lower amounts works as an antioxidant, protecting our own healthy cells and their component parts from damage. It also helps to regenerate other antioxidants like vitamin E so they can be used again. Vitamin C acts within the adaptive immune system, too. It improves the ramp-up of T and B cells in the presence of a pathogen. It also helps to stimulate antibody production. Given these wide-ranging roles, it's not surprising your immune system uses up so much more vitamin C when you're fighting something off.

Correcting a deficiency of vitamin C has been shown to reduce the incidence of infections, especially respiratory infections. And going above RDA levels can be beneficial for individuals with increased physical stress (see the section below: "Am I at Risk for Vitamin C Insufficiency?") or for those who have an infection as it may shorten its duration and reduce its severity.

WHERE TO FIND VITAMIN C

Vitamin C is found in many fruits and vegetables, especially kiwifruit, citrus fruits, strawberries, bell peppers, asparagus, and broccoli. (*Eating just two kiwifruit per day has been shown to improve immune cell movement and respiratory burst capacity.*) Some foods are also fortified in vitamin C. Vitamin C is partially destroyed by heat, so consuming some raw food sources is a good idea. Freezing preserves vitamin C, so frozen foods can sometimes contain higher levels of vitamin C than produce that has been picked early and had to travel long distances before appearing on grocery store shelves. High blood sugar interferes with our cells' ability to take up vitamin C—yet another reason to keep blood sugar well under control.

SHOULD I SUPPLEMENT WITH VITAMIN C FOR IMMUNE HEALTH?

Yes, as part of your daily multivitamin. In general, adults should choose a multivitamin with the full 100 percent of the RDA for vitamin C. More is needed during special circumstances: During a respiratory infection, a temporary increase in vitamin C intake to 2 grams per day may help shorten the duration of symptoms and help maintain adequate vitamin C levels. Between 1 gram and 2 grams per day may also be beneficial during extreme physical stress and in wound healing.

CAUTIONS

Doses above 1 gram per day may cause reversible diarrhea. If this occurs, lower the dose to a tolerated level. Vitamin C can increase absorption of dietary iron, so those with an iron overload condition called hemochromatosis should be cautious with their vitamin C intake. Higher doses of supplemental vitamin C (above 500 mg per day) may also increase the risk for calcium oxalate kidney stones in predisposed individuals.

AM I AT RISK FOR VITAMIN C INSUFFICIENCY?

Vitamin C insufficiency or deficiency is not uncommon, even in high-income countries like the US, Singapore, and New Zealand. Complete this questionnaire to find out if you may have insufficient levels of vitamin C.

Likely factors/signs	
Smoking	Yes ❑ No ❑
Occupational/ongoing exposure to environmental toxins	Yes ❑ No ❑
Heavy alcohol consumption (eight drinks or more per week for women and fifteen drinks or more per week for men)	Yes ❑ No ❑
High-intensity athlete	Yes ❑ No ❑
Work involving intense physical activity	Yes ❑ No ❑
Chronic inflammatory disease	Yes ❑ No ❑
Possible signs	
More frequent infections	Yes ❑ No ❑
Frequent cold sores	Yes ❑ No ❑
Poor wound healing	Yes ❑ No ❑
Frequent nosebleeds	Yes ❑ No ❑
Bleeding gums or reddened gum line	Yes ❑ No ❑
Gingivitis	Yes ❑ No ❑
Frequent bruises	Yes ❑ No ❑
Dry, wrinkled skin	Yes ❑ No ❑
Cracked lips	Yes ❑ No ❑
Tooth decay	Yes ❑ No ❑
Thin, brittle, or soft nails	Yes ❑ No ❑
Vision deterioration	Yes ❑ No ❑
Corkscrew hairs	Yes ❑ No ❑

If you answered yes to any of the likely factors or signs, or to three or more of the possible signs, add more vitamin C foods to your diet and consider increasing your maintenance level of supplemental vitamin C intake to 200 mg per day (for adults and children over eight years of age) as long as you have no history of iron overload.

VITAMIN D

Did your mother tell you to "go outside and get some vitamin D" as a child? If so, she was right. Vitamin D is unique in that it can be made from cholesterol in your skin, but only in the presence of sunlight, or more specifically UVB rays. UVB provides the energy necessary to convert that cholesterol into vitamin D. It's our very own form of "photosynthesis," something we normally think of only in relation to plants. (That's why vitamin D is often called the "sunshine vitamin.")

Vitamin D is best known for its role in bone health. However, vitamin D is in fact a supreme multitasker, with effects across the body. You'll often find vitamin D playing a regulatory role, which has earned it the designation of "hormone" in some scientific circles. Vitamin D is also an absolutely key nutrient for your body's defense. Most immune cells carry specialized receptors for vitamin D, indicating that those cells are finely attuned to "listening" to vitamin D's signals. Immune cells also contain the specialized machinery needed to convert skin-derived vitamin D to its most usable form, so that they always have a ready supply to hand. Very few other cells can do this! Here are some of the ways your immune system uses vitamin D:

- It is the major director of the production of the many AMPs your body produces, lending it a broad-spectrum "antibiotic" effect.
- It is important for maintaining adequate contact between adjacent barrier cells so that nothing gets through that shouldn't.
- It increases the effectiveness of your immune cells' oxidative burst.
- Through its ability to enhance immune cell communication, it helps mobilize immune cells to infected areas, improves the messaging between innate and adaptive immune cells, and influences the balance of "attack" and "hold back" signals.

Vitamin D insufficiency, at levels not severe enough to cause outright bone disease, is known to increase the risk and severity of several infections including respiratory infections, urinary tract infections, wound infections, and COVID-19. It is also associated with more severe outcomes from infectious diseases. By contrast, adequate levels of vitamin D are associated with improved protection against infection and better outcomes during infections. Vitamin D is also helpful in autoimmune diseases, allergies, and asthma.

WHERE TO FIND VITAMIN D

Vitamin D is not easy to source from food. Very few foods contain it. Liver, in particular beef liver, is one reasonable source. As are fatty fish and their oils (herring, salmon, and sardines, for example) and eggs from hens that have been supplemented with vitamin D. Some foods, such as milk and orange juice, are often vitamin D fortified. In an obscure twist, mushrooms exposed to sunlight can become vitamin D–rich.

An important source of vitamin D is sunlight exposure on your skin. This presents a conundrum, of course, since it's well known that excess sunlight can increase the risk for premature aging and skin cancer. However, Dr. Michael Holick, foremost expert on vitamin D with dozens of scientific publications to his name, advises that sensible sun exposure—just 5 to 15 minutes of sun exposure on your arms and legs three times per week between the hours of 10:00 a.m. and 3:00 p.m.—can usually provide sufficient vitamin D during the spring, summer, and fall. You will have to be sunscreen-free for this effect, though you should apply sunscreen after 15 minutes if you'll be in the sun longer.

SHOULD I SUPPLEMENT WITH VITAMIN D FOR IMMUNE HEALTH?

Yes, as part of your daily multivitamin (at your full RDA level). More may be needed during winter months and in special circumstances. In general, adults should choose a multivitamin with at least 100 percent of the RDA (600 IU) for vitamin D and follow the guidance for safe skin exposure outlined above. During winter months, when sunlight intensity and exposure is reduced, 1,500 to 2,000 IU of supplemental vitamin D is a good idea and is supported by the US Endocrine Society. Individuals with darker skin don't make as much vitamin D from sunshine because the increased pigmentation blocks sunlight. If this is you, consider taking supplemental 1,500 to 2,000 IU vitamin D per day year-round.

However, I routinely find reason to recommend supplementation with higher doses than even those I've just described. This is because many individuals have deficient or suboptimal levels and need short-term (or sometimes even long-term) higher dosing to achieve repletion. Insufficiencies are so common that I recommend, without question, that everyone test their vitamin D level. Vitamin D (specifically called 25-OH-D) tests are among only a few nutrient tests easily available from nearly all doctors (most other nutrients can be assessed only through specialized labs that are most often available only through qualified functional medicine or nutrition providers; see the Resources section if you're interested in finding out more). A preferred 25-OH-D result range is 40–60 ng/mL (100–150 nmol/L), as recommended by the US Endocrine Society.

CAUTIONS

Some research shows that signs of vitamin D toxicity can occur in some individuals when 25-OH-D levels exceed 100 ng/mL (250 nmol/L). It's extremely unlikely you would reach this range without taking tens of thousands of IU per day for many months. However, it's another reason to keep monitoring your levels through testing to be sure you're staying in the target range.

AM I AT RISK FOR VITAMIN D INSUFFICIENCY?

Likely factors/signs	
Vitamin D levels below 40 ng/mL (100 nmol/L)	Yes ❑ No ❑
Poor bone mineral density (osteopenia or osteoporosis)	Yes ❑ No ❑
Overweight or obesity	Yes ❑ No ❑
Possible factors/signs	
Dark skin (especially those of African descent)	Yes ❑ No ❑
Sun avoidance and/or regular sunscreen use	Yes ❑ No ❑
Living further away from the equator (especially at latitudes above 37 degrees north or below 37 degrees south)	Yes ❑ No ❑
Severe hair loss	Yes ❑ No ❑

Possible factors/signs (continued)	
More frequent infections	Yes ❑ No ❑
Yellow, slow-growing nails	Yes ❑ No ❑
Gingivitis	Yes ❑ No ❑
Muscle pain	Yes ❑ No ❑
Fatigue	Yes ❑ No ❑
Depressed mood	Yes ❑ No ❑
Poor wound healing	Yes ❑ No ❑

If you answered yes to any of the likely signs, you should supplement with 2,000 IU vitamin D per day regardless of the time of year and have your vitamin D levels checked since you may need a higher dose if your levels are low. If you also have poor bone mineral density, add vitamin K to help with calcium deposition into bones. If you answered yes to three or more of the possible signs and factors, maintain 1,000–2,000 IU per day of supplemental vitamin D and also request to have your vitamin D levels checked.

VITAMIN E

Fun fact: Vitamin E is found in higher concentrations in immune cells compared to other cells in blood. Many immune functions are better when vitamin E levels are replete—immune signals work better, immune cells (both in the innate and adaptive categories) perform better and proliferate more readily in response to pathogens, and our immune system stays responsive but balanced.

Vitamin E status becomes especially important as we age, and so most of the research showing immune benefit from extra vitamin E is in older groups. Here we see that it can boost T cell, neutrophil, and natural killer cell activity and improve natural resilience against respiratory tract infections and pneumonia. Older individuals who get extra vitamin E also generate a stronger protective response and immune memory after receiving a vaccine. You can find out more about how to help support your immune system in your later years in chapter 14.

WHERE TO FIND VITAMIN E

Vitamin E is a fat-soluble vitamin, so it is often found in combination with natural oils. Wheat germ, nuts (such as almonds, peanuts, and hazelnuts), seeds (such as sunflower, pumpkin, and sesame), nut and seed oils, and green leafy vegetables are good sources.

SHOULD I SUPPLEMENT WITH VITAMIN E FOR IMMUNE HEALTH?

Yes, as part of your daily multivitamin. In general, choose a multivitamin with 80 percent to 100 percent of the RDA for vitamin E. Most multivitamin supplements contain only the alpha-tocopherol form of vitamin E. However, there are three other tocopherols as well as four tocotrienols within the vitamin E family that each carry their own powerful immune benefits and are available as standalone supplements. As an (important) aside, food sources of vitamin E already contain a blend of the tocopherols and tocotrienols.

CAUTIONS

Choose a natural vitamin E form (rather than synthetic) for your supplement—look for the designation "*RRR*-α-tocopherol" (also referred to as "d-alpha-tocopherol") rather than the synthetic "*all-rac*-α-tocopherol." Synthetic forms, in large doses, have been found to potentially increase the risk for prostate cancer in men. Excess vitamin E may also increase the risk for bleeding since it acts as a blood thinner and so should be avoided before surgery.

AM I AT RISK FOR VITAMIN E INSUFFICIENCY?

Evidence indicates that 90 percent of American adults do not meet the estimated average requirement for vitamin E and that one-third of the population may have a marginal vitamin E deficiency.

Likely factors/signs	
Age over sixty years	Yes ❏ No ❏
Low dietary fat intake	Yes ❏ No ❏

Possible factors/signs		
Consumption of refined (milled) instead of whole grains	Yes ❏	No ❏
Tendency toward decreased bile flow or gallstones	Yes ❏	No ❏
Muscle pain	Yes ❏	No ❏
Muscle weakness	Yes ❏	No ❏
Neuropathy (nerve pain)	Yes ❏	No ❏
Coordination difficulties	Yes ❏	No ❏
Vision deterioration	Yes ❏	No ❏
Wrinkled skin	Yes ❏	No ❏

If you answered yes to either of the likely factors/signs or to three or more of the other possible factors/signs, focus on vitamin E intake from food sources, your multivitamin, and/or standalone supplement sources.

IRON

Iron is a critical nutrient for several fundamental processes that affect every cell in your body, and therefore your immune system, too. It is a required nutrient any time a cell reproduces itself, which of course immune cells have to do quickly and effectively when needed. It is also used to transport oxygen and generate the energy that all cells, including your immune cells, need to function. And it's for this reason that iron-deficiency anemia can really make you tired.

Other roles that iron plays are highly specific to your immune system: it is involved in forming the communications molecules used by your defense system as well as forming that helpful antiviral compound, interferon gamma. Similar to vitamin C, it's used as a pro-oxidant in your innate immune system's respiratory burst, but it is also part of an important antioxidant enzyme, catalase, that protects your own cells.

We know from looking at examples of iron-deficiency anemia that, as iron levels drop, immune cell activity diminishes, too. Science has observed that your barrier cells can lose their integrity, susceptibility to infections goes up, and vaccinations become less effective at prompting the development of immune memory.

An intriguing thing about iron is that it is also hijacked by most pathogens for their own nourishment and growth. That's right—iron is food for most infectious pathogens. So much so that your body has developed a unique way to deal with this nutrient during times of infection. When it needs to prevent pathogens from accessing iron, your body shunts iron into storage locations so that the circulating levels of iron drop. By ingenious design, immune cells act as some of those storage places, which provides sufficient levels of iron for immune defense, while limiting the availability to pathogens. This means, once again, that it's crucial to keep your body's iron stores at healthy levels *before* an infection, since once you are sick, your body deliberately tries to keep iron out of circulation.

WHERE TO FIND IRON

The easiest sources of dietary iron for your body to use come from animal foods, including beef, chicken, fish, eggs, and clams, as well as iron-fortified plant foods. Iron is also found in non-fortified plant foods, including beans, lentils, spinach, tofu, and cashews, but in a less available form. The absorption of this plant-derived iron is heavily influenced by other food components present at the same meal: vitamin C foods increase its absorption, while plant phytates (found in beans and lentils) and tannins in coffee and tea inhibit its absorption. Vegans and vegetarians can improve iron absorption from plant sources by soaking, sprouting, and/or fermenting their legumes, consuming tea and coffee away from mealtimes, and including vitamin C foods with their meals.

SHOULD I SUPPLEMENT WITH IRON FOR IMMUNE HEALTH?

General supplementation at 100 percent of the RDA is recommended for women in their reproductive years, who have a menstrual cycle. Otherwise, only supplement if an iron deficiency has been clinically identified and under the guidance of a qualified practitioner. In general, men and postmenopausal women should choose a multivitamin supplement that does *not* contain iron.

CAUTIONS

Iron supplementation during an infection may increase the availability for pathogen growth and should therefore be stopped temporarily if you become sick. Several relatively common hereditary diseases are associated with iron overload, and affected individuals often don't realize they are vulnerable. That's why iron supplementation should be limited only to the groups noted above and kept within recommended daily intake levels. Keep any supplements containing iron away from children; accidental overdose of iron-containing supplements is a leading cause of poisoning deaths in children under six years old.

AM I AT RISK FOR IRON INSUFFICIENCY?

Iron deficiency is the most common nutrient deficiency in the world, including in the USA.

Possible factors/signs	
General fatigue or low energy	Yes ❏ No ❏
Easily fatigued with exercise	Yes ❏ No ❏
Rapid heart rate/palpitations	Yes ❏ No ❏
Pale nail beds	Yes ❏ No ❏
Gray-tinged skin	Yes ❏ No ❏
Pica*	Yes ❏ No ❏
Regular high-intensity exercise	Yes ❏ No ❏
Frequent blood donation	Yes ❏ No ❏
Obesity	Yes ❏ No ❏
Chronic inflammatory disease	Yes ❏ No ❏
Parasitic infection	Yes ❏ No ❏
Vegan or vegetarian diet	Yes ❏ No ❏

*Pica is an eating disorder characterized by the compulsive consumption of nonfood items (or the desire to consume nonfood items). This can range from less harmful items like ice, to more harmful ones like soap, clay, or paint. Iron deficiency is one potential cause of this disorder.

If you answered yes to any of the above possible factors/signs it's a good idea to get your iron levels tested. This is a routine blood test that most practitioners will readily order.

SELENIUM

Selenium is not as frequently mentioned as other nutrients when discussing immunity, but it should be, especially when it comes to vulnerability toward viruses. It is a potent stimulator of antiviral interferon gamma as well as other antiviral molecules. Selenium is also needed for your immune system to produce T cells and antibodies, which work against viruses, bacteria, and other types of pathogens. It also helps your body make use of a compound called *glutathione*, considered a "master antioxidant" because it is found in substantial concentrations in nearly every single cell in your body and has the ability to regulate the balance of immune activity.

WHERE TO FIND SELENIUM

Good sources of dietary selenium are Brazil nuts (just two or three nuts can provide your whole daily amount) and meats (especially organ meats), eggs, cod, halibut, salmon, and oysters. Some plant foods, such as broccoli, garlic, and wheat, if grown in mineral-rich soils, can contain good amounts of selenium.

SHOULD I SUPPLEMENT WITH SELENIUM FOR IMMUNE HEALTH?

Yes, as part of your daily multivitamin. In general, adults should choose a multivitamin with 100 percent of the RDA for selenium.

CAUTIONS

Intakes above the Tolerable Upper Intake Level in supplement form, or even from dietary sources, have been associated with an increased risk for type 2 diabetes and some cancers. I have come across individuals who have overdosed over time by routinely consuming a handful of Brazil nuts every day.

AM I AT RISK FOR SELENIUM INSUFFICIENCY?

A selenium insufficiency, relatively common in the US and elsewhere, is closely linked with worsened viral infections and the reactivation of latent viruses in the body. So it's good to make sure you are getting enough.

Possible factors/signs	
Low thyroid function (even mild)	Yes ❑ No ❑
Reactivation of latent viruses (e.g., Epstein-Barr virus)	Yes ❑ No ❑
Infertility (in males)	Yes ❑ No ❑
Depression or aggressive behavior	Yes ❑ No ❑
Muscle weakness	Yes ❑ No ❑
Joint pain	Yes ❑ No ❑
Alzheimer's disease	Yes ❑ No ❑
Rheumatoid arthritis	Yes ❑ No ❑
White spots on nails	Yes ❑ No ❑
Hair loss	Yes ❑ No ❑

If you answered yes to any of the above, your selenium status may be insufficient. Pay attention to including selenium foods in your diet and ensure your multivitamin contains your RDA for selenium.

ZINC

Even though it comes last in any alphabetical list of immune-related nutrients, zinc is a powerhouse. And research supports the common practice of taking zinc to boost immune health: several high-quality clinical trials have demonstrated that, together with vitamin C, zinc can reduce the symptoms and shorten the duration of respiratory tract infections including common colds. In older individuals, zinc adequacy has been demonstrated to reduce the risk for, and severity of, colds, cold sores, influenza, and pneumonia. In infants and children, it has been shown to reduce the risk for, and severity of, colds, diarrhea, and pneumonia. And that's just what's been studied so far.

Zinc itself is naturally antimicrobial, which is why topical zinc-based creams and slow-dissolving zinc lozenges can help stall the growth of germs on skin, in wounds, and when you feel a sore throat coming on. It is also needed for cell membrane repair and so works to keep your barriers healthy and the healing of wounds efficient. It's a required nutrient for secretory IgA production and is (like vitamin C and iron) involved in both the germ-defeating pro-oxidant activities of your immune system as well as in antioxidant protection. It's also needed for natural killer cell activity, for phagocytosis, for immune cell communications, and interferon gamma production. It's a key nutrient for cellular replication and so is needed for immune cells to ramp up quickly, and for antibody production, in response to a harmful bug.

The thymus gland, an important immune organ where T cells are readied for active service, is very rich in zinc. Here, the master thymus hormone *thymulin* (which directs how T cells mature and what kind of T cells they become) is completely dependent on zinc for its function. Even a mild zinc insufficiency over time leads to less thymulin production, a smaller thymus gland overall, and the release of fewer T cells into circulation.

In a tangential but related role, zinc is also required for the extraction of other essential nutrients from the food you eat. Your digestive enzymes are all dependent on zinc to break down foods into their component nutrients so that they can be absorbed and circulated, and this is one of the earliest functions to deteriorate with inadequate zinc intake. The knock-on effects of even mild zinc insufficiency are therefore important and broad, since it impacts your uptake of other essential nutrients.

WHERE TO FIND ZINC

The most absorbable sources of dietary zinc are meat, eggs, and seafood (especially oysters). Relatively good plant sources are nuts, seeds, and legumes. However, these sources also contain phytates, which bind zinc and inhibit its absorption. Soaking, sprouting, and fermentation all improve zinc's availability from these plant foods and are important food preparation practices for vegans and vegetarians.

SHOULD I SUPPLEMENT WITH ZINC FOR IMMUNE HEALTH?

Yes, as part of your daily multivitamin. Choose a multivitamin with 100 percent of the RDA for zinc. Short-term use of doses higher than the RDA (but still within the Tolerable Upper Intake Level) can be beneficial, especially at the first sign of infection. See chapter 15 for more details.

CAUTIONS

While short-term use of zinc at doses higher than the RDA appears to be safe, long-term supplementation at these higher levels can lead to copper deficiency, since these two nutrients compete for absorption. Watch for cumulative zinc doses from multiple products used at the same time.

AM I AT RISK FOR ZINC INSUFFICIENCY?

The body has no storage system for zinc, and so you need to make sure you get enough regularly. Research has found that zinc inadequacy is common across the world, including in developed countries such as the US.

Likely factors/signs	
Heavy alcohol consumption (eight drinks or more per week for women and fifteen drinks or more per week for men)	Yes ❑ No ❑
Long-term use of zinc-depleting medications (e.g., some anticonvulsants and diuretics)	Yes ❑ No ❑
Impaired sense of taste and/or smell	Yes ❑ No ❑
Possible factors/signs	
Age over sixty-five years	Yes ❑ No ❑
Vegan or vegetarian diet	Yes ❑ No ❑
Cracked lips	Yes ❑ No ❑
White spots and/or white lines on nails	Yes ❑ No ❑
Nail ridging/grooving	Yes ❑ No ❑

Possible factors/signs (continued)	
Poor wound healing	Yes ❑ No ❑
Frequent infections	Yes ❑ No ❑
Irritable bowel/digestive dysfunction	Yes ❑ No ❑
In-home copper water pipes	Yes ❑ No ❑

If you answered yes to any one of the above likely signs and two or more of the possible signs, your zinc status may be insufficient. Pay attention to including high-quality zinc-containing foods in your diet and ensure your multivitamin contains your RDA for zinc.

OMEGA-3 AND OMEGA-6 FATS

You know from chapter 6 that a balanced level of fats is beneficial for immune health and that most of us get enough omega-6 fats in our diet from meats, poultry, eggs, and oils like safflower and sunflower, but not enough omega-3s. This can leave your immune system hampered when it comes to capping inflammation during an attack on a pathogen and to dialing down inflammation once the threat has gone. Consuming too few omega-3 fats also leaves you vulnerable to chronic inflammation and inflammation-related diseases. And this can potentially set the stage for the escalation of your next infection-targeted inflammation into more serious territory, increasing the risk of complications.

WHERE TO FIND OMEGA-3 FATS
Alpha-linolenic acid is found in flaxseeds, chia seeds, and walnuts and their oils. EPA and DHA are found in fish and seafood. You'll find more even detail on sources in part 3 as we review how to include these fats in your diet.

WHERE TO FIND OMEGA-6 FATS
Linoleic acid is found in nuts and seeds and their oils. It is also found in safflower oil, corn oil, and soybean oil. These are used in highly processed foods, which is why people who eat highly processed foods tend to

overconsume omega-6 fatty acids. I don't recommend sourcing your omega-6 fats from these industrialized oils.

SHOULD I SUPPLEMENT WITH OMEGA-3 OR OMEGA-6 FATS FOR IMMUNE HEALTH?

Multivitamins generally do not contain essential fatty acids. If yours doesn't, add 250 to 500 mg per day of EPA and DHA combined. Higher doses of omega-3 EPA and DHA (up to 3 grams of EPA and 1.5 grams DHA daily, approved and monitored by a qualified clinician), as well as the omega-6 GLA, can often be helpful for inflammatory conditions including autoimmune diseases. However, in general, most people do not need to supplement with any omega-6 fats.

CAUTIONS

High amounts of fish oil (over 1 gram of combined EPA and DHA per day) may decrease blood clotting (although the evidence for this remains weak and is evolving; see box, opposite). To be on the safe side, I recommend stopping fish oil before surgery and to discuss omega-3 supplementation with your physician, especially if you're taking a blood thinner like warfarin. Long-term use of high-dose EPA and DHA (4 grams per day) in older individuals may also theoretically decrease innate immune function by suppressing the initial inflammatory response, but again this hasn't been proven.

AM I AT RISK FOR ESSENTIAL FATTY ACID INSUFFICIENCY?

Omega-3 deficiency is a global issue—researchers have found average EPA plus DHA status to be "low" or "very low," i.e., levels associated with increased cardiovascular-related mortality, in most countries they studied.

Possible factors/signs	
Low fat diet	Yes ❑ No ❑
Low consumption of nuts, seeds, and fish	Yes ❑ No ❑
More frequent infections	Yes ❑ No ❑
Dry, scaly skin	Yes ❑ No ❑

Possible factors/signs (continued)	
Poor wound healing	Yes ❏ No ❏
Inflamed joints	Yes ❏ No ❏
Vision deterioration	Yes ❏ No ❏
Gallstones	Yes ❏ No ❏
Gall bladder removed	Yes ❏ No ❏
Neuropathy	Yes ❏ No ❏
Cognitive difficulties	Yes ❏ No ❏
Allergies and asthma	Yes ❏ No ❏

Omega-3 Fats and Surgery

Although it is commonly recommended to avoid omega-3 dietary supplements prior to undergoing surgery, an increasing body of evidence suggests that taking omega-3s before surgery may actually improve recovery by enhancing immunity and keeping inflammation manageable. Recently, too, a large (1,500-plus people) randomized and placebo-controlled clinical trial (i.e., the "gold standard" of medical research) found no risk of excess bleeding during surgery in individuals taking 8 to 10 grams per day for up to 5 days before surgery and 2 grams per day after surgery. These are huge doses that have been put to the test with no adverse effects on surgery outcomes.

These findings are starting to change the way the medical community looks at omega-3 fats and surgery. They are especially relevant for people who are at higher risk for sepsis following surgery, and who could therefore potentially benefit greatly from the protection of omega-3 supplementation.

Bear in mind that these studies are conducted in individuals who aren't otherwise routinely taking omega-3s. As you follow my guidelines, you'll be building up a good reserve of these fats in your cell membranes, ready to help you weather any surgical procedure. This ready-to-use reserve won't be hugely affected by stopping supplementation for a few days around surgery if, with your doctor, you decide to do so.

If any one of the possible factors/signs apply to you, you may be deficient in essential fatty acids. Make sure you're adding food sources to your diet and following the supplement recommendations above.

OTHER IMMUNE NUTRIENTS

There are other essential nutrients that have less well-known connections with your immune system but are still important. B vitamins—specifically vitamins B_1, B_2, B_3, B_5, B_6, B_9 (folate), B_{12}, and biotin—are essential nutrients for the release of energy from the food that you eat. And that energy powers every single cell within your body, including barrier cells and specialized immune cells. Folate also has an essential role in cell replication, making it indispensable for the rapid production of immune cells. Biotin, like several other nutrients we've covered, also has a role in keeping levels of inflammation in check. Copper has its own intrinsic antimicrobial properties and roles in cellular metabolism. Magnesium is also important. A few research studies have looked at the effects of magnesium deficiency on immune function and found it can lead to a drop in immune cells and response, as well as reduced barrier integrity.

Glutamine (not a vitamin or mineral, but a protein building block) also deserves a special mention, since it is an important building block for your rapidly reproducing barrier cells, and an energy source for immune cells when they are fighting an infection. During infection, the rate of glutamine use by immune cells at least equals that of the otherwise more commonly used glucose. Glutamine can also be converted into arginine for use in the respiratory burst process, and into glutamate for use in the formation of glutathione. Sufficient intake of these additional essential nutrients ensures there are no "leaky holes" in your nutritional immune support. Here's where you can get these in your diet:

Nutrient	Good food sources
Vitamin B_1	Whole-grain wheat and rice, pork, oats, sunflower seeds, turkey, lentils, carrots, oranges, fortified foods
Vitamin B_2	Beef or chicken liver, yogurt, milk, eggs, oats, spinach, mushrooms, fortified foods
Vitamin B_3	Beef liver, chicken, fish, oats, turkey, pork, peanuts, fortified foods
Vitamin B_5 (pantothenic acid)	Widespread in all foods
Vitamin B_6	Wild salmon, white potato with skin, turkey, chicken, fish, sunflower seeds, avocado, spinach, sweet potato, carrots, watermelon, banana, prunes
Vitamin B_9 (folate)	Lentils, beans, dark leafy green vegetables, broccoli, asparagus, liver
Vitamin B_{12}	All animal foods including meats, fish, seafood, eggs, and cheese
Biotin	Eggs (cooked, not raw), liver, salmon, avocado
Copper	Seafood, nuts, seeds, lentils, mushrooms, liver
Magnesium	Green leafy vegetables, whole grains, nuts and seeds, avocado
Glutamine	Bone-based stocks, chicken, fish, cabbage, dairy, tofu, lentils, and beans
Arginine	Nuts, meat, poultry, fish, dairy, eggs, grains

Look for 100 percent of the RDA for your B vitamins, biotin, and copper in your multivitamin. Supplemental vitamin B_{12} is especially important for vegans, since all dietary sources of this nutrient are animal-based. Multivitamins generally don't contain the full RDA for magnesium, since it is a large-sized nutrient; many contain no magnesium at all. Since around 50 percent of the US population is estimated to consume less than the recommended intake for magnesium, look for a multivitamin that contains at least 100 mg magnesium in each daily dose, or add a separate magnesium supplement alongside your multivitamin.

A NOTE ON NUTRIENT TESTING

Only vitamin D and iron levels are easily tested via standard labs that most practitioners will order. Standard labs also offer folate, vitamin B_{12}, magnesium, zinc, and selenium testing. Functional medicine and personalized nutrition practitioners may use specialized testing to assess other immune-related nutrient levels. This can provide helpful insight into what is known as *functional nutrient status*—the levels of a nutrient that are actually available for use in the body. In the Resources section, I've listed some of the labs that offer this kind of testing and how to find practitioners who can order them.

By now you should be constructing a pretty good idea of what you should *include* to build a resilient immune system—so let's now turn to some things we should *avoid* to keep our fragile system running smoothly: toxic chemicals and other harmful (usually man-made) substances in our environment.

To view the references cited in this chapter, please visit
www.immuneresilienceplan.com/science.

CHAPTER 8

Hidden in Plain Sight

The Impact of Invisible Environmental Toxins
on Your Immune System

As a population, we love our chemicals. The US produces or imports 27 trillion pounds of synthetic chemicals per year. That works out to be more than 240 pounds per person per day! Our daily living exposes us to myriad potentially toxic chemicals and metals through our food, air, water, personal care products, building materials, furnishings, and more. Just as infectious microbes are too small for us to see, so are these compounds. However, it doesn't mean they're not there. And there's no mincing words here: many of these have been shown to be able to derail our immunity. Worse, many of these chemicals are what's called "persistent" in the environment, meaning that they don't break down over time and continue to circulate through our soil, food, and water supplies. And when I say "chemicals," I'm referring to a wide spectrum of compounds including bisphenols (like BPA), phthalates, triclosan, parabens, flame retardants, perfluorochemicals (PFCs), and even heavy metals like lead, all readily found in plastics, preservatives, emulsifiers, pesticides, industrial chemicals, synthetic antimicrobial agents, and other sources.

Many of these environmental toxins are already flagged as public enemy number one because of their characterization as *endocrine disruptors*, which, like the name describes, disrupt healthy hormone activity in our bodies. *Endocrine* means "related to hormones" in medical lingo, anything from estrogen and testosterone to thyroid hormone and insulin. Even hormones that regulate appetite and satiety can be affected. For these reasons, endocrine-disrupting chemicals (EDCs for short) have been associated with many conditions including hormone dysregulation, reproductive harm, birth defects, reduced IQ levels, nervous system damage, obesity, and cancer.

What's less well recognized is that in addition to the disruption to your hormones, EDCs also target your immune system. In part because hormones affect immune responses, and in part because EDCs target and hinder other layers of your defense systems directly, such as your microbiota and barrier cells. The thymus gland, for example, essential for the development and maturation of our T cells, is highly vulnerable to the effects of EDCs. EDC exposure has been observed to lead to a shrinking of this gland, with direct impacts on the number of T cells that can be produced. EDCs have also been shown to prevent T cells from doing their job properly, which has the potential to dampen our innate immune defenses and predispose us to allergies later in life. Other science has shown that EDCs affect the development, function, and life span of all white blood cells.

The world's health authorities including America's Environmental Protection Agency (EPA) and the World Health Organization (WHO) recognize that EDCs are a significant human health problem that needs attention. However, regulators have yet to formally adopt definitive programs to address endocrine-disrupting chemicals, categorize them as hazardous, and implement policy to control them. And let's hope they do that soon: evidence has been accumulating over several decades that even small-dose, repetitive exposures may cause harm. This isn't enough to kill you outright, or cause visible harm in a short time period, but it can disturb our body's signaling systems—particularly the delicate hormonal, neurological, and immune systems and therefore contribute to the development of many chronic diseases, increase the risk for infection, and even reduce the effectiveness of vaccines. Research has shown that these everyday toxins can damage your defense systems and derail your immune resilience in a variety of ways:

- They can suppress healthy immune responses by damaging components of your defense networks.
- They can stimulate an unhealthy inflammatory immune response leading to chronic inflammation.
- They deplete antioxidants, leaving fewer available to quiet inflammation.
- They can dysregulate immune function leading to allergy, asthma, or autoimmunity.
- They can damage barriers by compromising tight junctions between cells.
- They can damage a healthy microbiota and promote dysbiosis.
- They can alter vaccine responsiveness, leading to reduced immune memory development and protection against future exposures.

One troubling effect of toxins, we are discovering, is the length of time they can remain in the body. The US National Biomonitoring Program, run by the CDC, keeps track of just a fraction (352 at last count) of the registered synthetic chemicals. It has flagged several toxins for their ubiquitous and long-lasting presence, including flame retardants in furniture, carpeting, and many other consumer products; bisphenol A (BPA) used in plastics; and stain-resistant and nonstick chemicals used in fabrics and cookware. These and other chemicals get inside our bodies—even if we don't work or live near major pollution sources—and *stay* there. They can remain in our systems, and we can pass them on: in one of the most extensive studies, researchers found that 80 percent of the chemicals present in maternal blood samples were also found in cord blood, indicating that they passed through the placenta and into the child before birth.

SURPRISING GAPS IN THE OVERSIGHT OF ENVIRONMENTAL TOXINS

Most of us assume that the chemicals in the products we use (like laundry detergents, household cleaners, shampoos, mattresses, breakfast cereals, disposable coffee cups . . . the list goes on and on) have been proven safe. Sadly, that's not the case. It may surprise you to know that:

- Many scientists at leading universities, health authorities, physicians, and environmentalists have criticized current regulations and government oversight as lacking the "teeth" needed to enforce meaningful safety standards.

- There's no requirement in the US for chemicals intended for industrial and consumer use to be tested before they are released into the marketplace. If adverse effects are suspected, the burden of testing and of proving harm lies with the regulatory agency.

- Determinations of chemical safety are made largely based on short-term animal studies and laboratory studies. Human observational data (data that is collected over time on people's exposure levels and their association with disease outcomes) are used, but collected only after exposure has happened.

- The US stands out for being more permissive in the use of synthetic chemicals than other parts of the world, allowing, for example, more than 70 pesticide products barred in other countries.

- The combined effect of multiple, simultaneous chemical exposures over time (as is most typical of our everyday life) has *never* been studied. And only very recently have scientists started to look beyond overt signs of toxic harm to the more subtle shifts that can disturb and interrupt essential biochemical systems like immunity. Some effects of early-life exposures are also now understood to appear only later in life, including increased vulnerability to infections, cancer, allergy, or autoimmunity.

While mounting evidence suggests there are many products made with chemicals that can cause insidious harm and derail your immune resilience, not all is lost. It is possible to steer clear of many of these toxins. Read your labels and stay informed. While we don't have better regulatory oversight it's crucial you are your own advocate. To help you get started, here is a brief lowdown on each of the immune-disruptive chemicals and how to all out rid your home of them as best you can.

BISPHENOL A (BPA) AND BISPHENOL S (BPS)

BPA was originally manufactured as a potential synthetic estrogen for medical use, and it's that hormone-like activity that is thought to be behind its effects on our body and immune system. The primary source of exposure to BPA is through our diet, when food and drink ingredients come into contact with plasticware, packaging, and equipment. Some other places you'll find BPA include automobile parts, CDs, food can linings, baby bottles, plastic dinnerware and food-storage containers, plastic drinks bottles, eyeglass lenses, dental adhesive and sealants, medical equipment and tubing, electronics, thermal paper receipts, sports equipment, and toys. Many of us get significant BPA exposure from one or more of these sources during routine daily activities.

So just how bad is this exposure? We know from scientific studies in animals and in human cell cultures that BPA is toxic to macrophages and neutrophil white blood cells, interfering with their ability to mount an effective innate immune response, emit warning signals, and perform phagocytosis. Researchers have observed, in animals, that this impairs the ability of that creature to defend itself against pathogenic bacteria and parasites. Its interference with interferon gamma signaling suggests it may also hamper our ability to ward off viruses. Adaptive immunity is also potentially affected since studies have reported reduced numbers of T cells linked with exposure. One human observational study reported that the amount of BPA in a mother's body is associated with higher risk for chest infections and bronchitis in her children—for each doubling of the BPA concentration, the risk for chest infections and bronchitis went up by 15 percent and 18 percent, respectively.

Following the public demand to remove BPA from consumer products, manufacturers have in large part responded by substituting alternative bisphenols such as BPS. Although there are far fewer studies that have been conducted on BPS, research indicates that BPS has similar immune toxicity to BPA. So be careful with any product labeled "BPA-free"—it may have BPS and other EDCs, and so it won't necessarily be any less toxic.

FLAME RETARDANTS

Flame retardants (known by their scientific name as *polybrominated diphenyl ethers*, or PBDEs) are widely used in household furnishings, building materials, and children's products including padded furniture, carpeting, tents, children's car seats, mattress pads, play mats, changing pads, nursing pillows, and children's pajamas. Older flame retardants are now banned in the EU and the US but persist in our environment since they don't degrade over time. Newer flame retardants, assumed to be safer, have not been well studied.

Some of the best-elucidated potential links between flame retardants and health are lower IQ scores and attention challenges in children. Animal studies also suggest that flame retardants may hamper the immune system's ability to fight a viral infection. In addition, they may increase the risk of infection complications, such as preterm birth, by driving up levels of inflammation in response to an infection. Flame retardants have also been studied for their harmful effects on thyroid hormones, which are essential for cellular function across the body and immune system.

HERBICIDES

Herbicides are very commonly used on residential, institutional, and commercial properties as well as on conventionally grown produce. The most controversial of this group is glyphosate, the main chemical ingredient of Roundup. It was first introduced in the 1970s and is now the most widely used weed killer across the globe. Yet research into the effects of this chemical is still limited, and some of the science that *is* increasingly available is concerning. One animal pilot study run by a collaborative group including experts from the University of Bologna, Italy, the Icahn School of Medicine at Mount Sinai, New York, and the George Washington

University, Washington, DC, showed that glyphosate can disrupt beneficial, immune-supportive gut bacteria at doses that are considered to be safe for humans by regulatory authorities. Another scientific paper predicted that around half of the beneficial species common to human digestive tracts may be harmed by glyphosate. Test tube and animal studies have also observed a detrimental effect of glyphosate on intestinal tight junctions. Both the microbiome and intestinal barrier are key factors in immune resilience, as you know, and so it seems possible that glyphosate could have a detrimental effect on immune function. This has yet to be directly studied. Several countries including France, Italy, and Belgium, and specific US states such as California and Connecticut, have legislation that restricts glyphosate use specifically due to toxicity concerns. More than $10 billion has also been paid out to settle claims that, at high doses, this herbicide causes cancer, especially non-Hodgkin's lymphoma.

PARABENS

Parabens are synthetic preservatives that are used extensively in consumer products like cosmetics, personal care products, pharmaceuticals, and long-life foods. They are added to prevent the growth of harmful bacteria and mold and to increase the shelf life of products. However, parabens have been observed in cell culture studies to be toxic to white blood cells, calling their safety into question. Those researchers involved in these studies raise the concern that paraben exposure may pose a risk to humans over the long term, especially with intensive exposure via multiple sources.

PERFLUOROCHEMICALS (PFCs)

You may want to think about what pan to use the next time you want to fry up some eggs. PFCs can be found in protective coatings such as nonstick, waterproof, and stain-proof coatings as well as in adhesives, flame retardant foams, and electrical wire insulation. Like many other synthetic chemicals, perfluorochemicals don't degrade over time—they persist in our environment. An unfortunate contamination in the US Mid-Ohio River

Understanding Relative Risk When Protecting Yourself from Pests That Carry Potentially Harmful Diseases

You may be surprised, given what I've shared here, but there are a few occasions when I think it's worth taking the risk in using certain chemicals. One of those instances is when there is a significant risk of contracting a harmful disease from pests, such as Lyme disease (and other infections) from ticks or West Nile virus from mosquitoes. This is especially relevant if you live in a high-risk area. Permethrin, a pyrethroid insect repellent, has been shown to effectively repel ticks and mosquitos and, in my opinion, is less of a risk than contracting a tick-borne illness that can lead to long-term, quality-of-life-altering effects. What that means is, if you're at high risk of exposure to potentially serious insect-borne illnesses, it's better to take the risk of the chemical insect repellant than risk the long-term consequences of the diseases.

There are ways to be extra careful with insect repellents, though. When I use permethrin, I apply it to my clothing rather than my skin. You can also find pretreated clothing that works for a few dozen washes. I also make sure to give extra support to my detoxification pathways while I use it (more on that later in this chapter). There are also lots of other non-chemical ways you can reduce your exposure to disease-carrying pests, such as wearing loose, long-sleeve tops and long pants and limiting exposed skin. To reduce ticks in your yard, make sure to clear debris such as wood and leaf piles that encourage rodents that can carry ticks (deer, although more commonly associated with disease-carrying ticks, are not the only species to act as tick transport). You can also place commercially bought "tick tubes" around your yard that contain permethrin-soaked cotton (I prefer this to spray applications since the pesticide is better contained). Whatever strategies you adopt, check yourself thoroughly for ticks if you've been outside in a known tick habitat, always. To combat mosquitos, make sure you eliminate any standing water around your yard—even water sitting on top of an overturned plant pot can be a breeding ground for these bugs. You can also consider planting mosquito-repelling plants such as lavender, marigolds, rosemary, geraniums, and citronella.

Given what we know about environmental toxins, I don't make these recommendations lightly. But the risks from these challenging diseases can be far worse and an ounce of prevention really goes a long way.

The good news is, however, that if despite best efforts you do end up with one of these illnesses, having strong immune resilience will help support recovery. And for long-term effects of diseases like chronic Lyme disease, many individuals I've worked with have dramatically improved their symptoms by using the principles in this book.

Valley water supply in the early 2000s helped researchers understand that perfluorochemical exposure likely leads to lower antibody production in humans, just as previous animal studies had suggested it could. They found that individuals who had higher exposure to the PFC leak were more likely not to achieve levels needed to provide immunity against the flu following immunization. Several other studies have suggested dose-related effects even when exposed to everyday environmental levels; those who have greater levels of circulating PFCs from everyday exposures can exhibit reduced antibody responses (including to vaccines), as well as more frequent fevers, cold symptoms, and gastroenteritis.

Even though severe leaks are rare, drinking contaminated water can still be a significant source of exposure; a 2016 Harvard T.H. Chan School of Public Health report found that PFC levels exceeded recommended safety levels in public drinking-water supplies in thirty-three US states, including Alabama, Arizona, California, Florida, Georgia, Illinois, New Jersey, New York, Pennsylvania, and Ohio, affecting 6 million people. (And this was only based off two-thirds of the total US water supply, since perfluorochemical levels aren't yet officially tracked in the remaining third.)

PESTICIDES

Pesticides are used extensively on residential, institutional, and commercial properties as well as on conventionally grown produce to protect plants and humans from harmful pests and disease carriers.

A large swath of synthetic chemicals have been used as pesticides over the last century, and several have been connected with altered immune function in humans. One organophosphate pesticide, for example, chlor-pyrifos (a phosphonothioate derivative), which is used on many crops including corn, soybeans, fruits, nuts, Brussels sprouts, cranberries, broccoli, and cauliflower, as well as in other applications such as on golf courses, has been shown in some studies to degrade immune barriers like the gut lining and skin. Another group of pesticides called pyrethroids have been observed to impair resistance against infections and potentially contribute to cancer, especially in those with already impaired immune function. Pyrethroids are found in household and commercial insecticides and pet products (shampoos and sprays). These and several other pesticides have been found to potentially damage T cells, natural killer cells, macrophages, and antibody-producing B cells.

PHTHALATES

Phthalates are plastic chemicals used for their flexibility, resilience, and stabilizing properties. They are commonly found in adhesives, detergents, pharmaceuticals, solvents, building materials, plastics, food packaging, food-processing equipment, tubing used for milking at dairy farms, and personal care products and cosmetics including shampoos, lotions, soaps, fragrances, makeup, hair spray, and nail polish. Since phthalates are only loosely bound to the substance they are in, they are readily released into their immediate environment. We women tend to have higher exposure because we tend to use more personal care products and cosmetics.

Phthalates have been found to increase harmful inflammatory signaling in laboratory-cultured human cells. Not only that, phthalates appear to inhibit our immune system's ability to produce antiviral interferons and the effective workings of our sentinel dendritic cells. Human exposure to phthalates has been shown to promote weight gain, impair blood sugar control, and interfere with the activity of thyroid hormones, all of which are known to worsen immune function. (I'll get into the connections between immune function and these underlying conditions in chapter 14.)

POLYCHLORINATED BIPHENYLS (PCBs)

In 1979, the US Environmental Protection Agency banned the commercial production of PCBs based on the animal and observational human studies available even at that time. However, because these chemicals degrade so slowly, we are still being exposed to them after all these years in everyday environments like our yard soil, drinking water, food, and older (pre-1979) buildings, appliances, and equipment.

Endocrine-disrupting PCBs have been associated with increased risk for infections including ear infections, respiratory infections, and even chicken pox. Animal studies demonstrate that PCBs may suppress antibody and white blood cell production, deplete vitamin A and vitamin D levels, and increase inflammation. If that were not enough, extensive animal and observational human evidence has also linked PCBs with several cancers as well as reproductive and neurological issues.

TRICLOSAN

Triclosan is a synthetic, broad-spectrum antibacterial compound that was long seen as helpful in the fight against harmful germs. However, in 2016 the FDA ruled that manufacturers must stop selling several consumer products (soaps, laundry detergents, toothpastes, deodorants, plastic kitchen utensils and toys) with triclosan, or its sister compound triclocarban. The reason—safety concerns such as bacterial resistance and endocrine-disrupting effects, and because evidence showed that these chemicals were no more effective than plain soap and water in preventing contagious illnesses. Worse, studies have found that triclosan directly disrupts an immune cell's ability to generate energy for essential functions, and it promotes inappropriately excessive levels of inflammation. Triclosan has also been shown to inhibit immune activity such as phagocytosis and the production of perforins and granzymes (those chemical weapons), and shortens the life of immune cells.

Despite the partial ban, triclosan is still allowed in some consumer hand sanitizers and wipes, toothpastes, deodorants, as well as antibacterial soaps used in health care settings. It is also incorporated into many textiles (including sportswear, footwear, bedding, and shower curtains), as well as food containers and cutting boards that are labeled "antibacterial."

TOXIC METALS

Lead is a well-known human toxin, and we've known for more than thirty years that it can suppress immune activity and reduce our resistance to infectious diseases. Contamination in water supplies has been much reduced but still occurs even in recently built houses that are connected to lead-containing municipal water pipes or have brass plumbing parts that are alloyed with lead. Lead has also been found in certain cosmetics, face paints, and some traditional herbal supplements. Mercury, another toxic metal, is a frequent contaminant in air pollution particles, fish, and can also be found in dental amalgams. Arsenic can leach from railroad ties and pressure-treated lumber (used in some instances for playground equipment, decks, and raised soil beds), and certain food crops can become contaminated. Rice is one kind of crop that has a higher level of arsenic if grown in contaminated soils (see the Resources section for an arsenic-free rice option).

We know that lead impairs macrophage function, skews the T helper cell response, damages your microbiota and the integrity of your gut lining, and increases the risk for inflammation-associated cell damage. Certain forms of mercury have been shown repeatedly in animal studies to be toxic to the immune system, inducing immunosuppression and other immune disturbances. Arsenic can impair our immune surveillance system by reducing our white blood cell count, and mounting evidence suggests the potential for arsenic exposure to lead to increased infection rates including respiratory and gastrointestinal infections.

CLUES OF TOXIN OVERLOAD

Certain conditions are associated with an increased toxic burden—an accumulation of low-dose exposures over time. The following have been linked with increased levels of toxicity, especially when there aren't any other obvious causes of the condition:

Immune	Asthma Allergies Chemical/odor sensitivities Autoimmune conditions Unexplained inflammation Fibromyalgia Recurrent infections Food sensitivities Low white blood cell count
Neurological	Cognitive or memory difficulties Mood, behavior, and addiction disorders Tremors Peripheral neuropathy Chronic headaches Poor sleep Fatigue Chronic neurological conditions such as autism, ADHD, depression, anxiety, Parkinson's disease, or Alzheimer's disease
Hormonal	Unexplained weight gain or loss Blood sugar dysregulation, insulin resistance, and diabetes Thyroid dysfunction Adrenal dysfunction Premature puberty Premenstrual syndrome Polycystic ovarian syndrome Endometriosis Fibroids Sperm dysfunction Infertility

Digestive	Constipation (poor clearance of toxins) Dehydration (poor clearance of toxins) Gut dysfunction Loss of appetite Metallic taste
Other	Osteoporosis Muscle or joint pain Heart disease Cancer Spontaneous abortion Birth defects Developmental disorders Liver disorders or abnormal liver function tests Kidney disorders or abnormal kidney function tests

If you have any of the above conditions, it may be that toxins are playing a role. And this is then one indication that your immune resilience may not be at its optimal level. For all of us looking for optimal immune resilience, reducing our exposure to harmful chemicals where we can is paramount. And that is just what we're going to look at next.

WHAT TO DO

Do you need a minute? Talking about toxins can be heavy. The reality, as you may well have already surmised, is that we can't eliminate our exposure to environmental toxins entirely. Many are persistent in our environment, and others will continue to be present as factors of our everyday modern life. But whether or not science eventually proves definitively that they cause harm, as consumers we have much better choices we can make.

I really can't emphasize enough that there is much we can do to reduce our potential risk. And the most absolutely important, fundamentally right place to start is to reduce how much we come into contact with toxins. After all, by reducing our exposure, we are fending off a large part of the problem before it even becomes an issue. It just makes good sense. In addition to reducing exposure, it's also important to continue to support your body's natural ability to detoxify. Let's look at these two steps.

1. LIVE AS "CLEANLY" AS REASONABLY POSSIBLE

Living clean in this context is not about living with fewer microbes, as your parents and older generations may assume. It's about living with fewer toxins around us to get in the way of our immune system doing its job. And it keeps the load more manageable for our detox organs to work their magic on the rest of our inevitable exposures. It's a different kind of clean than we think of when we're removing dirt and grime, especially since many "cleaning" products are ones we'll want to avoid!

In the following pages, we'll look at some of the areas where we tend to be most exposed to immune-damaging toxins. And in part 3, you'll learn more specific ways to avoid them.

FOOD

Processed foods: Synthetic food additives, commonly used by the processed food industry to improve attributes like shelf life, flavor, color, and texture, are not all received as benign food components by our body and our immune system. One example is the preservative tertbutylhydroquinone (tBHQ), which animal research suggests suppresses our immune response to flu infections and reduces the effectiveness of the flu vaccine due to its effects on T cells. Other additives can harm our immune system by affecting our microbiota, which you now know is a critical ally in our immune defense system: Dietary emulsifiers, such as carboxymethylcellulose and polysorbate-80, and artificial sweeteners like sucralose, saccharin, and aspartame promote the growth of bad bacteria. Polysorbate-80 is also able to stimulate unhealthy background inflammation, another factor that undermines immune resilience. Carboxymethylcellulose, carrageenan, and artificial sweeteners may interfere with proper blood-sugar regulation and promote higher levels of circulating blood sugar. Titanium dioxide is known to alter immune system responses, and research from Stony Brook University in New York even suggests that human cells exposed to titanium dioxide have twice the risk of developing a bacterial infection than they normally would.

Conventional vs. organic foods: Once upon a time there was plain "food." Then when chemical pesticides and herbicides came along, the industry needed a new way to describe them—the term *conventional* was born, although arguably it is organic foods, with thousands of years' history, that are actually the most conventional. One main reason to consider organic food is that it reduces your exposure to pesticides and herbicides. Several scientific studies in humans have demonstrated this. In one study of women in Idaho who reported eating *only* conventionally grown food before starting the study, switching their food consumption to be two-thirds organic plus one-third conventional for twenty-four weeks reduced the levels of pesticides circulating in their bodies by more than half. In a separate study in individuals across several sites in the US, moving to a 100 percent organic diet reduced levels of specific pesticides by up to 95 percent after just six days. Other studies have also found significant decreases in pesticide levels when switching diets from conventional to organic. These results are very promising.

Another good reason to choose organic plant food is for phytonutrient content. It turns out that plants seem to produce more of these important phytonutrients when they're left to defend themselves (without synthetic pesticides) against harmful pests—in fact, many of these act as natural pest deterrents for the plant. According to some reports, phytonutrient concentrations can be up to 70 percent greater in organic produce. As you know from chapter 6, these phytonutrient compounds have substantial roles to play in improving our immune response to infections and reducing our vulnerability to disease. Organic dairy and meats also tend to contain less saturated fats and more unsaturated fats, including higher amounts of immune-beneficial omega-3 fats, likely a direct reflection of the pasture-raising practices that are more common to organic livestock rearing. Not to mention they are less likely to be contaminated with antibiotic-resistant bacteria than conventionally raised meats, according to a Stanford University analysis. In part 3, I'll show you how to interpret organic labeling claims and how to prioritize which organic foods to choose.

Food packaging and cooking tools: Science has shown that making changes around food packaging, such as avoiding canned foods, substantially reduces our exposure to chemicals in plastic wrapping and the plastic-coated lining of food cans. A study in California, for example, showed that even just switching from canned foods to fresh, unpackaged foods for three days could cut the amount of BPA and phthalates in our blood by two-thirds. Just think what that could do over the longer term! Cookware is another place to limit your exposure: avoid cookware coated with a chemical nonstick surface, including pans, casseroles, grills, cookie sheets, slow cookers, and utensils, since these contain those perfluoro-chemicals that leach into foods during cooking.

Toxins in fish: Despite their healthy omega-3 fats, DHA and EPA, fish and seafood are also common sources of contamination, including with mercury, PCBs, and dioxins. There are ways to navigate this, though, so that you can still get the benefits of fish and seafood without the risk of toxins. States, territories, and tribes in the US provide local advice on the levels of contamination of fish caught in the waters under their jurisdiction. These can be found by going online to fishadvisoryonline.epa.gov. In addition, it is possible to choose fish that are both nutritious and lowest in mercury. In the Immune Resilience Diet chapter in part 3, you'll find those lowest-mercury fish to choose.

OUTDOOR AND INDOOR AIR

During the early stages of the COVID-19 pandemic, researchers from the Harvard T.H. Chan School of Public Health ran an analysis of data on air pollution across 98 percent of the US and death rates attributed to the SARS-CoV-2 virus. They found that those living in areas of the US with higher levels of air pollution were more likely to die from COVID-19 than those living in less polluted areas; in fact, for every 1 microgram per cubic meter increase in air particulate matter, there was a statistically significant 11 percent increase in COVID-19 deaths. Separately, but around the same time, two other scientific groups identified some possible reasons for this connection. At the Geisel School of Medicine at Dartmouth in New Hampshire, researchers found that fine particulate matter in air pollution seemed to be able to suppress vitamin D–triggered antimicrobial peptides (remember that important innate immune mechanism from chapter 3?). Those who also had a low vitamin D level *and* higher exposure to air particles might be experiencing a double whammy, they speculated. Then a collaborative group of scientists from Europe, Russia, and the US found that long-term exposure to air pollution particles contributed to immune suppression and increased levels of lung inflammation, not ideal for those exposed to a virus known to attack the lungs.

It's harder for us to immediately control the air quality outside, although we can all play a part in voicing concerns to local businesses and government. We can try to use our gasoline-fueled cars less, plant more trees, and switch to renewable energy sources. We can also do much in the short term to make our *indoor* air safer. Given that most of us spend more time inside than out, this can still have a large beneficial impact. Indoor air can become contaminated by outside air, if you live in an area with higher levels of air pollution, as well as from dust particles containing chemicals released from indoor building materials, furniture, carpeting, cleaning products, scented candles, and more.

WATER

Water treatment systems have the primary goal of removing harmful microorganisms such as parasites, viruses, and bacteria. This is so important, and it's not overstating it to say that reducing water-borne infectious disease through proper water sanitation has been one of the biggest public health successes of the last century.

However, today's water is also a source of most kinds of immune-harming environmental pollutants like toxic metals, pesticides, herbicides, fertilizers, flame retardants, PFCs, PCBs, microplastics, cosmetics, sunscreens, fragrances, as well as human and veterinary medications (including antibiotics). These enter our water supply via agricultural, industrial, and domestic runoff, accidental spills, and improper disposal and end up in surface water, underground water, wells, rivers, lakes, and reservoirs. Many aren't removed through standard water treatment. While extreme water contamination examples, such as the crisis of lead contamination in Flint, Michigan, in 2014–2015, are fortunately rare, other less extreme cases are relatively common. The EPA acknowledges that water is a known source of lead exposure for children in the United States, for instance, due to the corrosion of old water pipes and water distribution equipment. This despite the CDC's advisory that there is no safe level of lead exposure for children.

PERSONAL CARE PRODUCTS

Take a quick scan of the ingredient list on your shampoo, deodorant, skin moisturizers, nail polish, or toothpaste, and the chances are you'll see a laundry list of chemicals. Personal care products are a major source of potential toxins, including parabens, phthalates, BPA, triclosan, and heavy metals like lead. On average, people use nine personal care products per day, filled with dozens of different chemical ingredients. One quarter of us ladies use fifteen or more each day, adding up to hundreds of individual chemicals!

The problem is that we absorb a significant amount of those chemicals through our skin. And this absorption goes up further still when our skin is warmer, the longer we use the product, the larger the skin area we apply it to, when the product also contains alcohol, and when we apply the product to damaged skin. We also absorb some chemicals by breathing them in and ingest others from products such as lip balms and lipsticks.

Just as for other types of synthetic chemicals, US government regulators have been light in applying restriction: they have rejected just eleven ingredients as unsafe for use in cosmetics since modern regulation first began. By comparison, the European Union has banned hundreds of chemicals from use in such products.

HOME AND YARD CARE

Household cleaners are another major source of contaminants. These come into contact with our skin, and we also breathe them in directly or on dust particles. Phthalates, for instance, are commonly found in laundry detergents and other heavily fragranced cleaning products.

And then there are pesticides and weed killers, which up to 90 percent of us use inside and outside our homes to control insects, termites, rodents, fungi, and unwanted plants. EPA reports indicate that pesticide residues are widespread in indoor air, even if you haven't recently applied them indoors or nearby. This is because, in addition to traveling via air particles, indoor air contamination can come from house and yard care products kept in improperly sealed storage containers or from particles tracked into the home on shoes and clothing.

Reducing exposure is by far the best way to address environmental toxins. However, coming in a very close second is supporting your body's ability to remove chemicals it will still inevitably encounter. That is, through *detoxification*, your body's natural, in-built mechanisms that help eliminate and counter the potential effects of toxins.

2. DAILY DETOX SUPPORT

Although we tend to think of our liver, kidneys, and colon as our main detox organs (and they are of course important), detoxification is actually much broader than that: it is a fundamental process of *all* cells, which need to be able to deal with daily exposure to internal metabolic waste products and external toxins brought into the body. What's also less well known is that barrier cells in your digestive tract are especially good detoxifiers, especially in combination with a well-functioning microbiota—one more reason to keep those both healthy.

I like to think of the body's detox capacity as a bathtub. The level of water in the tub is your total toxic load (the cumulative level of toxins in your body, also referred to as your total body burden of toxins), and your body's natural ability to process and eliminate toxins is the drain hole at the bottom. As long as we keep the level of water in the bathtub manageable, it will drain well, and we won't have any problem. However, if we either put too much water in the bathtub at once or we have a smaller-than-normal tub or drain hole, then we run the risk of water spilling over. In other words, when we either have too much total toxin exposure or when our ability to detoxify is compromised, we can tip over into chronic health problems and a compromised immune system.

One more note before we dive in: detoxification isn't a dedicated event (although I'm not against a periodic cleanse!). Rather, when I'm working with clients, I try to help them realize that the best kind of detoxification

Your Detox Capacity Is Different from the Next Person's

There are many factors that influence how well we detoxify environmental chemicals, and so each of us ends up having our own unique level of detox capability. These include:

The genes we inherit: Because of the genetic hand we're dealt, some of us are better at detoxifying than others. For some of us, alterations (mutations) in genes that code for detoxification enzymes mean that they just don't function as well as they should.

Life stage: Our vulnerability to toxins is increased at several life stages, especially in utero and during childhood development. Even though science is very clear on this, current regulations don't account for these increased levels of vulnerability.

Nongenetic inheritance: Toxic insults on developing immune systems are now thought to be passed down to future generations via epigenetic inheritance (remember the new field of epigenetics we covered in chapter 6?), weakening their defenses against infections.

How well we take care of our detox capability: Our nutrient status, microbiota, the health of our barriers, how much fiber we eat, how much we sweat—all of these alter how well we're able to rid our bodies of the toxins we take in.

is *ongoing, daily detox.* We can do that by providing support in three areas: diet, circulation, and elimination.

DIET

Without a doubt, detoxification is a nutrient-dense process and therefore the best kind of diet for daily detoxification is one that provides those needed nutrients. Vitamins, minerals, proteins, omega-3 fats, and antioxidants are all used during the multi-stage processes that neutralize toxins and prepare them for elimination. Some even block their entrance: calcium, zinc, and iron, for instance, compete with lead for absorption from our intestines, so having sufficient levels of these minerals in your diet can reduce the amount of lead you absorb. Often, the vitamins, minerals, or proteins involved in detoxification processes are considered "spent," i.e., they are eliminated along with the toxin itself and cannot be reused for other functions. This means that additional nutrient repletion during or after detoxification is key.

Dietary fiber of both kinds is also important. The soluble kind of fiber for its ability to bind with many toxins and keep hold of them to be excreted in stool. And the insoluble kind to add bulk to the contents of your digestive tract to keep more bound toxins away from barrier cells that might inadvertently absorb them, and to help move things along and out of harm's way. Fiber, as you know, is also an essential food for the good microbes in your gut. Many of these beneficial microbes actually help you avoid harmful toxins in foods by neutralizing them before they are absorbed into your body.

Phytonutrients are useful, too, for their antioxidant role protecting our cells from daily brushes with toxins. Several phytonutrients can even bind with toxins to help excrete them from the body. Especially good choices for detoxification are those phytonutrients that come from green tea, onion, garlic, coriander/cilantro, and turmeric. Quercetin and NAC (N-acetyl cysteine), two supplements I recommend for immune health in general (see chapter 12), also aid detoxification by supporting liver function and protecting against the damaging effects of toxins.

The Immune Resilience Diet outlined in part 3 incorporates all these

Could Very Strict Fasts Hinder Immune Resilience?

Nutrition is so important for detoxification that I am concerned by severe forms of fasting that are sometimes promoted for detox purposes, such as a water-only fast lasting more than forty-eight hours. With such a fast, the body will soon start to lack the nutrients it needs for handling metabolic toxins and others released from fat stores (fat and bone are two places where your body prefers to sequester toxins, out of harm's way). Research suggests that withholding food for more than forty-eight hours may result in significant immune impairments. You can read more about safer forms of fasting that can actually be *beneficial* for your immune system in part 3.

dietary principles to help you support healthy detoxification alongside immune health.

CIRCULATION

Circulation is what helps mobilize those toxins we've taken on, readying them to be excreted and eliminated from the body. Several factors help with circulation:

Good hydration will always be important to help each cell detoxify, as well as to carry toxins through and out of the body. Exercise gets your blood and lymph moving, too, carrying nutrients to detox organs and toxins to where they can be eliminated. It also improves your resilience against the damaging effects of toxins by activating antioxidant enzymes and glutathione. Massage, especially one focused on the lymph system, boosts your body's ability to drain unwanted waste and toxins out of your organs so they can be sent for elimination. One of my personal favorites, an Epsom salt bath, may also help mobilize toxins so that they can be processed and passed out.

We tend to think of circulation in relation to movement when we are awake. But for detoxification, we also improve our toxin circulation and drainage when we sleep. Sleep, surprisingly, plays a vital role in detoxification. Many of our major detoxification systems are under the control of our body's circadian rhythms, the repeatable daily patterns of biochemistry that are most apparent in the difference between waking and sleeping. Science has shown that sleep is a time when certain lymph waves are most active and toxin clearance is highest. So make sure you're getting enough shut-eye, and that it's good-quality, restful sleep. We'll circle back to sleep, as well as exercise in the next chapter.

ELIMINATION

We excrete toxins primarily via our stool, urine, and sweat. Keeping these routes functioning well allows toxins to be easily released as needed. Constipation slows down the excretion of toxins from the body and actually gives the body more opportunity to reabsorb toxins—not what we want. Make sure you're getting enough water, as well as plant fiber in your diet to support a healthy flow of urine and allow you to "go" (pass a bowel movement) at least once a day.

Working up a sweat through exercise, a steam room, or a sauna all encourage the release and riddance of toxins. It's best to shower after any of those activities to rinse off excreted toxins so they aren't reabsorbed.

Now that you know where the worst chemical offenders lurk, I hope this empowers you to remain alert to what is in your food, your cleaning and beauty products, even in other everyday places. With the right knowledge, it is possible to reduce exposure, and to use diet and lifestyle practices to mitigate, even reverse, some of the effects of toxins. Our immune health depends on it.

———————————

To view the references cited in this chapter, please visit
www.immuneresilienceplan.com/science.

CHAPTER 9

Living a Good Life

The Importance of Your Lifestyle in Supporting Immune Health

don't understand . . . my diet is really good. I eat piles of vegetables, I source my meats locally from an organic farmer, I avoid processed foods and sugar like the plague. Why am I still getting arthritis flares?" This was the lament of Patricia, a lovely thirty-five-year-old woman who came to see me for help with her rheumatoid arthritis, a progressive autoimmune condition in which her immune system was mistakenly attacking her own joints. Patricia had read up on how diet can have a dramatic effect on the severity of autoimmune disease and had already done a marvelous job of cleaning up what she ate before she came to see me. Her symptoms had much improved overall, but she was perplexed as to why she continued to have episodic flares.

As we went over her background together, Patricia told me that she was a mom of three kids all under the age of eight (!), and she was inevitably up at least once a night to nurse her nine-month-old. She worked part-time as a visiting nurse, often juggling arrangements of school drop-offs and pickups, housekeeping, cooking, and caring for her aging mother, who lived in an assisted living facility thirty minutes away. Her husband was supportive but had a demanding job with a daily commute over an hour each way, so he was not home a lot.

"How do you manage your stress levels?" I asked. Patricia stared at me blankly. "I don't really have time to think about that," she returned, "though now that you mention it, I do feel pretty stressed out and exhausted most of the time." Patricia is a perfect illustration of how sometimes when we focus on diet alone we can miss other factors that contribute to a weakened immune system, or more specifically in Patricia's case, an upset immune system gone rogue due to stress and fatigue. When we started working on simple everyday steps that she could take to integrate stress management into her routine without making "managing stress" yet another "to do" on her list, Patricia was finally able to control the remaining flares. Yes, sleep was tricky still, as is inevitable with a young family, but Patricia also found ways to get help with some of the nighttime feeds and some time to sleep in on weekends when her mother-in-law and husband took on the early shift, enough to keep her feeling functional and able to cope without aggravating her autoimmune condition.

Most of us know that when we're stressed and not getting enough sleep (both often go hand in hand), we are more likely to catch any bug that's going around. But do we really understand just how important it is to keep on top of our lifestyle habits for good immune health? Science has clearly shown direct ties between exercise, sleep, stress, and even our connection with natural environments, and the effectiveness of our immune mechanisms. Let's take a look at how they can help—or hurt—your immune health (and later in the Immune Resilience Plan, you'll see how to apply the science in real life).

EXERCISE

I don't have to tell you how good exercise is for weight management and cardiovascular health, but moving your body on a regular basis also does wonders for your immune system. Specifically, moderate-intensity aerobic exercise, like brisk walking, active cleaning, yard work, light bicycling, or doubles tennis, succeeds in doing so in a number of ways. Many studies have shown that this type of exercise, when you do it regularly, improves measures of immune function including sIgA, interferon gamma, respiratory burst, and antibody capacity. It improves resistance against infection and reduces the intensity of symptoms if you do get sick. At the same time as boosting all this robust immune activity, moderate exercise decreases overall levels of inflammation and oxidative stress. Not least, several studies have demonstrated that regular aerobic exercise helps us better develop a memory response to vaccinations, blunts age-related declines in vaccine efficacy, and improves the overall level of immunity that vaccines confer. Sounds pretty compelling, don't you think? But that's not even all.

Moderate exercise helps with important internal movement. It helps your digestive system more effectively move food and microbes along. It aids circulation, delivering important nutrients and white blood cells to areas that need them, like your gut barrier and skin. It helps to clear toxins. Remember Andrea, who had a long-standing issue with athlete's foot? By simply incorporating some basic, regular exercise routines into her plan, she was able to help her circulation and immune system better fight the itchy condition that had plagued her for so long.

Exercise also does wonders for your sleep and your stress levels, which, as you'll learn later in this chapter, are highly important for immune resilience. And it improves your mood, which in my experience is critical for starting any kind of dietary or lifestyle change program (and it doesn't hurt to have as you stay on any program either).

The trick with exercise is to understand that there is a happy balance of getting enough exercise without overdoing it. We know that people who move too little have higher levels of inflammation, but so do people who move *too much*. For immune balance, exercise isn't about going all out all the time. And the reason is that exercise of any sort generates some muscle wear and tear, which manifests, in part, as oxidative stress. As long as that oxidative stress is at a level that can be countered by your antioxidant reserves, all is well. In fact, the practice helps you build even stronger antioxidant capability (and stronger muscles), which is what makes regular exercise anti-inflammatory over the long term. If oxidative stress exceeds those reserves, damage proceeds unchecked and leads to inflammation. So it really comes down to hormesis again: Moderate amounts of exercise within limits that your body can cope with trigger "healthy" levels of cellular trauma. However, when you push your muscles too much, the pro-oxidant, pro-inflammatory compounds they produce end up being more than your antioxidant reserves and healing mechanisms can cope with.

Science tells us that bursts of intense exercise or high levels of training, especially the kind that leaves your muscles overly sore and needing a day or more to recover, can increase inflammation in your body, suppress your immune surveillance systems, and increase the risk of developing an infection if you happen to also be exposed to a harmful germ. Even high-intensity interval training (HIIT)—an increasingly popular fitness program that combines short bursts of intense exercise with periods of lower-intensity exercise or rest—has been shown to be potentially detrimental to immune resilience. Some research has found that HIIT programs may lead to reduced circulating white blood cell count whereas moderate-intensity training can favorably improve white blood cell counts. More research is needed to confirm these findings, and they stand somewhat at odds with other studies that report HIIT can improve measures of brain, heart, and metabolic function. But it sheds interesting light on this currently popular form of exercise.

So remember the "Goldilocks" rule here: the "just right" amount of exercise helps your immune system—not too little and not too much. Overdoing it in your fitness training can be just as harmful as being too sedentary and immobile.

There's one more consideration to take into account—and that is that "moderate exercise" is a moving target. It can differ from one person to the next, and from one person one month to the same person in six months' time, depending on the differences in their level of fitness. Over time, with a gradual increase in exercise intensity, your muscles can adapt to what's being asked of them without producing high levels of inflammatory compounds. This is why, with regular moderate exercise over time, you can build muscle strength and endurance. In part 3 you'll learn how to tell if you're getting the right amount of exercise and find ideas for how to incorporate movement into your daily and weekly routines.

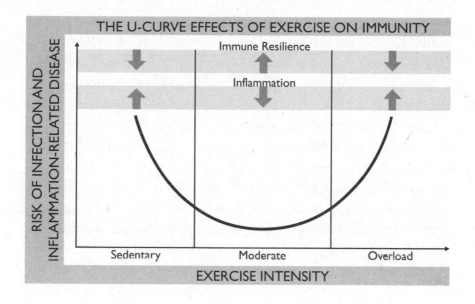

SLEEP

Another thing your mom may well have told you is that "sleep is the best medicine." Sleep is considered a natural, commonsense remedy for many illnesses. And our bodies often seem to need more sleep when we're ill. If you've ever wondered if there's science behind that, your instincts would be correct.

Sleep is not a passive condition. Even though your "lights may be out," your body and brain are highly active in pursuits that can be described mainly as organizing, cleaning, rebuilding, maintaining, and patrolling. Studies of sleep deprivation demonstrate just how much anything that interferes with healthy sleep leads to decreased immunity and increased vulnerability to infection. Military recruits, for example, who slept less than six hours per night during thirteen-week training periods were four times more likely to catch a cold or the flu than those who slept seven to nine hours per night, according to one research study. Even those of us mere mortals who care for infants and small children during the night (yes, you parents!), work long hours or night shifts, or even travel regularly between time zones can put ourselves at risk with poor sleep habits: sleeping five hours or less per night on a regular basis has been observed (in us regular people) to lead to an increased risk for respiratory infections and pneumonia when compared with sleeping seven to eight hours nightly. Habitual shorter sleep duration is also associated with more frequent episodes of cold, flu, and gastroenteritis.

Poor sleep and insomnia are also linked with higher levels of inflammation. This has been studied in human trials where elevated blood inflammation markers were measurable after shortened sleep—less than seven hours—even after just *one* night. It has also been observed in night-shift workers and is thought to be why prolonged sleep deficiencies are associated with diseases that have an inflammatory component, like heart disease, stroke, diabetes, Alzheimer's disease, and cancer. In mice, researchers have observed that persistent sleep disruption that mimics jet lag patterns not only increases inflammation but also accelerates immune cell aging. In addition to warding off infections, dialing down inflammation, and protecting your immune system from aging, sleep seems to be important for developing immune memory. Sleeping just four hours per night for four days before and two days after getting the flu shot, as described in one study, meant that those sleep-deprived individuals produced only half the amount of flu antibodies compared with those who slept a more normal 7.5 to 8 hours. Other studies looking at the effects of sleep deprivation on other vaccines found similarly detrimental effects on generating immune memory.

COULD MELATONIN BE THE KEY TO SLEEP'S BENEFITS?

Toward the end of the day, as light exposure fades, deep in your brain your small, pea-shaped pineal gland produces and releases melatonin, a neurotransmitter that not only regulates sleep timing but is also an important regulator of your immune function. Melatonin may be a significant reason why sleep and immunity are so closely linked. In fact, your immune system seems to consider melatonin so important for immune activity that your T cells and B cells even have their own equipment for producing it so that they don't always have to rely on the pineal gland (say, when it's not night-time and they need to kick quickly into gear). Animal studies also suggest that melatonin might be an important key to sleep's effects: mice who are kept under constant light so that they produce less melatonin, or who are given melatonin-blocking medications, are found to mount an ineffective antibody response to pathogens and have a smaller overall thymus gland compared with mice who don't.

Melatonin helps to turn on many critical immune processes like the formation and activity of white blood cells, phagocytosis, respiratory bursts, and antibody production. It boosts our levels of interferon gamma and other antiviral compounds to aid our resilience against viruses, and it regulates immune communication through its effects on cytokines. Melatonin is also an efficient anti-inflammatory and antioxidant agent, able to dampen pro-inflammatory signals, reduce the toxicity of environmental chemicals, and neutralize the oxidative damage that our immune system inadvertently creates as it fights a germ. In this capacity, it helps your immune cell population (and other cells like barrier cells in your gut and your skin) resist the aging effects of free radicals. No wonder we're told to get our "beauty sleep."

SLEEP AND OTHER DEFENSE MECHANISMS

Sleep is also intimately connected to the other critical pillars of your immune system: your barriers and your microbiota. Sleep disturbance such as in sleep apnea or insomnia can alter the makeup of your gut microbiota, leading to dysbiosis and dysbiosis-associated inflammation. Increased gut permeability, promoted by both the imbalance of microbes as well as the fact that circadian rhythms also control gut barrier integrity, allows more inflammatory microbial compounds to enter circulation and exert negative effects systemically on your immune system.

Another barrier that you want to keep healthy is disrupted by lack of sleep: your blood-brain barrier. This barrier separates your internal "brain space," or central nervous system, from the rest of your body and is designed to filter nutrients, toxic compounds, and of course pathogens from this vital organ. Infections that do penetrate your central nervous system, such as meningitis, while rare, are much more likely to be serious or even life-threatening. A growing body of research also indicates that the health of your gut—its barriers and microbiota—is connected with the health of your blood-brain barrier. When the former goes downhill, so does the latter. The reasons for this are thought to be due to higher levels of circulating gut-derived inflammatory compounds that occur when your gut is compromised, and which trigger immune hyperactivity at the blood-brain barrier or even in your central nervous system directly.

All said, the science is compelling: I could go on about the studies—there are reams of them—but they all point to how important it is to catch enough zzz's.

STRESS

Melatonin is to sleep and its effects on our immunity what cortisol is to stress. Cortisol is your primary stress hormone. Originally designed to protect you from serious threats such as a predator, cortisol, along with adrenaline, redirects the body's resources toward what it considers essential for short-term survival. Adrenaline increases your heart rate and ups your blood pressure, pumping blood to your muscles in anticipation of having to run for your life. Cortisol increases your blood sugar, released from short-term reserves and redirected from nonessential functions, in preparation for the increased energy needs of your muscles and brain.

Nowadays, you're hardly likely to encounter such a hazard, but that doesn't mean you don't experience stress. Intermittent, stressful situations are a normal part of life. Being laid off from work, getting a divorce, bereavement, or even happy occasions such as getting married are among some of the top ten most stressful modern life events that most of us experience at some point. More minor, everyday events, like getting an unexpectedly large bill in the mail, having a disagreement with your spouse or a coworker, taking an exam, or even triaging your kids' before-school morning routine can also get your cortisol and adrenaline pumping.

The physical effects of stressful situations are usually short-lived. However, some of us with ongoing stress can end up in a near-constant alarm state. And that's when stress becomes chronic and problematic for your health and your immune system. High-pressure jobs, destructive relationships, and financial difficulties without an obvious solution are some of the more common potential causes. Telltale signs of chronic stress included fatigue, sleeplessness, irritability, and—you guessed it—frequent infections and illnesses.

Like many of the other systems you're reading about in this book, stress is all about balance and about working within your tolerance levels. Hormesis comes into play here, too, because not all stress has a negative effect; in fact, some stress is good. Moderate amounts of stress—say, positive, healthy challenges that you are able to cope with, can help you improve your performance and overcome obstacles. Giving a public presentation or running a race are usually instances where a manageable amount of stress can help you deliver a better outcome. Scientists call this *eustress*. Similarly, when you have the right amount of stress in short bursts, say the amount naturally triggered by the physiological stress of an infectious bug, it helps your immune system mount an effective attack and neutralize the threat. However, when you have *too much* stress—more than your system can cope with—things can start to go awry.

Stress that exceeds your body's coping mechanisms, especially when this occurs continually over a period of time, can ravage your defense system, your barriers, and your microbiota, leaving you vulnerable to infection and immune-related diseases. This kind of stress is termed *distress*. The relationship between distress and your immune system is characterized by suppression, cortisol resistance, and dysregulation. Let's look at each of these.

IMMUNE SUPPRESSION

As well as being an activation hormone, cortisol is also your body's natural glucocorticoid hormone (a type of steroid). In that role it is immunosuppressive and anti-inflammatory. This is the reason its pharmaceutical glucocorticoid peers, like medical hydrocortisone and prednisone, are used to control inflammation and other harmful immune activity that occurs in asthma, autoimmune disease, vasculitis, and arthritis. Your body also uses natural cortisol to ensure inflammation doesn't exceed safe levels. In short, that brief burst of cortisol may ramp things up, but it also helps you keep your cool.

On the other hand, an immune system that is excessively or chronically exposed to cortisol can become too suppressed. And this can make you more vulnerable to infections—either new ones or ones that have been lying dormant, waiting for this very moment. (Reactivation of latent infections, incidentally, is also a known potential side effect of glucocorticoid medications.) Research, once again, provides evidence for this effect: One study of army cadets undergoing their first six months of training observed that those who had higher levels of cortisol were more likely to experience a reactivation of a dormant viral infection. Other human studies support the potential for stress to reduce immunity to either latent or new infections, including herpesviruses and Epstein-Barr virus, or to new ones. Researchers also point to indicators of impaired immune function in some people, like reduced natural killer cell activity, longer wound healing, lower secretory IgA and interferon gamma, as well as a diminished ability to quickly ramp up immune cell production when a harmful bug comes along. Some of these effects may also explain why stress appears to interfere with vaccine effectiveness in some individuals studied. Chronic stress has also been linked to cancer in part because of the suppression of those components of our immune system that normally root out and kill emerging cancer cells.

CORTISOL RESISTANCE

Cortisol resistance means that, after prolonged exposure to cortisol, your immune cells start not to listen to it. They become less responsive, "resistant," to its effects. To those cells it's like the cortisol signal is dialed down, quieter, harder to hear. This is a well-studied phenomenon in the context of glucocorticoid medications, but is also an increasingly appreciated result of chronic stress. When your cells no longer "hear" cortisol's message clearly, your immune system loses an important mechanism by which it controls the inflammatory response. This is likely a major reason why individuals with higher cortisol resistance tend to have higher levels of inflammation and are known to be more likely to get stronger symptoms when exposed to, say, a common cold virus.

IMMUNE DYSREGULATION

Paradoxically, stress can exacerbate immune diseases like asthma, autoimmune diseases, and allergic reactions, even though logic might otherwise suggest that these immune dysfunctions should also be suppressed. Science doesn't yet have all the answers here, although early evidence points to the effects of cortisol and adrenaline on the balance of helper T cells and regulatory T cells, suggesting that, in vulnerable individuals, stress may be a triggering or contributing factor to ongoing immune disease activity. Certainly, in many individuals I've worked with who have such immune-related diseases, like Patricia, stress can be a very large contributing factor.

As with exercise, each of us has a different ability to cope with stressors. Even though stressful situations may tend to suppress immune function and increase infection risk in most people, some individuals actually demonstrate *improved* immune responsiveness when going through the same experience. It just goes to underscore that what stimulates a beneficial *eustress* effect in one individual might cause a harmful *distress* in another. Later on, in part 3, we'll review ways that you can not only reduce your exposure to stressful situations but also improve your stress resilience. That is to say, you'll be raising the level at which a harmful stress response is triggered, improving your ability to turn *distress* situations into *eustress* ones, and supporting your immune resilience to boot.

NATURE

As rural environments are increasingly absorbed by urban spread, many of us get farther and farther away from natural environments, spending more time indoors at home, in cars, in schools or offices, at indoor sports centers, cinemas, and shopping malls. One of the most interesting investigations of just how much natural vs. man-made environments can influence immune resilience dates back to World War II. During the war, Finland was forced to cede large portions of the Karelia region to the then Soviet Union. People living in the Finnish Karelia transitioned to more urban living after the war, fueled by greater economic growth. By contrast, those in the Russian Karelia (which was completely closed to visitors until the 1990s) maintained traditional ways of living, highly connected with their natural environment through small livestock holdings and homegrown food. By the late twentieth century, significant disparities in immune diseases were apparent; those living on the developed Finnish side were much more likely to acquire the diseases of modern living, including allergies, whereas on the Russian side, allergies were hardly present at all.

Although researchers investigated for hereditary origins, genetics did not seem to explain the differences at all. Instead, they theorized that the environment was the factor that made the greatest impact and, more specifically, the greater exposure to natural environments on the Russian side that harbored a different set of more diverse microbial species. Those on the Russian side possessed a greater variety of antibodies to various pathogenic germs, and the more of these they had, the less likely they were to have developed allergic disease. The research team concluded that contact with a diverse natural environment with abundant types of bacteria and other microorganisms may help support immune tolerance and protect against immune dysfunction.

Of course, I'm not suggesting that you deliberately try to infect yourself with potentially harmful organisms. However, the lessons appear to be clear: the more that your immune system is able to have "healthy," hormetic encounters with germs (either with friendly microbes or by mounting a successful defense to pathogens), the more resilient and balanced it becomes. Research in the US has also found, just as the Karelia data show, that greater exposure to infections is associated with a lower probability of having allergies and asthma. It's from these kinds of studies that scientists have formulated what's known as the "hygiene hypothesis," which argues that our declining exposure to germs is part of the reason for the rise in these diseases.

Unexpected Benefits of a Pandemic Lockdown

The COVID-19 pandemic did have the unexpected benefit of reversing the trend of limited exposure to natural environments for the first time in decades, as many of us started to explore our local parks and natural areas seeking some break from the monotony and claustrophobia of our own four walls. My hope is that this redirection is something that we can all maintain, since, perhaps surprisingly, spending time in nature has a significant impact on your immune defenses and resilience.

More lessons about the relationship between nature and your immune system can be learned from Japan, where the concept of *shinrin-yoku,* or "forest bathing," was first coined. Forest bathing became popular in the 1980s in Japan, where it offered a calming antidote to the work-related burnout of those participating in the country's economic tech boom and as a way to promote the protection of forests. Over the last several decades, research has delved into the physiological effects of forest bathing and found some surprising connections, including improved immune cell function and reduced inflammation.

In one study, a simple two-hour leisurely forest walk taken by healthy individuals led to increases in their levels of natural killer cells and to those cells' ability to release perforins and granzymes (remember those chemical weapons described in chapter 4?). When the researchers had those same participants go for two more two-hour forest walks the next day, these measures all increased further still, reaching an average 50 percent increase in natural killer cell activity compared to before the experiment began. The effects were still present more than seven days later, suggesting surprisingly long-lasting results. Similar results have been reported in several other studies, ranging from just one and a half hours of forest immersion to up to a week's worth of twice-daily forest walks.

The Impact of Ecological and Climate Changes on Infection Risk

Infectious diseases have long been associated with climate conditions: Temperature and humidity, for example, have always affected the risk for catching mosquito- and tick-carried diseases in hot and humid areas like Africa, and for catching colds and flu in colder parts of the world. With the steady rise of global temperatures and extreme weather events, daunting changes are taking place on our planet. Warmer climate conditions increasingly favor microbial growth. Scientists have reported weather-related impacts on the spread and severity of diseases such as hand, foot, and mouth disease, fungal diseases, tick-borne Lyme disease, and parasitic Leishmaniasis. Vector-borne illnesses such as those carried by mosquitoes and ticks are expected to continue to rise with the effects of climate change. This means, according to the CDC, that we can expect increases in incidence and geographic spread of Lyme disease and West Nile virus. Scientists at the Mayo Clinic College of Medicine and Science have predicted that Lyme disease rates will increase by over 20 percent in the next few decades if the latest official climate forecasts are realized.

Mold is another potential problem. Weather-related events and floods have increased the risk for mold growth in affected buildings (as well as the spread of other harmful germs such as aquatic *Vibrio* bacteria). Although hard to prove definitively, most public health professionals acknowledge there is a likely connection between mold exposure and immune health: For susceptible individuals, chronic low-level mold exposure can cause airway symptoms, including difficulty breathing, and asthma symptoms. It may even cause lung infections.

The increase in severe weather incidents, like hurricanes, will also likely mean more instances of environmental chemical contamination as chemical storage locations are breached by flood waters or debris. During Hurricane Katrina, which has been called "the most devastating natural calamity in US history," numerous spills from oil refineries and compromised waste dumping sites in states along the Gulf of Mexico contaminated surrounding soil and waterways. Researchers from the Natural Resources Defense Council (NRDC) found many instances of "dangerously high levels" of industrial chemicals and heavy metals in soil sediment redeposited in many areas around New Orleans, including arsenic, which in some locations exceeded EPA safety limits by a factor of 30, and banned pesticides presumed to have leaked from waste dumping grounds.

On the other end of the spectrum, areas such as the western United States are experiencing increased drought conditions and longer, more dangerous wildfire seasons. Warmer, drier conditions mean that fires spread more easily and are harder to put out. In addition to the negative health effects of smoke exposure we already know of like asthma, chronic obstructive pulmonary diseases (COPD), and other respiratory illnesses, researchers from the Harvard T.H. Chan School of Public Health also discovered that thousands of COVID-19 cases and deaths may be attributable to air particle pollution caused by wildfires. They found that time periods with the highest air particle circulation matched with a subsequent amplification of COVID-19 cases and deaths for up to four weeks afterward. This translated to an average of 11.7 percent more COVID-19 cases and 8.4 percent more COVID-19 deaths for every $10\mu g/m^3$ increase in fine particulate matter in the air. In the most affected counties, these increases reached 71.6 and 65.9 percent, respectively. What is especially notable is that the researchers argued that these effects likely weren't just due to the inflammatory stress on the respiratory system along with simultaneous exposure to SARS-CoV-2. Instead, they pointed to other emerging COVID-19 research, also from Harvard scientists, suggesting that the increased vulnerability could also be due to weakened mucous membranes, increased lung barrier permeability, and weakened macrophage and antiviral interferon activity in response to air pollution, all of which compromise immune defenses against this and other pathogens.

Last but not least, rising overall temperatures, with earlier spring and longer fall weather, is increasing the quantity and duration of pollen exposure. The renowned journal *The Lancet* has published on how this will most likely continue to drive further increases in the rates and severity of allergy and asthma.

Our health is inextricably connected to the world around us. Climate, and other human-driven environmental changes, will lead to a new, more challenging reality for our immune systems to confront. Taking steps to stem, and even reverse, these changes, through actions that improve the stability and health of natural habitats, is simply an extension of building immune resilience inside each of us. It should be part of any immune resilience activity.

Beneficial effects on natural killer cells have in some cases lasted for up to one month. Another interesting observation in these studies: levels of measurable inflammatory markers and stress went down (including cortisol, heart rate, and blood pressure), suggesting that simply walking in a forest environment is an effective anti-inflammatory and stress-reducing activity. Even lowered blood sugar levels have been reported.

Scientists aren't yet sure exactly what it is about the forest environment that has these dramatic effects. Yes, it could be the biodiversity of microbes, but researchers also speculate that other potential mechanisms may be at work. This might include reduced air pollution and heat, the visual, auditory, and tactile relaxation cues, the gentle exercise, and even potentially the essential oils released from the trees and that circulate in the air in the lush, wooded environment. Phytoncides, specific wood essential oils that volatilize into the air and are inhaled while walking in forests, have in laboratory test tube studies demonstrated an ability to increase human natural killer cell function similarly to the effects seen in actual human studies.

Whatever is behind this connection, life on earth evolved over millennia immersed in natural surroundings that contained a huge diversity of organisms. The exponential growth in the human population, rapidly expanding urbanization, pollution, and climate change have led to dramatic declines in species biodiversity and access to natural environments. Perhaps one of the ways that we can support immune balance and resilience is to look to reestablishing those original connections. Getting back to nature often just "feels right."

You'll see, as we embark on part 3, that having a healthy immune-supportive lifestyle is nearly as important, if not equally so, as our diet. It's time to find out how to put this all into practice.

<hr>

To view the references cited in this chapter, please visit
www.immuneresilienceplan.com/science.

Your Immune Resilience Plan

CHAPTER 10

The Immune Resilience Diet

Your Foundation for Immune Health

absolutely love food. And I love to eat. I love the ritual of it, punctuating the day with a regular rhythm. I love the backdrop it provides for connecting with family and friends, and I love how food is such a tool for health and how it can even be medicine. That's why diets to me should never focus on restriction. They should feel abundant, joyful, exciting, and purposeful. And my hope is to impart some of that "spice of life" feeling in this section, too.

It's a good thing to love food because it is one of the biggest levers for health and immune resilience that you have at your disposal. Even though I routinely use nutritional supplements in practice, this is not at the expense of whole foods. In fact, there are several attributes that you can harness to your advantage when using your kitchen pantry and refrigerator as your culinary immune pharmacy:

- *Sophisticated.* Whole-food meals contain tens, hundreds, sometimes thousands of nutrients and phytonutrients in just one bite. The vast majority of phytonutrients are not even available in supplemental form. No supplement can match that sophistication and broad impact.

- *Synergistic*. Foods have synergistic effects. For example, black pepper increases the absorption of several other important compounds. Fats increase the absorption of many phytonutrients. Chromium and magnesium found in whole-grain rice (but not white rice) improve the utilization of the carbohydrate that rice contains and help keep blood sugar within normal limits. Vitamin C regenerates vitamin E, and both work best in tandem with other antioxidants.

- *Steadfast*. The very fact that we eat at least three times per day provides a constant and dependable means by which to support immune function. By choosing immune-supportive foods, we benefit from a whole complement of effective immune boosters throughout each day.

- *Safe*. Getting your nutrients from a balanced, healthy diet where foods are used in traditional quantities is considered extremely safe (except for those with food allergies, the triggers for which must of course be avoided). This is not always the case with dietary supplements, especially when consumed above those amounts normally found in foods and in some synthetic forms.

- *Scalable*. Supplements can get quite pricey. Especially when you stick to the higher-quality brand names such as the ones I recommend. There's good reason for that, as I'll explain later on in this section. Foods, however, are usually a much more economical, and therefore scalable, way to achieve the immune support we're looking for.

The foods I recommend in this chapter are based on hundreds of scientific research studies that have uncovered amazing connections to those factors that impact our immune health. As you'll discover, the Immune Resilience Diet is a plant-based but not necessarily plant-exclusive eating plan that is a flexible and powerful way to create an optimal foundation for immune health. It can fit in easily with your current eating philosophy, whether you are vegan, vegetarian, or omnivore. And it is chock-full of delicious food options that leave you satisfied and your immune system soundly supported. Let's dive into what to eat.

I created the following chart to show how to balance what you eat across different food groups. It's a little more detailed than the USDA's MyPlate and other food charts you may have seen, but that's for a very good reason: it ensures that no important category gets left out, including nuts and seeds, oils and fats as a whole (not just dairy), legumes, herbs and spices, and fermented foods. As you read on, I'll explain just how each of these groups helps your immune system and offer practical guidance on which specific foods to choose.

The Immune Resilience Plate

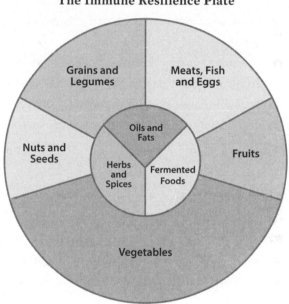

VEGETABLES

As you can see from the Immune Resilience Plate, vegetables are king! Abundant, colorful veggies should make up 40 percent of your food intake for optimal immune resilience. That's nearly half of what's on your plate for breakfast, lunch, dinner, and snacks. Yes, of course, this can vary somewhat and what we're really looking for is an average over time, with regular exposure at least on a daily basis. For most adults, this equates to 7 to 9 cups of vegetables (measured raw, but can of course be subsequently cooked) per day. These will provide a dense source of vitamins, minerals, phytonutrients, and fiber that will nourish your microbiome and provide vitamins, minerals, and phytonutrients for your immune system.

The vegetables below are listed by color group to emphasize that we need to eat a diverse, colorful array of vegetables that will give us a broad set of phytonutrients. Remember, these are the immune-benefiting plant components that are responsible for the bold colors of plant foods. Aim for a good rotation of vegetables incorporating all the color groups to maximize the variety of phytonutrients you're getting. Note: The list below represents those vegetables that are more commonly found in American grocery stores. However, I fully acknowledge that there are many traditional foods found in the US and around the world that are not listed here. If you use in your cooking more traditional whole foods that are rich in fiber and phytonutrients, they're likely excellent choices, too.

Choose from this abundant list of colorful options:

Red: red beets, red peppers, red potatoes, radishes, radicchio, rhubarb, tomatoes.

Yellow/Orange: yellow beets, butternut squash, carrots, yellow and orange peppers, yellow potatoes, pumpkin, rutabaga, yellow summer squash, sweet corn, sweet potatoes, yellow tomatoes, winter squash, yam.

Green: artichokes, arugula, green asparagus, beet greens, broccoflower, broccoli, broccoli rabe (rapini), Brussels sprouts, Chinese cabbage, green cabbage, celery, collard greens, cucumbers, dandelion greens, endive, escarole, grape leaves, green beans, kale, lambsquarters, leeks, lettuces, mustard greens, okra, green olives, peas, green peppers, scallions, sea vegetables (e.g., kelp, kombu, nori, wakame), snap peas, snow peas, spinach, sprouted greens, Swiss chard, turnip greens, watercress, zucchini.

Blue/Purple/Black: purple asparagus, purple cabbage, purple carrots, eggplant, purple Belgian endives, black olives, purple peppers, purple potatoes, red onions, black salsify, shallots.

White/Brown: bamboo shoots, cauliflower, celeriac, chicory, daikon radish, fennel, garlic, ginger, hearts of palm, horseradish, Jerusalem artichokes, jicama, kohlrabi, mushrooms, white/yellow onions, parsnips, white potatoes, turnips, water chestnuts.

HERBS AND SPICES

Culinary herbs and spices are the second food category whose importance in immune health I want to emphasize, even though they take up just a fraction of the space on your plate. These little phytonutrient bombs are immune regenerative and balancing, anti-inflammatory, barrier restoring, and even antimicrobial. However, the quantity of phytonutrients you'll get from any given product depends on several factors, including whether it is fresh or dried, pre-ground or whole, how long it's stored for, at what temperature, and how much light it's been exposed to. I use fresh herbs and spices wherever possible since vitamin and phytonutrient content can decline quite rapidly during storage (those fresh herbs languishing in your refrigerator, for instance). This means that sometimes quick-dried or freeze-dried herbs end up having more phytonutrients than their fresh-but-long-stored counterparts. Grinding dried spices from their whole forms as you need them helps retain the most phytonutrients, although I appreciate that's not always practical. In addition, keeping your dried herbs and spices in a dark, dry, and cool place helps them retain their potency. Avoid humid storage places and replace dried products frequently and for certain as they expire to avoid potential rancidity and mold. You'll find a list of my favorite dried herb and spice brands in the Resources section.

Herbs and spices can be used directly in cooking and sprinkled over finished dishes. They are great for jazzing up your meals, giving a totally different lease on life to the foods they're paired with. Herbal teas are also an excellent choice and have a long history of medicinal use. If you're interested in brewing medicinal-strength teas (which I highly recommend), you'll find instructions on page 304.

Culinary herbs: basil, bay leaves, capers, chervil, chives, cilantro, curry leaf, dill, fennel leaf, lemongrass, marjoram, Mexican oregano, mint, oregano, parsley, rosemary, sage, savory, tarragon, thyme.

Culinary spices: aniseed, annatto, asafoetida, cardamom, celery seed, chilies, cinnamon, cloves, coriander seed, cumin seed, dill seed, fennel seed, juniper berries, mustard seed, nigella seed, nutmeg, paprika, pepper, star anise, sumac, turmeric, vanilla pods.

Herb/spice teas: black tea, chamomile tea, cinnamon tea, dandelion tea, echinacea tea, elderflower tea, fruit tea, ginger tea, green tea, hawthorn tea, hibiscus tea, honeybush tea, jasmine tea, lemon balm tea, marshmallow root tea, mint tea, nettle tea, oolong tea, passionflower tea, raspberry leaf tea, rooibos tea, rosehip tea, rosemary tea, thyme tea, tulsi tea, turmeric tea, uva-ursi tea, valerian tea, verbena tea.

FERMENTED FOODS

Human use of fermented foods can be traced all the way back to the Neolithic age, beginning around 10,000 BCE. The preserving process gave much longer life to plant foods that would otherwise only last a few days. Cabbage kept in a cupboard, for instance, will last a few weeks if you're lucky. But ferment it into sauerkraut and it will keep for several months! During the 1950s and '60s, many fermented foods fell out of favor as refrigeration and processed canned foods became convenient and fashionable preservation alternatives. But as a result, many of us have lost the significant health and immune benefits that these foods provide.

There are three main types of food fermentation: lactic acid, acetic acid, and alcoholic fermentation. Lactic acid and acetic acid fermentation are the ones most preferable for immune health. During lactic acid fermentation, *Lactobacillus* organisms feed on sugars and starches in the food, quickly forming lactic acid, a natural, low-pH preservative that inhibits the growth of harmful bacteria. The total number of bacteria present in the fermenting food drops very quickly during the first forty-eight hours of fermentation, after which lactic acid bacteria (beneficial species that can survive in this new environment), especially *Lactobacillus plantarum*, become the dominant organisms. Glutamic acid (glutamate) is also produced during this process, which creates an "umami" flavor and makes fermented foods especially delicious. Glutamate, incidentally, is readily converted to glutamine by immune cells which you now know is an important source of energy during illness.

Acetic acid fermentation involves the fermentation of sugars to first ethanol (alcohol) and then to acetic acid. The most well-known products of acetic acid are vinegar and kombucha. Vinegar has been found to possess antimicrobial, antioxidant, digestion-supportive, and blood-sugar-lowering properties. Kombucha, a type of traditional fermented tea, has similar potential properties that haven't been well studied in humans but that animal studies suggest also include ones that are antimicrobial, antioxidant, and blood-sugar lowering. When raw or unpasteurized, kombucha contains live probiotic organisms.

Fermented foods that are still "live" contain a rich abundance and diversity of beneficial microbes. Some of the probiotic strains in fermented foods are the same as those you'd find in a supplement, but there are many, many more that currently exist only in fermented food form. And while many over-the-counter probiotics have 1 billion to 3 billion colony-forming units (CFUs, the common measure for quantifying probiotics), fermented foods can have far more. Good-quality yogurts can have over 40 billion CFUs per serving, and kefirs (a kind of fermented milk) on the order of hundreds of billions of CFUs.

The practice of having a small amount of fermented food with each

More Ways to Tend to Your Microbial Allies with Food

While fermented foods are great for introducing live beneficial organisms into your upper digestive tract, it's wise to complement them with *prebiotic* foods. Prebiotic foods are those foods with extra-high amounts of fibers that "feed" the healthy microbes in your gut. Especially 25 feet down your digestive tract—the distance it takes to reach your colon, where the vast majority of them reside. Research has shown that you can make significant changes to the balance of microbial species living in your colon even after just twenty-four to forty-eight hours of changing what you eat—so it's never too late to get started. Here are some of the best prebiotics you can choose that will keep your microbiota super happy and working in lockstep with your immune system:

- *Vegetables:* chicory root, dandelion greens, garlic, Jerusalem artichokes, jicama, leeks, onion, seaweeds.
- *Legumes:* beans, chickpeas, lentils, split peas.
- *Fruit:* apples, bananas, nectarines, peaches, pomegranate, watermelon.
- *Whole grains:* barley, oats, rye, wheat.
- *Nuts and seeds:* cashews, chia seeds, flaxseed, pistachio nuts.
- *Other:* honey.

Tips for Incorporating Prebiotics into Your Diet
- Switch from refined grains to whole grains for bread, pasta, and rice.
- Set up a jar with a combination of crushed nuts and seeds and keep it handy for sprinkling over salads, soups, breakfasts, or yogurts.
- Add chickpeas or beans to your salads (each ½ cup is approximately one-quarter of your daily fiber needs).
- Make legume-based dinners two to three times per week.
- Snack on cut vegetables and hummus, or fruit.
- Have fresh fruit for dessert.
- Have whole fruits instead of fruit juice (which doesn't have fiber).

Help! Eating Prebiotic Foods Gives Me Gas
The gas that comes from eating higher fiber, higher prebiotic foods is produced by the microorganisms in your gut. This can sometimes be

very painful, as the gas presses out on the intestinal lining as it tries to find a route to escape. Most often, this happens when we change our diet too quickly. If you haven't been eating a lot of plant foods, especially prebiotic foods, it's best to add them into your diet gradually over seven to fourteen days. This gives your gut microbes time to adapt without causing excessive gas.

If that still doesn't work for you, and especially if you have other symptoms combined with a fiber intolerance, such as chronic reflux, bloating, constipation, and/or diarrhea, this may indicate an underlying issue. One possibility, which I see with some frequency in clinic, is an overgrowth of bacteria in the small intestine (called small intestinal bacterial overgrowth, or SIBO). This overgrowth means that there are too many bacteria, even beneficial ones, hanging around. When this is the case, eating fiber causes too much microbial activity and symptoms such as gas, bloating, reflux, diarrhea, and/or constipation. (If this happens to you, it's best to work with a gastroenterologist, qualified nutritionist, or functional medicine provider who knows how to address it.)

meal helps you curate your own healthy microbiota. It has also been shown to reduce the incidence and duration of respiratory infections as well as providing other immune support. The list of possible fermented foods is practically endless, especially when considering traditional recipes from different cultures around the world. However, these are my preferred choices from those more commonly found in American stores. And if you are inclined to make your own (which I highly recommend), one of the easiest recipes to start with is sauerkraut (see page 335).

Fermented milk products: buttermilk, crème fraiche, kefir, sour cream, quark, yogurt.

Fermented grains and legumes: miso, natto, sourdough bread, stinky tofu, tamari, tempeh.

Fermented drinks: kombucha, kvass.

Fermented vegetables and fruits: raw apple cider vinegar, black garlic, kimchi, sauerkraut, umeboshi plums, and many more such as fermented ginger, beets, cucumbers, olives.

A note of caution: Anyone with a weakened immune system should ask their doctor's advice before including fermented foods since, in rare cases, contaminated fermented foods can lead to infection.

HERE'S HOW TO GET THE MOST FROM YOUR FERMENTED FOOD CHOICES

- *Check the label to see if the food contains live cultures*—usually these foods are the ones that you find in the refrigerated section of your local grocery store and are sometimes labeled "lacto-fermented" or "live." Many pickled foods don't actually contain live bacteria since they are simply processed in vinegar. Some fermented foods, like yogurt and sour cream, are re-pasteurized after fermentation, which kills the beneficial bacteria. Those won't have the benefits you want.

- *Make sure the fermented food is either unsweetened or doesn't contain excessive levels of sugar* (no more than 4 grams of sugars per serving, ideally. That's equivalent to 1 teaspoon of table sugar). Yogurts and kombucha are some of the worst offenders here. Watch out for other undesirable ingredients such as dyes or food additives.

- *Make sure it passes safety checks.* For commercial preparations, look for a reputable company that adheres to federal and state regulations for fermented foods. For home preparations, make sure you follow the directions closely (as much as I love to improvise with recipes, this isn't the moment to do so) and if it doesn't taste pleasant or "right," just ditch the batch and start again.

NUTS AND SEEDS

Nuts and seeds are a naturally dense source of minerals and essential fats—both omega-3s and omega-6s—so these are featured prominently in the Immune Resilience Diet. It's usually harder to get enough omega-3 fats in your diet so I've put an asterisk (*) next to those nuts and seeds in the list below that are especially good sources of these essential fats. If you don't eat fish (one of the best sources of omega-3 fats), you'll need to pay special attention to these non-fish sources and consider a supplemental form of EPA and DHA.

Since nuts and seeds are so nutrient dense, you don't have to eat large quantities to get the benefits: one to two servings per day is sufficient. To measure a serving, simply scoop them into the palm of your hand and fold your fingers over them to make a loose fist. That's one serving.

Nuts: almonds, Brazil nuts, cashews, chestnuts, hazelnuts, macadamias, peanuts (actually a legume), pecans, pine nuts, pistachios, walnuts*.

Seeds: cacao, chia seeds*, flaxseeds*, hemp seeds*, poppy seeds, pumpkin seeds, sesame seeds, sunflower seeds.

WHOLE GRAINS AND LEGUMES

The second largest segment of your diet (along with meats, fish, and eggs) should comprise whole grains and legumes. (The only exception to this is if you have any glucose dysregulation such as insulin resistance or diabetes; see chapter 14 for more details on how to adapt this diet for those conditions.) Grains in their whole form and legumes are full of nutrients, fibers, and phytonutrients. Switching to whole grains instead of consuming refined grains has a rapid effect on your microbiome and immune system. Research participants who made this change over just a few weeks experienced

Lectins in Food

Lectins are natural carbohydrate-bound proteins that are biologically widespread across almost all species including plants, animals, and tiny microorganisms. Lectins have become more prominent in popular nutrition thinking in recent years, since some nutrition and wellness advocates claim that they can cause inflammation, increased intestinal permeability, and symptomatic reactions to foods. By this logic, certain conditions may be worsened with higher consumption of lectins. But, given that many traditionally healthy diets like the Mediterranean and Okinawan Diets contain high levels of lectins in foods such as grains, legumes, and nightshade vegetables (tomatoes, peppers, and potatoes), can they really be all that bad? For the most part, the answer is no.

What's important to know is that as yet no human clinical trials have demonstrated any harm from food-based lectins, when properly prepared. This means soaking and boiling beans, for instance. Sprouting and fermentation go even further to reduce lectin content in grains and legumes. These are all practices widely used in traditional diets. Conversely, consuming some legumes in raw form (e.g., kidney beans) is known to cause acute food poisoning—an effect attributed to the specific type of uncooked lectins they contain. But as long as you avoid the raw versions (not a typical way to eat them for sure!), you avoid the problem.

Another reason not to give up on lectin-containing foods is that lectins have antimicrobial activity against harmful organisms. That means there's potential here for lectins to play a role in supporting a healthy microbiota and protecting against digestive infections. There's also some suggestion from animal studies that lectins may inhibit cancer growth. Certainly, there's more for science to uncover about these intriguing compounds.

A last note about lectins: Some people do genuinely feel better when they reduce high-lectin foods in their diet. If you find this is the case for you, I might suggest there are several possibilities as to what is going on. First, if your digestion or microbiota are compromised in some way, you may not be able to handle higher lectin foods well since they also tend to contain higher amounts of fermentable fiber. The typical symptoms that might follow their consumption tend to be concentrated in the digestive system and may be improved by targeting digestive function or microbial balance. Second, if you experience non-intestinal symptoms after consuming high lectin foods (like brain fog or joint pain), you may be experiencing an effect that is mediated via an unhappy (dysbiotic) microbiota that releases more LPS (lipopolysaccharides) after consuming foods higher in carbohydrates and fiber. As you've learned, these can be absorbed into your blood and trigger inflammatory reactions around the body. Improving the health of your gut microbiota may resolve an LPS-triggered reaction. And third, there are some early data showing that, in rare situations, some individuals with autoimmune disease may generate antibodies to lectins. In this case, there may be a "true" reaction to the lectin itself that provokes an immune cross-reaction toward your own cells, therefore fueling an autoimmune process. While the latter is still largely theoretical, it may turn out to be the only real reason to avoid some lectins specifically.

positive effects on their microbiota, increased SCFA production, improved memory T cell measures, and improved bowel movements. For vegans and vegetarians, a balanced combination of both whole grains and legumes (or legumes and nuts/seeds) is essential for obtaining the full complement of amino acids, the building blocks of proteins.

Whole grains and legumes are best cooked after they have been soaked and even sprouted if you can. Sprouting is the process by which seeds are germinated and start to grow into a new plant. During sprouting, the outer layer splits and a young new shoot emerges. Sprouting actually enhances vitamin and phytonutrient levels, reduces starchiness, and further improves digestibility (helpful if you find you get gassy from eating beans).

Whole grains: amaranth, barley, brown rice, buckwheat, bulgur, corn, farro, kamut, millet, oats, quinoa, rye, sorghum, spelt, teff, wild rice, wheat.

Legumes: black beans, black-eyed peas, cannellini beans, chickpeas, fava beans, Great Northern beans, kidney beans, lima beans, lentils, lupins, mung beans, navy beans, pinto beans, peanuts, soybeans.

HOW TO SOAK AND SPROUT SEEDS, GRAINS, AND LEGUMES

Soaking and sprouting seeds, grains, and legumes is an age-old practice across many cultures that helps improve their digestibility and helps harness the nutrition that's locked up inside them.

To soak these foods, first make sure you have a clean batch: go through the dry seeds, grains, or pulses and pick out any debris. Rinse them thoroughly. Then soak them in a bowl with roughly two to three times the quantity of water to grain for up to twenty-four hours. The grains/legumes will absorb a great deal of that water and swell in size. Smaller varieties, like seeds or lentils, will be sufficiently soaked in four to six hours. Larger ones like dried cannellini or garbanzo beans may need the full time.

Once the soaking stage is complete, drain, and rinse again. You can either use the seeds/grains/legumes now or proceed to the sprouting stage. To sprout the grains/legumes, place them back into your soaking bowl and loosely cover with a cloth. Keep them in a dark place at room temperature. Once again, sprouting time varies; some will sprout in just a few hours but others will need to be left overnight or even a few days before they begin to send out a shoot. If you're nursing a multiday sprout, be sure to rinse the grains/legumes with fresh water each day and drain well before returning them under cover. Multiday sprouts run a higher risk of contamination with pathogenic species like *E. coli*, so be sure to keep everything as clean as possible and avoid eating raw sprouts if you have a compromised immune system. Once you see small shoots, you can either decide to cook them then or continue to sprout until you have stalks of 2 to 3 inches that produce a pair of first leaves.

Soaked and sprouted grains and legumes should always be cooked before eating. Soaked or sprouted seeds may be eaten raw.

EATING SOY?
HERE'S HOW TO MAKE SURE IT'S GOOD QUALITY

Certain cultures have a long history of soybean consumption, including the Okinawan community, known for their high number of centenarians. However, the way they prepare soy is dramatically different from the majority of soy in our processed food chain. Their soy is minimally processed, traditionally pesticide-free, and soaked, cooked, and then fermented into a completely different kind of end product that is richer in antioxidant phytonutrients and far better for your microbiota. In the US, by contrast, 94 percent of soybean crops are genetically engineered to tolerate herbicides. This varietal is therefore more liberally sprayed and retains a greater residue of herbicide than other non-genetically engineered crops. This soy makes its way into animal feeds and into foods prepared for human consumption, especially processed foods that use cheaper ingredients.

You can avoid such soy products and find the healthier versions in the US if you know what to look for: organic tempeh, miso, natto, tamari, and shoyu are all good options.

MEATS, FISH, AND EGGS

Animal foods, fish, and seafood are an excellent source of protein, which as you know now is key to a happy immune system, as well as essential immune-supporting minerals like iron and zinc. Fish is also a direct source of those important longer-chain omega-3 fats, EPA and DHA. Eggs, too, can be enriched with omega-3 fats and are high in iron, vitamins, minerals, and phytonutrient carotenoids derived from the hen's diet.

However, think of these animal foods as "accessories" to your meal, not as the main event. Too much meat in comparison to plant foods pushes up levels of inflammation and leaves us short on fiber and phytonutrients. High meat diets are also associated with accelerated aging, which affects your immune resilience as much as your body's other systems. Conversely, small amounts of good-quality meat consumed in the context of a fiber- and phytonutrient-rich diet does *not* push up inflammation and provides a good source of nutrition.

Did you know? Those of us in the US consume the most meat per capita of any country in the world: around 214 pounds per person annually. In the European Union, meat consumption is dramatically less, at 153 pounds per person per year. In China, annual meat consumption averages 124 pounds, and in Japan it is just over 66 pounds. That's less than one third the US consumption. Residents of communities that have the highest percentage of centenarians share a common trait of eating low amounts of meat. Most don't eschew it altogether, but they treat it as a condiment, rather than the center of their plate. And so, too, should we.

Meats: beef, bison, chicken, duck, goat, goose, lamb, pork, quail, rabbit, turkey, venison.

Fish (lowest in mercury)*: anchovies, Atlantic croaker, Atlantic mackerel, black sea bass, catfish, cod, flounder, haddock, hake, herring, mullet, Pacific chub mackerel, perch, pickerel, plaice, pollock, salmon, sardine, shad, skate, smelt, sole, tilapia, trout, tuna (light, including skipjack), whitefish, whiting.

Seafood (lowest in mercury)*: clam, cockles, crab, crawfish, eel, lobster, oysters, scallops, shrimp, squid.

Eggs: chicken, duck, goose, quail.

* Mercury contamination is an issue with fish and seafood. All the major US authorities, including the EPA and FDA, and state-level advisories caution against overconsuming fish that are high in mercury, while simultaneously advocating that fish continue to be important in a healthy diet. I have listed here only the fish and seafood that are lowest in mercury and can be safely eaten two to three times per week. Note that king mackerel, marlin, orange roughy, shark, swordfish, tilefish, and bigeye tuna are highest in harmful mercury, and so should be avoided altogether. A current list of recommendations can be found at epa.gov/fish-tech.

FRUITS

Fruits are an excellent addition to your diet, in moderate amounts (because of their natural sugar content), two to three servings per day. One serving equates to, for example, one orange, one kiwi, or ⅓ cup of berries. I mention these three because they are some of my favorite choices for immune health. Berries are rich in very powerful phytonutrients called anthocyanins, and citrus and kiwi contain high levels of vitamin C as well as their own suite of active phytonutrients like hesperidin and naringenin, which science has shown are active in deterring harmful invaders.

Red: red apples, blood oranges, cherries, cranberries, red grapes, pink/red grapefruit, red pears, pomegranate, raspberries, strawberries, watermelon.

Yellow/Orange: yellow apples, apricots, bananas, cantaloupe melon, cape gooseberries, grapefruit, golden kiwifruit, lemons, mangoes, nectarines, oranges, papayas, peaches, yellow pears, persimmons, pineapples, tangerines.

Green: green apples, avocados, green grapes, honeydew melon, kiwifruit, limes.

Blue/Purple/Black: blackberries, black currants, blueberries, elderberries, figs, purple grapes, plums.

White/Brown: white nectarines, white peaches, brown pears, plantains.

OILS AND FATS

Oils and fats are key elements of a healthy diet and just as important for immune resilience. Fats are a vital component of cell membranes, which play very active roles in our immune defenses, from being barriers to engulfing microbes through phagocytosis. They also act as a repository for fats that form both pro- and anti-inflammatory compounds that your immune system uses to balance between attack and rest modes. Another important role for fats and oils is as phytonutrient enablers: many phytonutrients are fat soluble, and therefore *require* some fat to aid their absorption. As you learned in chapter 6, fat consumption is all about balance: aim to keep saturated fats to one-third of your total fat calorie intake or less (up to 10 percent of your total calories). This means that good-quality sources of animal fats such as organic, unprocessed butter, ghee, and coconut oil aren't off the table—they're just moderated. Then make up the other two-thirds with monounsaturated and polyunsaturated fats. Within the polyunsaturated category, omega-3s and omega-6s are essential fats that we must all source through our diets. It's generally harder to get more omega-3s in your diet than omega-6s, so focus on getting those in a little every day. One thing to know is that highly polyunsaturated oils like flaxseed and chia seed oil are prone to oxidation, which renders them harmful rather than helpful to your immune system. Always keep these fragile oils in a dark, cool place, such as the refrigerator, and preferably drizzle them on foods *after* cooking to avoid potential heat damage.

Saturated fats: Fats—butter, chicken fat, coconut oil, duck fat, ghee (see the recipe on page 354), goose fat, lard, tallow; and foods—coconut, eggs, poultry, and meats.

Monounsaturated fats: Oils and fats—almond oil, avocado oil, canola oil, chicken fat, duck fat, goose fat, hazelnut oil, lard, olive oil, macadamia nut oil, sesame seed oil, high oleic sunflower oil, tallow; and foods—almonds, avocados, cashews, eggs, hazelnuts, macadamia nuts, olives, peanuts, pecan nuts, pistachios, poultry, pumpkin seeds, sesame seeds, sunflower seeds.

Polyunsaturated fats
  Omega-3: Oils—canola oil, chia seed oil, cod liver oil, flaxseed oil, hemp seed oil, walnut oil; and foods—chia seeds, dark leafy greens (especially arugula, Chinese broccoli, collard greens, grape

leaves, spinach, sprouts, and turnip greens), pasture-reared animal foods, hemp seeds, oily fish, flaxseeds, walnuts.

Omega-6: Oils—almond oil, hemp seed oil, pumpkin seed oil, sesame seed oil, sunflower oil, walnut oil; and foods—almonds, eggs, hemp seeds, pumpkin seeds, sesame seeds, sunflower seeds, walnuts.

Did you notice that several fats appear in more than one category? This is because when you eat any liquid oil or solid fat, you are *always* eating a combination of different fats. Yes, some oils and fats are known for being predominantly one kind or the other, but the reality is that these foods provide different categories of fats at the same time.

Choosing the Right Cooking Fat

Given that some fats (especially the polyunsaturated kinds) can be more easily damaged by heat, knowing which are safest for cooking is important. Butter, ghee, coconut oil, and animal fats have the highest smoke points and are therefore safe for stovetop and oven cooking. Avocado oil and olive oil are also relatively heat-resistant and are fine to cook or bake with at moderate temperatures. In all situations, I recommend avoiding extremely high heat cooking as much as possible. I'll explain in more detail in the next section, but one reason for this is that every oil has a natural smoke point, beyond which it starts to oxidize and denature. It's best to keep cooking temperatures low to moderate.

SUPERHERO FOODS

One of the most eye-opening experiences I had back when I started studying nutrition was, "Wait a minute. There are specific studies on the effects of individual foods?" I realized that these foods really are not just pretty on a plate—they do some highly specific things in your body that scientists observe and report on. Below is a comprehensive list of foods that are packed with nutrients and ingredients scientifically proven to be "super-hero foods" for your immune resilience.

Allspice. *Antimicrobial. Antioxidant. Anti-AGE (advanced glycation end products). Anti-inflammatory.* Allspice contains eugenol, which is antimicrobial, anti-inflammatory, and analgesic (pain relieving). Since it is so potent, eugenol is best used at low doses, which makes its common use at low levels in cooking ideal.

Apples. *Anti-allergy. Gut barrier health. Healthy microbiota. Vitamin C.* "An apple a day keeps the doctor away"—this adage rings true when we consider that apples are high in vitamin C, as well as a soluble fiber called pectin that feeds the good bacteria in your gut, which in turn use it to produce butyrate—that important compound that nourishes your gut barrier and tones your immune response. Apples are also a good source of quercetin, which (as you'll learn more about in chapter 12) is also supportive of gut barrier health, dials down inflammation, and helps reduce environmental allergies. These compounds tend to be concentrated in its peel, making it a good idea to eat whole apples (preferably organic), cored but unpeeled.

Apple cider vinegar (raw). *Antimicrobial. Antioxidant. Anti-inflammatory. Digestive support. Healthy microbiota. Blood sugar balancing.* Vinegars are mildly acidic, which helps to control the growth of harmful bacteria. Raw apple cider vinegar has been fermented and therefore contains those beneficial microbial species that can survive in a more acidic environment. It also contains beneficial antioxidants that help keep inflammation levels down. Several studies suggest that, when ingested as food, it can also improve blood sugar control to help keep levels of blood sugar out of a harmful range. Diluted, it can also be applied topically to skin and scalp.

Basil. *Antimicrobial. Antiparasitic. Antiviral. Antioxidant. Anti-inflammatory. Congestion relief.* Basil leaves are an astounding one-fifth essential oil. They contain the phytonutrient eucalyptol, which makes basil a natural expectorant and so great for the relief of congestion in nasal passages and lungs. Basil constituents have been shown to have blocking effects against *Giardia* and other parasites. Its oils are also used as a natural repellent against germ-carrying insects.

Bell peppers (sweet). *Antioxidant. Vitamin C. Vitamin A. Healthy microbiota. Blood sugar balancing.* Sweet bell peppers are an excellent source of fiber and phytonutrients including beta carotene, quercetin, and apigenin. Two-thirds cup of chopped sweet red bell peppers can provide 100 percent of your daily requirement for vitamin C and 60 percent of your daily vitamin A requirement.

Blackberries. *Antiviral. Antiparasitic. Antioxidant. Anti-inflammatory. Blood sugar balancing. Calming. Detoxifying.* Two of the most prominent active constituents of blackberries are ellagic acid and anthocyanins, which are thought to be behind many of their beneficial effects. While they are nutritionally quite similar to their cousins, blueberries, blackberries tend to have more vitamin C (over double by some reports) and other vitamins, minerals, and phytonutrients. Though this may be because modern blueberry breeds are selected to be sweeter and larger, diluting their benefits somewhat compared with wild blueberry and blackberry varieties.

Black pepper. *Antiviral. Antibacterial. Antifungal. Antioxidant. Anti-inflammatory. Anti-allergy. Anti-autoimmune. Immune balancing. Potentiates other phytonutrients.* Black pepper contains a phytonutrient called piperine. Early studies on piperine indicate it may stimulate innate immune cells and dial down aberrant adaptive immune activity. It also protects immune cells against injury caused by toxins. One particularly interesting role of piperine is that it increases the absorption of several other phytonutrients from the digestive tract into circulation, such as those found in turmeric and green tea.

Cardamom. *Antimicrobial. Antibacterial. Antifungal. Anti-inflammatory. Immune responsiveness. Digestive support.* Cardamom, a member of the ginger family, is a good decongestant, attributed to its 5 percent eucalyptol content, the same constituent found in eucalyptus leaves. It also has demonstrated antimicrobial properties, including to drug-resistant strains of bacteria, and is traditionally used for diarrhea, nausea, vomiting, and infections of all kinds. Cardamom also aids white blood cell production when the immune system is challenged and enhances the activity of natural killer cells.

Celery seed. *Antibacterial. Antioxidant. Anti-inflammatory.* Celery seed is strongly antioxidant and is known to tone down proinflammatory immune activity. It is also traditionally used for urinary tract infections since it reduces the ability of pathogens to adhere to the lining of the urinary system. It may also act as a diuretic, helping to flush out unwanted germs that might cause infection.

Chamomile tea. *Antimicrobial. Anti-inflammatory. Anti-allergy. Barrier stabilizing. Congestion relief. Wound healing. Calming.* Chamomile is a useful gentle antimicrobial that both inhibits the growth of bacteria and fungi and breaks up the protective biofilms they hide behind. Chamomile tea has been shown to be effective for upset stomachs, as an oral rinse against periodontitis, and as a topical compress to aid wound healing. Sipping hot chamomile tea can be helpful in dealing with the respiratory symptoms of colds and flu. Chamomile blocks histamine release, making it a good choice for most allergy sufferers. However, since it comes from the same botanical family as ragweed, ragweed allergy sufferers need to be cautious with chamomile, which can sometimes exacerbate their allergy symptoms.

Chia seeds. *Antioxidant. Anti-inflammatory. Healthy microbiota. Omega-3s. Barrier stabilizing. Blood sugar balancing.* Chia seeds are rich in plant-derived omega-3 fats as well as antioxidants and fiber to dial down inflammation and nourish your allied gut bugs. Chia seeds absorb a considerable amount of water and expand as they do so, slowing the release of carbohydrates in the digestive tract. This can help us reduce cravings for the wrong kinds of foods and better regulate blood sugar.

Chili peppers. *Antimicrobial. Antibacterial. Antiviral. Anti-inflammatory. Anti-autoimmune. Healthy microbiota. Blood sugar balancing.* When studied in a lab environment, the compound *capsaicin*, found in hot chili peppers, inhibits the growth of several potential pathogens, including *Porphyromonas gingivalis* (a cause of periodontal disease), *Staphylococcus aureus* (which can cause infections in several sites including the digestive tract, airways, skin, and urinary system), and *Streptococcus pyogenes* (which causes strep throat). Recently, research has suggested that capsaicin-containing foods may also be beneficial for autoimmune diseases.

Chives. *Antimicrobial. Antifungal. Antioxidant. Anti-inflammatory. Healthy microbiota.* Chives belong to the same family of plants as garlic, onion, scallions, and leeks but impart a milder flavor and are easily grown. The sulfur compounds in chives and its relations are thought to be one reason why they have antimicrobial activity.

Cinnamon. *Antimicrobial. Antiviral. Antifungal. Antiparasitic. Antioxidant. Anti-inflammatory. Congestion relief. Anti-nausea. Anti-diarrhea. Improves circulation. Blood sugar balancing.* Cinnamon is known to inhibit the growth of harmful microbes that can attack the mouth, and respiratory and digestive tracts, without impeding beneficial probiotic bacteria. It also slows the digestion and absorption of carbohydrates from the digestive tract and supports insulin's action in helping glucose get into cells, making it good for keeping blood sugar levels lower.

Citrus fruit. *Antimicrobial. Antibacterial. Antiviral. Antioxidant. Anti-inflammatory. Immune responsiveness. Vitamin C.* Citrus fruits like lemon, lime, and orange are most often appreciated for their vitamin C content. Less well known are their phytonutrient components with names like naringenin and hesperidin; these have additionally useful effects including blocking the activity of several pathogens and improving immune responsiveness. Many of the phytonutrients are concentrated in the peel, making it worth steeping citrus fruit slices (preferably organic, with the peel still attached) in hot teas and using the zest in cooking.

Cloves. *Antimicrobial. Antifungal. Anti-inflammatory. Congestion relief. Analgesic (pain relief). Improves circulation. Immune balancing. Immune responsiveness. Barrier stabilizing. Wound healing. Blood sugar balancing.* Clove has a long history of use for digestive and oral infections, as well as in wound care and as a natural insect repellant. It contains around 70 percent or more eugenol, a potent phytonutrient responsible for its antimicrobial, antioxidant, decongestant, and pain-relieving properties. The high concentration of this compound means that clove is best used sparingly since it can cause irritation when overused.

Coconut and coconut oil. *Antibacterial. Antifungal. Antioxidant. Anti-inflammatory. Anti-allergy. Immune responsiveness.* The medium-chain fatty acid lauric acid and its derivative monolaurin, found in coconut oil, act as natural antimicrobials, including against *Candida*. Virgin coconut oil may also improve immune cell (specifically macrophage) activity. You'll need to source an unrefined virgin coconut oil without additives, and that hasn't been altered by heat or chemical extraction methods, to harness its higher content of phytonutrients and vitamins A and E and sidestep the harmful components introduced via industrial processing. Use in balance with unsaturated and polyunsaturated fats such as olive and flaxseed oils.

Coriander (cilantro) leaves. *Antimicrobial. Antioxidant. Anti-inflammatory. Detoxifying. Healthy microbiota. Blood sugar balancing. UV protection.* Cilantro is an all-around powerhouse working on several aspects of our biology that impact immune function. One of the applications I use it for most is detoxification support, since cilantro is known to bind unwelcome toxins, including lead and mercury, in the digestive tract so that they can be safely eliminated rather than absorbed.

Coriander seed. *Antibacterial. Antiparasitic. Antifungal. Anti-inflammatory. Healthy microbiota. Digestive support. Blood sugar balancing.* Coriander seed has a long history of traditional use for many medicinal purposes. Coriander seed improves insufficient stomach acid secretion and aids digestive motility, helping to promote both the chemical and movement barriers that make up part of your first line of defense.

Cruciferous vegetables. *Antibacterial. Antiviral. Antioxidant. Anti-inflammatory. Detoxifying. Healthy microbiota. Anti-allergy. Blood sugar balancing.* All cruciferous vegetables contain sulforaphane, that powerful phytonutrient which, as you saw in chapter 6, can alter the very expression of your genes to dial down inflammation and reduce the effects of aging on your immune cells. The family of cruciferous vegetables includes arugula, bok choy, broccoli, Brussels sprouts, cabbage, cauliflower, kohlrabi, radish, rutabaga, turnip, and watercress.

Cumin seed. *Antibacterial. Antifungal. Anti-parasitic. Antioxidant. Anti-inflammatory. Blood sugar balancing.* Cumin seed has antimicrobial properties in part through its ability to inhibit the biofilm layer produced by certain pathogens that otherwise protects their growing colonies. It is also known to interfere with the synthesis of pro-inflammatory compounds in the body and so plays a role in keeping levels of inflammation in check.

Dark chocolate. *Antioxidant. Anti-inflammatory. Blood sugar balancing.* People are always happy to find out that dark chocolate is on the list of immune superfoods! And that's because true cocoa contains beneficial phytonutrients that improve blood sugar management and lower inflammation. The trick is finding chocolate that isn't also high in sugar and undesirable additives. For that, check out your local health food store or Thrive Market online, listed in the Resources section at the back of the book.

Fermented foods. *Anti-microbial. Antibacterial. Antiviral. Anti-inflammatory. Immune responsiveness. Digestive support. Barrier stabilizing. Healthy microbiota. Anti-allergy. Blood sugar balancing.* Fermented foods that still are "live" contain a rich abundance and diversity of beneficial microbes (see box on page 201)—more than any probiotic supplement—which as you know are essential allies to our immune defense system. The practice of having a small amount of fermented food with each meal is traditional in many cultures around the world and has been shown to reduce the incidence and duration of respiratory infections as well as providing other immune support. Examples of fermented foods are found on pages 183–184.

Fish and seafood. *Antioxidants. Anti-inflammatory. Immune balancing. Immune-supportive nutrients (omega-3 fatty acids, selenium, zinc). Barrier stabilizing.* When we think of nutrients in fish and seafood, we primarily think of those long chain immune-supporting omega-3 fats, EPA and DHA, which help keep inflammation balanced and enable many immune functions. One advantage that fish and seafood have over consuming these fats as supplements is that they also contain natural antioxidants that protect those delicate fats from oxidation, as well as immune-supportive nutrients.

Flaxseed and flaxseed oil. *Antioxidants. Anti-inflammatory. Immune balancing. Omega-3 fats. Healthy microbiota. Barrier stabilizing. Blood sugar balancing.* Flaxseeds are one of the best plant sources of

Examples of Probiotic Species Found in Fermented Foods

Several of these are species you might recognize from probiotic supplements. But, as you may also notice, fermented foods contain additional beneficial species that have yet to be formulated as supplements.

- Bifidobacteria (general)
- *Bifidobacterium bifidum*
- *Bifidobacterium lactis*
- *Lactobacillus acidophilus*
- *Lactobacillus argentinum*
- *Lactobacillus brevis*
- *Lactobacillus bulgaricus*
- *Lactobacillus coryniformis*
- *Lactobacillus curvatus*
- *Lactobacillus delbrueckii*
- *Lactobacillus fallax*
- *Lactobacillus mesenteroides*
- *Lactobacillus paraplantarum*
- *Lactobacillus pentosus*
- *Lactobacillus plantarum*
- *Lactobacillus rhamnosus*
- *Lactobacillus sakei*
- *Lactococcus species*
- *Leuconostoc citreum*
- *Leuconostoc gasicomitatum*
- *Pediococcus cerevisiae*
- *Saccharomyces species*
- *Streptococcus thermophilus*

the omega-3 fat, alpha-linolenic acid. In their whole or crushed seed form, flaxseeds also contain active phytonutrients called lignans and fiber that both support the growth of healthy gut microbes and have wider effects against inflammation and excess blood sugar.

Garlic. *Antimicrobial. Antibacterial. Antiviral. Antifungal. Antiparasitic. Antioxidant. Anti-inflammatory. Immune responsiveness.*

Detoxifying. Healthy microbiota. Improves circulation. Blood sugar balancing. Wound healing. Garlic has cysteine-containing organosulfur compounds that give it its odor, flavor, and biological activity. Consuming even just one to two cloves of garlic per day can both enhance immune responsiveness and detoxification and reduce excess levels of inflammation. Garlic has antimicrobial activity against a wide range of bacteria, viruses, fungi, and parasites, too. It also increases your body's production of glutathione. A tip for getting the most immune benefits from your garlic: Let chopped or crushed garlic sit a few minutes on the countertop before eating or using it in cooking to allow more of the active beneficial compounds to develop.

Ghee. *Anti-inflammatory. Immune balancing. Immune responsiveness. Barrier integrity. Sleep support. Anti-stress.* Ghee is a relevant immune superfood because it is a direct dietary source of butyrate, one of the most well-researched short-chain fatty acids produced by beneficial gut microbes. Butyrate is known to help maintain a healthy gut lining and to support immune balance, dialing down excessive inflammation and aberrant immune activity. Early studies even suggest it can enhance sleep quality and reduce stress, possibly through its effects on inflammation. Ghee is often sold in health food stores, and I have included a recipe for making your own from butter on page 354.

Ginger. *Antimicrobial. Antibacterial. Antiviral. Antifungal. Antiparasitic. Antioxidant. Anti-inflammatory. Immune balancing. Barrier stabilizing. Digestive support. Healthy microbiota. Pain relieving. Blood sugar balancing. Anti-autoimmune. Anti-asthma.* Ginger is a great immune all-rounder! It has several biologically active compounds including gingerols and shogaols that are responsible for its wide-ranging and impressive effects. Ginger has a long history of culinary and traditional medicine use and is easily incorporated into Indian and Thai dishes, sushi plates, and in hot teas. See more about ginger in the supplement section below.

Green tea. *Antimicrobial. Antibacterial. Antiviral. Antioxidant. Anti-inflammatory. Healthy microbiota. Barrier stabilizing. Blood sugar balancing.* Green tea should be high on your list of immune superfoods for its robust anti-inflammatory action and, through the theanine it contains, its ability to boost glutathione levels and regulate stress. Its overall anti-aging effects protect your immune system just as they protect other essential body systems. It even helps protect your skin barrier against the aging and immune-suppressing effects of UV light. Green tea has also been demonstrated to help counter the effects of a poor diet, revamp the gut microbiota, and improve barrier integrity throughout the body.

Holy basil (tulsi) tea. *Antimicrobial. Antibacterial. Antiviral. Antifungal. Antiparasitic. Antioxidant. Anti-inflammatory. Immune balancing. Immune responsiveness. Anti-anxiety. Sleep support. Detoxifying. Blood sugar balancing. Anti-allergy. Wound healing.* Holy basil, also known as tulsi, is in the same plant family as basil, but is a completely different species. It has a wide range of immune benefits including improved natural killer cell and T cell responses, and an enhanced ability to fight off viral infections. For this reason, it's often used against respiratory infections like colds and flu. Holy basil has also been demonstrated to be a potentially useful intervention to counteract modern lifestyle concerns and conditions including inflammation, insulin resistance and diabetes, stress and anxiety, sleep disturbances, and toxin exposure.

Honey. *Antimicrobial. Antioxidant. Anti-inflammatory. Anti-allergy. Barrier stabilizing. Wound healing.* Scientists have documented the broad-spectrum antimicrobial activity of several types of honeys against common pathogens and some drug-resistant species such as MRSA. The best known of these medicinal honeys is manuka, which appears to be especially effective against *Staphylococcus aureus* and MRSA. However, other traditional and minimally processed honeys, especially dark, raw honeys whose coloration indicates higher quantities of phytonutrients, have also demonstrated equivalent antimicrobial effects. *Caution: Honey should never be given to infants younger than one year old. Raw honey should be avoided during pregnancy and lactation. Use in moderation due to its sugar content and avoid if you have prediabetes or diabetes.*

Jerusalem artichoke (sunchoke). *Antioxidant. Anti-inflammatory. Immune balancing. Healthy microbiota.* Jerusalem artichokes are actually not a type of artichoke at all. Rather, they are the edible tuber of a type of sunflower plant. Jerusalem artichokes are especially high in a type of prebiotic fiber called inulin, which when eaten is very nourishing to healthy gut bacteria and helps to reduce bad gut bacteria.

Kiwifruit. *Antioxidant. Anti-inflammatory. Healthy microbiota. Blood sugar balancing. Vitamin C.* One kiwifruit has between two and three times the vitamin C content of an orange! Human research has shown that kiwifruit consumption may improve congestion and sore throat symptoms related to respiratory infections and reduce gum inflammation related to gingivitis. Kiwifruits also improve the number of beneficial microbes in the digestive tract.

Mint. *Antibacterial. Antiviral. Antifungal. Antiparasitic. Antioxidant. Anti-inflammatory. Digestive support. Congestion relief. Pain relieving.* Mint leaves contain menthol, eucalyptol, rosmarinic acid, and many other phytonutrient compounds that provide effective antimicrobial and sinus-clearing action. Peppermint has the highest menthol content but can be too strong for some. Spearmint is an alternative, milder mint.

Mushrooms. *Immune balancing. Immune responsiveness. Healthy microbiota.* There are so many different types of edible mushrooms that are increasingly available to buy at grocery and health food stores. Many are well known for their medicinal effects (see also the listings for shiitake mushroom, oyster mushroom, and white button mushroom). Among other things, mushrooms are an excellent source of glucans, which act on several different parts of the immune system, including the innate and adaptive branches, as well as on the gut microbiota.

Oats. *Anti-inflammatory. Immune responsiveness. Barrier stabilizing. Healthy microbiota. Detoxifying. Blood sugar balancing.* Oats contain beta-glucans, which have direct immune tuning activities (including increasing helpful immune cell activity and levels of secretory IgA antibodies), improve the integrity of the gut lining, and provide a source of nourishment for beneficial gut microbes. The fiber in whole-grain oats also helps to regulate blood sugar and improve natural movement in the digestive tract. Look for whole-grain oats to be sure to get the full complement of beta-glucans, other fibers, and phytonutrients.

Olives and olive oil. *Antimicrobial. Antioxidant. Anti-inflammatory. Immune balancing. Immune responsiveness. Vitamin C. Vitamin E. Blood sugar balancing.* The monounsaturated fatty acids that predominate in olives and olive oil are important for maintaining a balanced intake of different healthy fats. Olives and their unfiltered oils are also rich sources of phytonutrients that have additional benefits, including increasing the levels and diversity of beneficial gut microbes and enhancing secretory IgA activity. Olive oil is also a good source of vitamin E and is demonstrated to improve vitamin C and E levels through its own antioxidant activity that spares these important immune nutrients.

Oregano. *Antibacterial. Antiviral. Antifungal. Antiparasitic. Antioxidant. Anti-inflammatory. Blood sugar balancing. Wound healing.* In clinical practice I use oregano oil to help individuals with problematic dysbiosis and infections. However, the oral oil preparations, while effective, are strong and can sometimes irritate the digestive tract; so for general use, I prefer to stick to the culinary herb and use the essential oil only in steam inhalation (see page 303 for more information).

Oysters. *Antioxidant. Anti-inflammatory. Immune balancing. Immune responsiveness. Digestive support. Zinc. Iron. Vitamin D. Omega-3s.* Oysters are an astoundingly rich source of immune-supportive zinc. So much so, that you need only eat two oysters to get your full daily requirement for this mineral! They are also a good source of vitamin D (one of the few foods that contain it), iron, and selenium. It's for this reason that I like to sneak a couple into my breakfast omelet, as you'll see in the recipe on page 320.

Oyster mushroom. *Immune balancing. Immune responsiveness. Healthy microbiota. Anti-allergy. Blood sugar balancing.* In a study of children with recurrent respiratory infections, glucans derived from oyster mushrooms reduced the frequency of respiratory illnesses including lung infections. In a separate study of athletes, those same glucans were able to protect against post-exercise-induced dips in immune function. The blood sugar–regulating effects of oyster mushrooms have also been demonstrated in individuals with type 2 diabetes.

Parsley. *Antimicrobial. Antibacterial. Antiviral. Antifungal. Antioxidant. Anti-inflammatory. Digestive support. Detoxifying. Anti-allergy. Anti-autoimmune.* Parsley is rich in a phytonutrient called apigenin, which, along with other parsley constituents, has noteworthy activity against pathogenic microbes and supports our immune systems. Common harmful bugs, including *Staphylococcus aureus*, *Escherichia coli*, *Pseudomonas aeruginosa*, herpes simplex, and *Candida*, are susceptible to its effects, as is *Streptococcus mutans*, a problematic bacterium that hangs out in the mouth and is responsible for the development of dental caries. Parsley has also been shown to calm the activity of immune cells that become unruly in allergic and autoimmune disease.

Raspberries. *Antibacterial. Antioxidant. Anti-inflammatory. Detoxifying. Barrier stabilizing. Lowers blood sugar.* Like their other berry cousins, raspberries contain concentrated amounts of phytonutrients including anthocyanidins, quercetin, and catechins. You'll also find vitamin C, beta-carotene (a vitamin A precursor), and the antioxidant glutathione in these tiny bursts of juiciness. When tested against common food-borne pathogens like *Salmonella* and *E. coli,* raspberries have antimicrobial effects thought to be due to their ability to disintegrate the bacteria's outer membranes. Although we are most familiar with red raspberries, black raspberries are also available and I am excited about the research emerging on this particular kind that suggests they can increase natural killer cell activity and inhibit cancer cell growth. Grab them if you find them!

Red onion. *Antimicrobial. Antiviral. Antioxidant. Anti-inflammatory. Healthy microbiota. Detoxifying. Anti-allergy. Blood sugar balancing.* Onions of all kinds have immune benefits; however, I particularly recommend red onions, and as a close second shallots, for their higher concentration of the phytonutrient quercetin. Quercetin offers antimicrobial, anti-inflammatory, gut-healing, and anti-allergy benefits (more on quercetin in the supplement section below). Onions are also rich in prebiotic inulin fibers which nourish healthy bacteria.

Rosemary. *Antimicrobial. Antioxidant. Anti-inflammatory. Immune balancing. Congestion relief. Pain relieving. Anti-anxiety. Anti-allergy. Anti-asthma. Blood sugar balancing.* Rosemary is one of my favorite herbs for cooking and as an essential oil for congestion symptoms, stress relief, and memory support. I also use cold rosemary "tea" as a facial toner to support skin barrier integrity and microbial balance. Rosemary is rich in rosmarinic acid and luteolin, two phytonutrients that have been demonstrated to favorably alter genetic expression with the potential to turn back our biological aging clock and rejuvenate our immune system.

Sea vegetables. *Antiviral. Antioxidant. Anti-inflammatory. Healthy microbiota. Detoxification. Omega-3s. Blood sugar balancing.* Sea vegetables like brown algae, kelp, dulse, and nori can be great additions to your Immune Resilience Diet, in moderation. They contain concentrated phytonutrients and trace minerals and have been shown to inhibit many kinds of viruses. They are excellent at absorbing heavy metals, which can aid in preventing unwanted absorption and facilitating their elimination. However, their toxin-absorbing ability also means that they can absorb heavy metals from the environment in which they are grown, making it extra important to choose ones from clean sources that have been tested and verified as contaminant-free. Sea vegetables are also very high in iodine, an essential nutrient but which in excess can sometimes disrupt thyroid function. So, while there are many benefits to sea vegetables, I recommend consuming them only in small amounts and not every day.

Shiitake mushroom. *Anti-inflammatory. Immune balancing. Immune responsiveness.* Shiitake mushroom is known to improve markers of immunity. In human studies, it has been shown to increase T cell and B cell responsiveness, natural killer cell activity, interferon gamma production, and secretory IgA production, all while decreasing excess inflammatory signals.

Soy. *Antioxidant. Anti-inflammatory. Immune responsiveness. Healthy microbiota.* Good-quality soy has anti-inflammatory effects likely derived from its phytonutrient isoflavones, genistein and daidzein, and its prebiotic fibers. Poor-quality soy, on the other hand, has been shown to have potential pro-inflammatory outcomes. The concern about soy being a phytoestrogen and promoting harmfully high estrogenic activity in the body is sometimes raised; however, this oversimplification is incorrect. Soy's weak estrogenic activity means that when it attaches to our cells' estrogen receptors it exerts only a mild stimulation. This means it can both help correct an internal estrogen deficiency *and* block the attachment and activity of stronger estrogen compounds (like estradiol and estrogen-mimicking EDCs) that can be problematic in excess. In postmenopausal women, whose estrogen levels are lower than those in premenopausal women, consuming good-quality soy phytonutrients has been shown to improve B cell populations and therefore influence immune responsiveness. For tips on choosing good-quality soy see page 189.

Thyme. *Antibacterial. Antiviral. Antifungal. Antiparasitic. Antioxidant. Anti-inflammatory. Anti-stress. Congestion relief. Wound healing.* One of the main phytonutrients in thyme is thymol, known for its antimicrobial effects. Thyme has a history of traditional use against the flu and other respiratory viruses (where it also helps reduce congestion), as well as against *Candida* species.

Turmeric. *Antimicrobial. Antibacterial. Antiviral. Antifungal. Antiparasitic. Antioxidant. Anti-inflammatory. Immune responsiveness. Healthy microbiota. Anti-allergy. Blood sugar balancing. Wound healing.* Turmeric is a great all-around immune superfood known for being antimicrobial against pathogens but also for supporting beneficial bacterial strains such as bifidobacteria and lactobacilli, and for reducing inflammation. Curcumin, a constituent of turmeric, is understood to be the main reason for these effects, although science is still exploring the other compounds turmeric contains. (See the section on curcumin supplements on pages 245–46.)

Walnuts and walnut oil. *Antioxidant. Anti-inflammatory. Immune responsiveness. Barrier integrity. Healthy microbiota. Sleep support. Omega-3s. Vitamin E.* Walnuts are the nuts with the highest alpha linolenic acid (ALA) content, an essential type of anti-inflammatory and protective omega-3 fat and one which your body can use to produce other omega-3 fats like EPA and DHA. They are also a good source of fiber, vitamin E, magnesium, L-arginine, and phytonutrients, all of which, as we saw in part 2, are important immune-related nutrients. Walnuts even contain reasonable amounts of melatonin, our immune- and sleep-supportive hormone.

White button mushroom. *Anti-inflammatory. Immune responsiveness. Healthy microbiota. Blood sugar balancing.* The humble white button mushroom, while not perhaps as impressive in its range and potency of immune effects as its "medicinal" cousins, is still worth your attention. Especially since it's so accessible and affordable. It has been shown in human studies to increase levels of secretory IgA, that important broad-spectrum chemical defense at each of your body's barriers. It also helps to tone down inflammatory lipopolysaccharide signaling, potentially decreasing overall levels of inflammation.

Winter squash. *Antioxidant. Anti-inflammatory. Healthy microbiota. Vitamin A. Vitamin C. Blood sugar balancing.* A bountiful source of alpha- and beta-carotene, which convert to vitamin A and vitamin C, as well as fiber. Available just as the fall cold and flu season kicks in, winter squashes such as butternut, acorn, delicata, and spaghetti squashes, as well as pumpkins, are great immune support foods.

To view the references cited in this chapter, please visit
www.immuneresilienceplan.com/science.

CHAPTER 11

Food Principles to Live By

Navigating Day-to-Day Food Choices

N ow that you know what types of foods to eat, we will dive into the ancillary (yet impactful) principles to incorporate as you zero in on the immune-supportive foods in the preceding chapters. These include buying and food preparation practices that I recommend, which make a surprising difference in how well this way of eating will work for your immune system (as well as for your budget). I'll also cover some of the important kinds of foods to *avoid* and explain why (and how) you might want to consider fasting to strengthen your immune system. Last but not least, we'll take a reality check when it comes to what to expect when changing your diet, and how and when it's okay to bend the rules to accommodate, well . . . life.

PRINCIPLE 1: CHOOSE THE BEST QUALITY FOODS YOU CAN

I define high-quality foods as foods that maximize what you want and minimize what you don't want. And I'm not comparing quality *between* different foods here; I'm talking about the *same food* that can come from different sources and travel through different handling processes before it arrives on your plate. Here are some examples that demonstrate why quality matters:

- Produce that is grown locally doesn't have to be picked before it fully ripens, and doesn't have to travel or spend long periods in storage before it gets to you. This helps maximize its nutrient value—of both vitamins and minerals and phytonutrients.

- Grass-fed or pastured animal foods have higher levels of anti-inflammatory polyunsaturated fats and lower levels of the more pro-inflammatory saturated fats than conventional animal foods. For example, omega-3 fats in organically reared animals can be nearly 50 percent higher than in those that are conventionally reared. It's thought that the high grazing and foraging-based diets of organic standards are the main reason for this difference.

- The level of phytonutrients you'll find in olive oil is closely related to its preparation and processing. Extra-virgin olive oils have substantially more than refined olive oils, especially when unfiltered. Similarly, less refined oils from nuts and seeds, which are carefully processed (i.e., with low heat and chemical free) to retain the integrity of any fragile polyunsaturated fats and phytonutrients, have beneficial effects in your body and on your immune system. Chemically extracted, heat-treated, and ultra-refined oils, on the other hand, can be damaging.

- Canola oil that is industrially produced undergoes chemical extraction where it is dissolved in hexane, filtered, and deodorized using heat. During this process, vitamin E and phytonutrients are largely removed. The fragile polyunsaturated fats can oxidize and harmful trans fats can be formed. And pesticide and hexane solvent residues can remain in the final product. Cold-pressed organic canola oil, by contrast, omits chemical contamination and preserves the integrity of its valuable oil components.

- Dairy products from conventional cows in the US often contain harmful contaminants used during the farming process. This includes antibiotics, used to control the tendency for disease to spread in cramped feed-lot conditions, and growth hormones, used to increase milk production. A recent study conducted by Emory University found residues of both of these in conventional milk, as well as controversial restricted-use pesticides. By comparison, none of the organic milk samples they tested contained any of these contaminants.

QUALITY LABELS TO LOOK FOR

Here are my top terms to look for when buying foods. Any one of these on their own isn't an automatic guarantee of optimal quality, but they do go a long way to giving you the most of what you want—nutrient and phytonutrient density—and minimizing what you don't—processed and pro-inflammatory compounds.

USDA Organic: People who consume a primarily organic diet have lower detectable levels of chemicals in their body, making it worth aiming for. The USDA Organic designation indicates that the farm and producer meet specific standards, including using only organic feed for animals and never giving animals hormones or antibiotics. Genetically engineered foods are not allowed in organic food production, either as seeds or in animal feed. Organic plant food farms must grow only in soil that has been free of chemical fertilizers, herbicides, pesticides, and a long list of other items for at least three years prior to harvest. One important thing to know is that becoming *certified* organic is an expensive undertaking, beyond the reach of many small farms who otherwise follow equivalent best practices but can't afford to go through the certification process. Getting to know your local producers can be a way to find and support local farmers who can offer produce that's just as good as its certified alternatives.

Made with Organic [Ingredient]: When a product states it is made with an organic ingredient, this means that at least 70 percent of *that ingredient* must be organic. While these products don't qualify for the full USDA Organic seal, they can still be a useful way to increase your organic food range.

Non-GMO Project Verified: Non-GMO Project offers an independent verification program that helps consumers choose products that do not contain GMOs (genetically modified organisms). *Non-GMO Project Verified* means *either* that a product was produced without ingredients that have been genetically engineered and therefore contains only ingredients that are natural to our environment or have been achieved through traditional cross-breeding methods, *or* that a product contains minimal GMO ingredients (less than 0.9 percent). Although there isn't definitive proof that genetically modified foods are not safe, the reality is that we don't have independent long-term human data to indicate that they are. GMO foods can have higher levels of chemical contamination from herbicides. Many consumers, myself included, choose to opt out of GMO foods whenever we can.

Local: While there is no oversight of a distance that defines "local" when it comes to food production, choosing produce that is grown closer to home can often mean you're getting a better nutritional (and flavor) profile than if you're choosing a food that has had to be picked before ripening and transported in airplanes to get to you. My favorite way to shop "local" is at farmers' markets, where you get the added benefit of being able to talk to the growers themselves about their farming practices and ethics.

American Grassfed: This designation is overseen by the nonprofit American Grassfed Association and is given to farms where cattle are fed only grass and are raised on pastures. Farmers must avoid antibiotics, growth-promoting hormones, and GMOs, and minimize the use of pesticides. Diet and rearing environment make a big difference to the nutritional composition of meats, as I mentioned above: pasture-based diets and the ability to roam outside mean that animals are leaner overall, and have a higher proportion of anti-inflammatory fats.

Raised Without Antibiotics: Antibiotics are routinely used in conventional livestock and fish farming to control the spread of disease. Some producers, however, opt not to use antibiotics and can label their products as such even if they don't qualify for the full "organic" designation. Choosing animal products that have been reared without antibiotics (or that are labeled organic) is one important way for consumers to help minimize the risks of antibiotic contamination and resistance.

Wild Caught: A term that generally applies to some fish or seafood, *wild caught* indicates the product was caught in a lake, ocean, or other natural body of water. In general, wild caught varieties have a better nutritional profile with more omega-3 fatty acids and less saturated fats and can often contain fewer man-made contaminants since they eat a natural diet. The deeper color of wild salmon is due to higher amounts of an antioxidant called astaxanthin that wild varieties contain. Farmed fish have in the past been more likely to be contaminated with PCBs from their feed and to have been given antibiotics to fend off the disease promoted by crowded conditions. These days, however, it's possible to find better farmed fish options such as those that are certified by the Aquaculture Stewardship Council (ASC certified), which works to control the use of antibiotics and chemicals, and ensure sustainability.

Extra-virgin: The USDA regulates the use of the term *extra-virgin* for olive oil, ensuring that all olive oils carrying this label have been extracted without heat or chemical solvents. There is no regulation of the term *extra-virgin* for other oils, although you can look for labels such as "expeller-pressed" or "cold-pressed" to indicate processing methods that don't use chemical solvents.

PRINCIPLE 2: KEEP IT COST-EFFECTIVE WITH SAVVY SHOPPING AND MORE

I know what you're thinking: *All this high-quality food can get supremely expensive.* And you're not wrong that these foods cost more. Here are a couple of ways I, personally, tackle that and which I share with those who come to me for advice:

Head to the freezer aisle: The only exception to my "buy local" recommendation above is for foods that are picked ripe and then quickly frozen. The quick-freezing process protects the cellular and molecular integrity of the food, so that it doesn't get broken down too quickly. Flash-frozen foods usually retain high levels of many nutrients even if they then travel some distance before arriving in your local store's freezer department, often topping the nutrient levels in fresh produce (that has traveled), or canned fruits and vegetables, at a much lower cost.

Know which conventional fruits and vegetables you can still buy without the pesticide risk: One easy rule of thumb is to prioritize eating organic versions of produce where you consume the skin or outer part of the food too (like berries or lettuce) and relax the rules for produce that sits within a removable skin (like bananas or avocado). Washing conventional produce with a scrubbing action has also been shown to remove a significant amount of pesticide residue. Another good point of reference is the Environmental Working Group's (EWG) Dirty Dozen and Clean Fifteen rankings of conventional produce, published each year based on data released by the USDA. Those that make the Dirty Dozen list are ones that carry the highest pesticide residues and are therefore the ones that you'll want to always try to buy organic (strawberries, spinach, and apples, for instance, frequently make this list). Those that are on the Clean Fifteen list (like avocado, onions, and pineapple), however, are ones that you could buy conventional with minimal concern for pesticide residues. You can find the most recently published lists at ewg.org.

Find your local farmers: Most grass-fed meats and organic produce in the US are still produced by small-scale farming operations. You can often find better pricing by going directly to the farm or shopping at farmers' markets. Some farms will sell frozen butchered meats and poultry in bulk. One of the best things I ever did was to acquire a separate, modest freezer to accommodate my direct-from-the-farm meat purchases.

Remember, you're reworking your ratios of animal food intake: There's a good chance that by adopting the Immune Resilience Diet, you'll be reducing your meat intake, often the most expensive ticket item on your shopping list. The savings you'll achieve by shifting away from higher meat intake levels should go some way (if not all the way) to covering the higher cost of the meat you do still eat. Many plant foods are much less expensive: whole-grain rice, whole-grain millet, lentils, chickpeas, sweet potatoes, carrots, celery, onions, broccoli, apples, and cantaloupe melon are some of my favorite budget buys that are very pocketbook friendly.

Grow your own: I don't know how much of a green thumb you have, but mine is always rather less green than I'd like it to be. Still, I usually manage to grow plenty of herbs, which are so valuable for your immune health, tomatoes, peppers, and cucumbers. Of everything I've ever grown, I'd say that the herbs are by far the best economically (herbs in the store can get expensive!) and the easiest for anyone to get started with. All you need is a sunny indoor spot, somewhere you'll remember to water them, and a little organic fertilizer.

Make your own: Switching from prepared foods to home-cooked foods can also reduce cost. I appreciate that this doesn't work for everything, since the food industry has been able to make many unhealthy, processed foods so undeniably cheap. However, it does help reduce the cost of higher-quality foods. Preparing a large batch of sauerkraut at home, for instance, is much less expensive than buying a premium, live version in a health food store (and you can find an easy recipe on page 335). Besides, now you have a ton more reasons to be discerning in your food choices, given how much they can affect your immune system. And remember I said that a distressed immune system is connected to nearly every chronic disease out there via its capacity for aberrant inflammation?

Recognize that you're underwriting your future quality of life: Making an investment in your health has never had such a large payoff—for its effects on immune resilience and for reducing the risk of all kinds of chronic diseases. And as one of my long-time clients, Emily, explained: "When it finally dawned on me that eating this way was an investment in my future health—better productivity, less time off work, more time spent on fun activities, and fewer medical bills—I couldn't imagine eating any other way. I had been spending more time and effort keeping my plants well cared for than I had ever considered spending on my own health. Not anymore . . . this way of eating has become second nature and protecting my immune health makes me feel great to boot!"

PRINCIPLE 3: PREPARE FOOD WITH IMMUNE HEALTH IN MIND

Cooked vs. raw: Unless you have a heavily compromised immune or digestive system, it's a good idea to include some raw foods in your diet, especially easily digestible ones like fruits, sprouts, herbs, and salad items. These raw foods provide good amounts of insoluble fiber, phytonutrients, and vitamins. However, we should eat raw foods in balance with cooked foods, which are easier for your body to digest and harness nutrients from. After all, cooking starts the process of breaking up plant cell walls, making the nutrients inside more accessible. Several phytonutrients are actually more available for your body to absorb *after* cooking. This is the case for lycopene in tomatoes and carotenoids in carrots, bell peppers, and spinach. Cooking also tends to increase the soluble fiber content of foods, the kind that feeds your microbiota. In general, a balance of about 60 percent to 70 percent cooked, 30 percent to 40 percent raw works well for most people. More raw food than that can be taxing on your digestive system and make it harder to extract all the nutrition you need from foods.

Gently does it: When it comes to preserving the nutritional content in food, "gently does it" are the words to live by. Vegetables retain more nutrition when they are lightly cooked in moist heat, like steam. Generally, you'll want to look for the peak in color—when that broccoli turns its brightest shade of green and well before it goes gray-looking. Cooking vegetables in water that is then discarded also leads to significant nutrient losses. You can avoid this by steaming or by consuming the cooking liquid too (such as in a soup or casserole). Avoid very high temperature cooking like grilling, searing, or broiling whenever possible, since browning foods, especially meats and bakery items, leads to the formation of those harmful AGEs, which damage your cells, promote inflammation, and can increase the risk for several cancers. If you do occasionally use a high-temperature method, soak the meat in an acidic marinade such as lemon juice or vinegar, and add a strong antioxidant herb like mint, green tea, sage, or rosemary, all of which have been shown to help reduce AGE formation.

PRINCIPLE 4: KNOW WHAT TO LIMIT OR AVOID

Sugars and other simple carbs: Simple carbohydrates to avoid as much as possible include refined grains like white flour, pizza dough, pasta, pastries, sweet desserts, white rice, starchy potatoes, and added sugar. Sugar can be especially sneaky, as it is added into all kinds of foods that you may not expect, including salad dressing, savory dishes, snacks, and drinks. In fact, added sugar is estimated to be present in three out of every four packaged foods you might pick off the shelf. Once you start looking, you'll see sugar everywhere! The number one, hands down, most effective way to avoid added sugar is to choose whole foods that don't come in packets and that don't even need ingredient labels. What you see is what you get from these foods. I'm talking plain vegetables, fruits, beans, lentils, nuts, seeds, eggs, meats, and fish. For packaged foods, you'll have to read labels to look for the grams of sugars in the Nutrition Facts box and for sugar in the ingredient list. It's not always that easy, though, since sugar goes by a slew of different names, making it much easier to hide. Check out my handy list on page 220 for the different ingredient names for sugars to avoid or limit.

Here are some must-know facts and tips about sugar to keep you where you need to be:

- 4 grams of sugar is equivalent to 1 teaspoon. So if a label states that the food contains 24 grams of sugars per serving, that's equivalent to 6 teaspoons! Aim to limit added sugars to 5 grams or less per serving.
- Skip a food altogether if there are more than 10 grams of added sugars per serving.
- Ideally, don't exceed 12 grams of added sugars over the course of the day. For children it should be half that amount.
- Occasional indulgences are okay, such as for birthday celebrations. But this should be a once- or twice-a-month treat at most.
- If you have blood sugar regulation issues, you will want to be even more careful with your intake of refined carbs. You'll find those adjustments in chapter 14 in the section for prediabetes and diabetes.

The Many Names for Sugar

All these names refer to different types of sugar. Finding any of these ingredients on food labels should make you suspicious of that food's sugar content:

agave syrup/nectar	galactose
barley malt	glucose
beet sugar	golden syrup
blackstrap molasses	high fructose corn syrup
brown rice syrup	honey*
brown sugar	invert sugar
caramel	lactose
cane sugar	maltodextrin
carob syrup	maltol
castor sugar	maltose
coconut sugar	malt syrup
confectioner's (powdered) sugar	mannose
corn syrup	maple syrup
corn sweetener	muscovado sugar
crystalline fructose	rice syrup
date sugar	saccharose
dehydrated cane juice	sorghum syrup
dextrin	sucrose sugar
dextrose	Sucanat
ethyl maltol	syrup
evaporated cane juice	treacle
fructose	turbinado sugar
fruit juice	yellow sugar

*Note that, while a good-quality raw honey can have beneficial immune properties (see page 203), it can still add to the total simple carbohydrate content of your diet and should only be consumed in careful moderation.

Ultra-processed foods: The best way to identify ultra-processed foods is to check whether the ingredient label contains any of the ingredients that characterize these foods. Often these will be hard-to-pronounce ingredients that are nothing you'd recognize from home cooking, like potassium bromate, propyl paraben, and butylated hydroxytoluene (BHT). Common types of ultra-processed foods include mass-produced convenience foods such as breakfast cereals, cereal bars, pre-prepared meals, packaged snacks, baked goods, sweetened yogurts, ice creams, sodas and sports drinks, as well as fast-food meals and a large number of other restaurant foods. You'll have most success at avoiding ultra-processed foods by sourcing from small-batch, farm-to-table producers and restaurants, and, of course, from buying whole-food ingredients to cook at home yourself.

Industrialized vegetable oils: These are the cheap, highly refined, and usually chemically extracted oils that are most often used in ultra-processed foods. Corn, cottonseed, peanut, safflower, and soybean oils are commonly produced this way. The trouble with these oils is first that they are high in the more pro-inflammatory omega-6 fats that we are all consuming too much of in relation to anti-inflammatory omega-3 fats. In addition, the delicate polyunsaturated omega-6 fats that these oils are rich in aren't intended to be used at high cooking temperatures, because that dramatically increases their rate of harmful oxidation. In processed foods, vegetable oils are often used in deep frying and other high-temperature cooking methods that make them even more inflammatory.

Artificial sweeteners: You're most likely to inadvertently consume artificial sweeteners in sweet-tasting processed foods, especially those that are labeled as "diet" foods. Artificial sweeteners to avoid are as follows: sucralose (Splenda), saccharin (Sweet'N Low), aspartame (NutraSweet or Equal), acesulfame K (Sunett and Sweet One), and neotame (Newtame). Instead of listing them by name, labels may identify them as non-nutritive sweeteners, noncaloric sweeteners, or sugar substitutes.

Coffee and black tea: The evidence for regular coffee and black tea consumption is mixed. On one hand, coffee and black tea have concentrated amounts of phytonutrients that have been shown to be beneficial in many ways (including by lowering inflammation). However, high levels of caffeine consumption are associated with higher levels of cortisol release in response to stress, meaning that excess caffeine can worsen a chronic stress situation and may eventually lead to immune suppression. Here's

What Is Glycemic Value and Why Is It Useful to Know?

For optimal immune health, we want to focus on foods that are lower in their glycemic value. Glycemic value is a measure of how fast a particular carbohydrate source raises blood sugar levels. Typically, this is expressed as the glycemic index or glycemic load of a food. The glycemic *index* compares foods measured by an equal amount of carbohydrate content. The glycemic *load* also considers how much carbohydrate there actually is in each typical serving and can therefore be a better predictor of a food's actual effect in your body. This adjustment for carbohydrate content is why a food such as carrots can have a high glycemic index, but—because there is actually relatively little carbohydrate content per serving (carrots are high in fiber and water)—a low glycemic load. Because it is able to account for serving size in this way, I prefer using glycemic load values over the glycemic index.

Several factors influence your glycemic response to a food: more refinement and processing, a greater surface area, longer cooking times, and low fiber content all increase glycemic responses. A healthy microbiome will also temper your glycemic response to a food. Combining carbohydrates with some fat or protein helps to slow its digestion and reduce spikes in blood glucose.

Tip: How to eat potatoes in a low glycemic way. Some starchy vegetables like potatoes contain high amounts of very accessible carbohydrate that the body sees similarly to sugar and can give us a higher glycemic spike than we want. For potatoes, this might be mashed potatoes, French fries, or potato chips. However, if unprocessed, whole-food potatoes are prepared by first cooking and then allowing them to cool to a refrigerated temperature before eating, they will convert that high glycemic starch into resistant starch. Now you have a food that the body responds to completely differently. The resistant starch can be an excellent source of nourishment for your microbiota and is digested and absorbed much more slowly, generating a lesser glucose response.

where I stand—if you tolerate one to three cups of coffee or black tea per day without it impacting your sleep or anxiety levels, then that's likely fine, even potentially beneficial. If you don't currently drink coffee or black tea, there's no need to start, though. You can get plenty of phytonutrients from other caffeine-free teas and food sources.

Tip: If you're drinking more than three cups of caffeinated tea or coffee per day, or if you notice side effects, it's time to cut back. I recommend doing so slowly, since caffeine withdrawals can trigger headaches and malaise. Switching to lower-caffeine options such as green tea or oolong tea can help and are even very beneficial. Look for alternative ways to energize yourself naturally such as taking five minutes to walk outside, stretching, or drinking a tall glass of water.

Alcohol: There's no doubt that excess alcohol is harmful for many reasons, one of them being its adverse impact on defense systems. Too much alcohol, especially when it becomes a regular habit, can reduce stomach acid (recall that this is an important first line of defense against germs you unknowingly swallow), damage your gut barrier and increase permeability, reduce important clearance movements in the digestive tract and the beating of cilia in the lungs, cause dysbiosis, reduce white blood cell numbers, increase inflammation, promote immune-related nutrient deficiencies, and increase wound recovery time. Yikes! Heavy alcohol consumption (eight drinks or more per week for women and fifteen drinks or more per week for men) is associated with increased risk for serious infectious disease and cancers, as well as the more well-known liver and pancreatic diseases.

The latest US data show that more than 40 percent of us consume more than the recommended guidelines for alcohol intake. Alcohol consumption has been rising notably in certain pockets of our population, such as in women. To reduce the risks related to alcohol consumption, limit your alcoholic drinks to one per day for women and two per day for men. One drink equates to 12 ounces of beer, 5 ounces of wine, or 1.5 ounces of distilled spirits or liquor.

Wheat: Wheat may be a surprising addition to this list as a food to limit, especially since it's included in the whole-grains section in the previous chapter. But there's a good reason why. As a society, we have developed an overdependence on wheat. Pastries for breakfast, sandwiches for lunch,

Food and Skin Issues

Remember Julia? She had eczema issues and recurrent, drug-resistant skin infections on her legs and arms. As you might suspect, diet was a major focus of our work together and the Immune Resilience Diet was our foundation. Onto that we layered a two-week sugar "detox" (no added sugars at all and a temporary hold on higher-carbohydrate foods such as grains, legumes, and most fruits, to break the cravings cycle). In this case, I suspected that some foods may have been irritating Julia's skin barrier, potentially worsening her problems, so we also added an elimination diet, which can be a helpful tool to identify whether there are any problem foods your body can't tolerate well. It's something best done with a qualified practitioner, although the widely available book *The Elimination Diet,* coauthored by the excellent Tom Malterre, is a useful primer.

It wasn't a walk in the park, as Julia will attest to—these dietary shifts really did their work on resetting her microbiome, and as those unwanted microbes died off, the compounds they released made Julia feel pretty lousy and her cravings intensified for a while. She held strong, though, and kept symptoms manageable through some gentle detox strategies: supplementary probiotics and activated charcoal, light exercise, and sauna. Two weeks later she reported her cravings were miraculously gone. She was feeling lighter, more energized, and incredibly motivated. Her skin was improving already; there was less redness and intensity of irritation.

Time for the next layer: we added some supplemental support with a multivitamin and mineral, fish oil, some extra vitamin D (her labs indicated a deficiency), vitamin C, and a probiotic (oral probiotics have been shown to improve measures of skin integrity). I recommended Julia try alternating between two types of baths each day: one with 8 drops of tea tree oil added, and one with raw honey and oatmeal (see the recipe on page 359). I also gave her a combination herbal product to try out topically on infected areas.

Two months later, things were going well. The patches of affected skin had shrunk dramatically. From the elimination diet we identified eggs and soy as foods that increased skin cracking and itchiness. Removing those foods had made a big difference, and so she continued to exclude them. We relaxed the restrictions on carbohydrate foods such that she could incorporate moderate amounts of whole grains, legumes, and fruits. To help her body manage that carbohydrate load, she agreed to implement a gentle form of fasting, restricting her daily eating window to between 8:00 a.m. and 6:00 p.m. Julia also decided to get a carbon water filtration system for her drinking water and begin a home evaluation for lead (she found lead-based paint and lead in some of her glazed ceramic dishes). We reviewed other sources of environmental exposures, and Julia started the process of shifting over to more immune-friendly versions of her personal care and home cleaning products.

After five months Julia's skin was more than 80 percent improved. She was ecstatic! And so were her doctors. And when I reached out to Julia to write up her case for this book eighteen months later, she reported that she was symptom free "most of the time." And, equally important, "I know what to do when I do get a flare."

"I couldn't be happier," she shared. "You have restored my confidence in my ability to manage my own health and resilience, even in the face of a seemingly impossible infection."

pasta for dinner, crackers in between—wheat sneaks in everywhere. And wheat contains a particularly immune-provoking protein called gluten. When we combine this with the overstressed immune systems that many of us have (with high levels of inflammation, a leaky gut barrier, and a dysfunctional microbiota), we have the perfect storm for our immune system to start reacting to that gluten.

The groundbreaking work of Dr. Alessio Fasano, chief of pediatric gastroenterology and nutrition at MassGeneral Hospital for Children, expert on celiac disease and other gluten-related disorders, has demonstrated that in increasing numbers of people, gluten can be a powerful trigger of gut barrier permeability and a spectrum of immune reactions, from celiac disease to wheat allergy and gluten sensitivity. And that these gluten-related immune reactions can underlie immune disorders, including autoimmunity and inflammatory diseases, especially in individuals who might be genetically predisposed.

The bottom line is, a revved-up, irritated (inflamed) immune system tends to look for something to attack. And it's most likely to attack something it sees a lot of. Far better for your immune system is to keep wheat consumption in balance with other types of grains and with other kinds of foods in general. If you don't have any current health issues, this is the best strategy. If you do have a current health issue, such as autoimmune thyroid disease, I often recommend a trial period where gluten is avoided entirely (see pages 286–287).

PRINCIPLE 5: CONSIDER A FORM OF INTERMITTENT FASTING

At this point, you should have a good idea of what to eat for immune health. But did you know that *not eating* can also impact your immune system? In a good way. I'm talking, here, about fasting.

Forms of fasting have been part of the human experience for millennia. Sometimes by choice, as in religious practices, and sometimes unavoidably during periods of famine or war. It's only really within the last seventy years that food availability has been as secure as it is now. Three regular meals per day plus snacks and calorie-rich beverages were just not possible for our (recent and distant) ancestors. And probably because of the sheer ubiquity of food, we tend to overeat rather than undereat. The concept of fasting—what, no food for *how* long?—is frankly pretty daunting to most of us.

Yet fasting has regained a lot of attention recently. And not in a way that is about extreme fasts or starving yourself at all. This is carefully controlled, mild to moderate fasting. In a recent survey, around 10 percent of Americans aged between eighteen and eighty practice regular gentle fasting, making it more popular than "clean eating" and other types of diets. And there's good reason why dietary influencers are promoting it to their public audiences: studies have shown that this kind of fasting can help combat several conditions including neurodegenerative disease, high blood pressure, rheumatoid arthritis, obesity, type 2 diabetes, and cancer. Fasting also appears to be specifically good for your immune system.

A MODERN PROBLEM: EXCESS FOOD

One of the biggest reasons why fasting works is because it cuts through our modern problem of excess eating. After you eat a meal, your cells are exposed to high levels of circulating sugars (broken down from the carbohydrates you eat) and free fatty acids (the component form of fats). These are used by your cells for energy, which is helpful. However, they are a double-edged sword. When your cells are exposed to *excess* amounts of circulating sugars and fats, they also turn on their pro-inflammatory responses, increasing levels of oxidative stress and cellular damage. Too much food is simply stressful for your cells, reduces their ability to function well, and promotes cellular aging.

When you eat, your pancreas also produces insulin. Insulin's job is to help your body get the glucose provided from carbohydrates at that meal as well as the free fatty acids into your cells so they can be used to produce energy. Insulin also promotes the storage of excess glucose as glycogen (but there's limited room for that) or fat. When we consume too much of any macronutrient (carbohydrate, protein, or fat), we send the insulin system into hyperdrive. Being in hyperdrive for too long (typically years or decades) can wear out your pancreas, making it eventually unable to produce sufficient insulin at all—this is how type 2 diabetes develops. Protein, too, stimulates insulin release, which is why long-term high-protein diets have also been associated with an increased risk for type 2 diabetes. Too much fat and our cells can't "hear" insulin so well and your pancreas has to produce more and more insulin just to keep the status quo. Not least, too much inflammation from the higher circulating glucose and fats (or from other sources like a dysbiotic microbiota) interferes with your cells' ability to hear insulin's signals too.

Still with me? The bottom line is, our body really doesn't like to receive more food than it can manage. It's a primary driver of inflammation, aging, and their associated diseases. So, whether you want to incorporate fasting or not, avoiding overeating is a must.

HOW TO TELL IF YOU'RE OVEREATING

Do any of the following apply to you? If so, there's a good chance you may be eating more than your body wants you to.

- You eat very quickly and don't realize you're full until you're very full.
- You feel weighed down after eating.
- You eat when you're not hungry or beyond the point at which you feel satisfied.
- Keeping a favorite snack in the house means you'll probably eat it all in one sitting.
- You often multitask while you eat, such as at your desk or in front of the TV.
- You're still eating like you're in your teens and twenties, even though you're forty or older. Our metabolism slows as we age and so we actually need to eat less over time.
- You're worried about having a big appetite.
- You're steadily gaining weight without wanting to (although weight gain can be driven by several things—not just diet).

I'm often asked if it's a good idea to count calories. Calorie counting is a tool I only rarely use in clinic. Unless someone is really having a hard time regulating how much to eat, needs to gain weight, or finds significant motivation in calorie targets, I usually find it much more effective to work on our in-built food and appetite regulators. One of the most effective ways to keep appetite under control is to eat the *right foods*. Remember: junk foods create ongoing cravings and blunt satiety signals. Getting back to whole foods (nutrient dense and high in fiber) is the most effective way to bring back equilibrium in food intake.

However, if you *do* want to check your calorie needs, any one of the diet tracking apps are another option to help you do that. You can also use the online tool available at calculator.net/calorie-counter.html.

WHAT HAPPENS DURING FASTING?

Fasting breaks this cycle of overeating, inflammatory stress, and over-stretching your insulin production. When we give our body some time away from the constant bombardment with food, amazing things have a chance to happen—inflammation goes down, and real cellular rejuvenation and resilience building occurs, as several studies have demonstrated, including in humans. Cells in all areas of the body, including immune and barrier cells, demonstrate improvements in function after fasting. Furthermore, they are better able to withstand other insults that are thrown at them. Metabolism also improves, whether the fasting is accompanied by weight loss or not.

One key behind these benefits of fasting is the beneficial stress (hormesis again!) that it inflicts on the body that then triggers an adaptive response to improve human resilience and survival. During a fast, cells go from "feast" to "famine" mode, and as sugars start to run down, cells break down fats and proteins for fuel. Fast for long enough and you'll also start to produce compounds called *ketones*. These are a long-conserved alternative fuel source that was essential for our species' survival during hard times. Some individuals following lower-carbohydrate diets can actually generate some ketones simply from the absence of eating between meals or overnight, but for most of us it takes a fast of twenty-four hours or more to start generating ketones. Ketones are quite strongly anti-inflammatory, known to block an otherwise potent inflammation master switch called the NLRP3 inflammasome.

"Famine" mode also appears to be "recycle and repair" mode. Older, damaged cell parts are removed as part of that breaking-down process and, intriguingly, mechanisms of repair are activated. For example, in investigations of individuals observing Ramadan, a religious fasting practice that involves abstaining from eating during daylight hours, increases in DNA repair factors have been observed. In a separate, deliberately designed fasting experiment, where participants abstained from eating during daylight hours on two days out of every week for twelve weeks, impressive rejuvenation-like effects were seen on older participants' immune systems: by the end of the fasting practice, the immune cell counts of those aged fifty years and older were seemingly "restored" to match those of the younger participants in the study. Animal studies have also provided exciting evidence that fasting can trigger the recycling of a significant portion of "old and tired" immune cells and intestinal barrier cells. These are then replaced with brand-new versions once the fast is over and food is available again.

In addition to its effects on inflammation and immune cell rejuvenation, fasting also has a significant effect on your gut microbiota, your important allies in immune defense. With less ability to withstand food deprivation, microbial populations in the digestive tract are significantly culled during a fast. It's likely that this intermittent "pruning" of the microbiota is helpful in preventing overgrowth and enhancing the dominance of beneficial symbiotic strains over pathogenic ones. This reduces the chance of a problematic strain taking hold and growing, and keeps your microbiota happy and healthy.

This is all to say that fasting may well pay off in resistance to infections, as well as other immune-mediated diseases, though the research in humans is still in its earliest stages. One study has shown that a periodic "fasting mimicking diet" may reduce symptoms of the autoimmune condition multiple sclerosis in individuals who are particularly severely affected by relapses. Another study in individuals with asthma showed that fasting for twenty-four hours reduced levels of airway inflammation. And a study in mice that were fasted on alternate days for twelve weeks found they were better able to fend off *Salmonella* infection than the mice that did not fast beforehand. The researchers observed fewer *Salmonella* bacterial counts in the animals' intestines and a higher antibody response. These are just some of the early but impressive studies that indicate that fasting might just be the closest to an immune "refresh" we can get.

COMMON FORMS OF FASTING

Below are some of the most common evidence-supported ways to fast, listed in order from easiest to implement to most advanced (in my view, at least). All of these have shown benefits for metabolic health, weight maintenance, and immune health. When choosing a fasting program, a lot comes down to personal preference and tracking your response (for instance, I track symptoms, weight changes, as well as markers of metabolism and inflammation, depending on the goals for each individual I work with). Also consider your life routine, since it's a good idea to reduce physical activity on days where you are restricting calories.

Time-restricted eating: Time-restricted eating (sometimes called "time-restricted feeding") limits eating to only a certain number of hours each day. It does not involve restricting calories. Unless you're a night owl who likes to raid the refrigerator at one in the morning, the chances are you're already doing a basic overnight fast. That makes this the easiest starting point if you're new to fasting. To increase your fasted state, you can try extending your fasting hours to between twelve and sixteen hours per day. That decreases your eating "window" to, say, 7:00 a.m. to 7:00 p.m., or 10:00 a.m. to 6:00 p.m. An extended overnight fast can be used long-term as long as overall nutrient needs can still be met.

Fasting two days per week (the 5:2 diet): The 5:2 diet involves eating a normal diet (in your case, an Immune Resilience Diet) for five days per week, and then on two days per week limiting your calorie intake to 500 calories for women and 600 calories for men. The fasting days don't have to be consecutive days. A 5:2 diet can also be used long-term as long as overall nutrient needs can still be met.

Alternate-day fasting: Just as it sounds, alternate-day fasting involves fasting every other day and eating a normal diet (or the Immune Resilience Diet) on the non-fasting days. Some versions of alternate-day fasting advocate consuming no calories on your fasting days; however, this isn't sustainable long-term. Other versions allow 500 calories on fasting days, which is better for beginners and makes it easier to stick to the diet. I recommend doing alternate-day fasting for no more than four weeks at a time, paying attention to overall nutrient needs.

Fasting Mimicking Diet: The Fasting Mimicking Diet is a dietary program developed by Dr. Valter Longo, the director of the Longevity Institute at the University of Southern California–Leonard Davis School of Gerontology, Los Angeles. Dr. Longo is one of the foremost researchers in the area of fasting, longevity, and immune health. The Fasting Mimicking Diet is a five-day meal program that comes boxed and ready to use and provides your body with calorie-restricted meals that mimic the effects of a fast. Dr. Longo's results are very promising (he is behind several of the studies mentioned earlier in this section on fasting including the reversal of multiple sclerosis symptoms and immune cell regeneration) and my experience so far has generated good results. The Fasting Mimicking Diet is intended for intermittent use only. You can check the website prolonfmd.com for the latest recommendations of how often to use the Fasting Mimicking Diet since they are continuing to evolve based on Dr. Longo's research.

FASTING SAFELY

When deciding to fast, there are additional things to know to ensure it is practiced safely.

Nutrition still counts: First, fasting should not involve a continual state of undernutrition. In fact, undernutrition and protein malnutrition are the dominant causes of immunosuppression across the globe and will have the opposite effect to what you want. Poor nutrient intake has been observed to lead to impairments in immunological memory cells, a state of low-grade inflammation, increased intestinal permeability, dysbiosis of the intestinal microbiota, and the perpetuation of chronic infections. It's important that we pay attention to micronutrient-dense foods and overall micronutrient nutrient intake during and/or surrounding a fast. And we should not "overdose" on fasting.

Fasting may suppress immunity temporarily: While fasting may have long-term benefits for the immune system, in the short term it may reduce immune activity. Here's how this apparent contradiction works: During a fasting period, circulating immune cells in the body can decrease in numbers. The effect is temporary; when we start eating again, new immune and barrier cells are regenerated. But your immune systems may be temporarily more vulnerable during a fast. What this means for us is that if you are fasting, you should do so when you're not at a higher risk for catching an infection (such as during a local outbreak).

Focus on what you eat after the fast: The period after a fast when you start to eat food again is when the body does the majority of its rebuilding work. Not to mention your microbiome, which will enter its own rebuild mode, too. This isn't the time for a celebratory binge on ice cream and pizza. What you eat will replenish the nutrients your body will draw on during its renewal and that will shape your gut microbe populations. This is the time to stick closely to the Immune Resilience Diet to see you through that rebuilding process.

Who should not fast: Fasting is not recommended for individuals who are underweight, undernourished, who have low muscle mass or frailty, who are pregnant or nursing, who take medications that need to be consumed with food, whose medications reduce blood sugar, or for children and adolescents. Anyone with an active eating disorder or disordered eating tendencies should not undertake fasting. Anyone who is under intense physical stress such as laborers and athletes should not fast. I also recommend that menstruating women should not fast intensely during the week prior to getting their period and the first few days of their period, since their body can be more vulnerable to stress during that time. Always get your physician's approval before beginning any fasting program.

Can We Get the Same Effect as Fasting with a Ketogenic Diet?

Diets that severely restrict carbohydrate and promote higher fat intake can also lead to the production of ketones and to their use as a cellular fuel. These are another group of popular diets that are collectively labeled as "ketogenic diets." The biochemistry of fasting actually looks metabolically very similar to nutritional ketosis, with higher circulating levels of fats and ketones, and lower blood sugar and insulin. *(cont.)*

Similar to fasting, nutritional ketosis has been shown in animals to improve certain measurable characteristics of cells of the immune system. It can also reduce the signs of cellular aging. This may offer substantial immune protection. Researchers at the Yale School of Medicine, for example, have reported that putting laboratory mice on a ketogenic diet before exposing them to a pathogen (in this case, a flu virus), helped those mice generate a more robust, protective immune cell response and kept the virus from spreading in their body (compared with mice fed their regular diet). The ketogenic diet also seemed to help the cells in the airways of those infected mice better maintain their barrier function, helped avoid weight loss during the infection, and led to improved survival rates. Interestingly, when the same researchers tried out a high fat plus high carbohydrate diet (the diet most like a Western, processed food diet, as you know), or supplemental oral ketones administered on top of the regular diet, there wasn't any protection evident, suggesting that it was the metabolic adaptation of ketone production, *plus* lowered insulin and glucose, that was effective.

Incidentally, you'll often see headlines blasting high-fat diets for their negative health effects, as shown in this or that latest study. Don't confuse those with a properly constructed ketogenic diet even though it is also high in fat. Most often, when you look at the type of diet used in those studies, you'll find it is a high fat *plus high refined carbohydrate* diet. They'll also usually lack fiber and phytonutrients. This is not at all a well-constructed ketogenic diet, and these misrepresentations problematically muddy the water when it comes to understanding the effects of different therapeutic diets.

As with fasting, we do not yet have conclusive evidence about the use of ketogenic diets for immune resilience. But the early science and my experience with its careful, select use in clinical practice is very promising, especially for hard-to-shift metabolic and inflammatory disorders, weight-loss resistance (where calorie restriction alone isn't enough), and certain instances of cognitive decline. When I do use a therapeutic ketogenic diet in practice, however, it is also under close supervision, in concert with an individual's physician, and in a way that still maintains a high intake of plant-based fiber and phytonutrients—no carnivore-style menu in my keto diet. And I ensure that an individual's cholesterol levels are tracked, since ketogenic diets can raise LDL cholesterol levels in some people.

PRINCIPLE 6: KEEP IT REAL
(I.E., KNOW HOW TO KEEP YOUR SANITY)

WHAT TO EXPECT WHEN CHANGING YOUR DIET

It all depends on where you're starting from, of course, but changing what you eat can be tough. There are old habits to break, new ones to form, new skills to learn. And that rather uncomfortable feeling of giving up something that perhaps gives you temporary feelings of pleasure—like sugar. Sugar has such "claws," doesn't it? And you're not just imagining it: research has shown that sugar and sugar-sweetened foods create a psychological dependence. Removing sugar from a baseline sugar-rich diet can trigger behaviors akin to addiction withdrawal. No joke.

In addition to rewiring our neuronal brain circuitry into hedonistic desires for hyperpalatable foods, sugar and high-fat-plus-refined-carb ultra-processed foods also control us via our microbiota. When we eat these foods, we promote the growth of bad bacteria in our guts, who, as long as we keep feeding them what they want, stay relatively happy. Once we take that away, they get upset. Without their preferred source of food, they start to wither and break down. But as they do so, they release toxins that stimulate our immune system's inflammatory pathways and make us feel bad.

The good (or at least better) news is that these effects are reversible. Yes, sugar and ultra-processed foods can be unpleasant to break away from, but after just a few days, cravings start to diminish. During this time, it's best to keep all sources of sugary foods, processed foods, and refined grains out of sight and out of immediate reach. Out of your house altogether is best! Make sure you have lots of healthy foods to keep you satiated and your energy levels steady. Get your sleep, exercise, and do your best to avoid big stressors and minimize situations (tiredness, irritability, anxiety, low moods) that can undermine your break away from sugar. If you need some extra support for cravings, I have found it can help to supplement with N-acetyl cysteine (NAC), 1,200 mg twice per day to get past that cravings "hump" or if you feel cravings resurfacing again.

DO I NEED TO EAT LIKE THIS ALL THE TIME?

No. Perfect adherence to any dietary plan is near on impossible. It's important to know that if you can eat according to the Immune Resilience Diet at least 80 percent of the time, you'll likely be able to make allowances for deviations for important occasions without any problem. And actually, when we set the bar too high, we tend to undermine our own efforts—any slipup feels like a failure and dampens our enthusiasm for getting back on the diet again. When you're eating the abundant levels of vitamins, minerals, fiber, and phytonutrients that you'll find on this eating plan, you can feel confident that this absolutely solid base will carry you through any minor, occasional blips. We know, for instance, that you can improve your glycemic response to foods simply by improving the *context* of the diet you're introducing them into. Eating adequate amounts of fiber-rich foods on a regular basis, for example, improves your ability to tolerate one serving of a refined carbohydrate compared with someone who is eating that same refined carbohydrate serving on top of a diet that is already full of processed, sugary foods. Fiber and phytonutrients, too, when combined with a serving of refined carbohydrate, significantly reduce the impact of that carbohydrate on blood sugar levels. So if you are in a situation where you can't choose a better alternative than a processed restaurant meal, add a cup of green tea, dried herbs, or some strawberries to offset some of that meal's inflammatory effects. It's been proven to help.

KNOW WHEN TO BE FLEXIBLE

We all need some flexibility in our lives, especially to be able to navigate social and work situations that involve food, as well as when we travel. One of the growing problems with popular restrictive diets is that for some of us, they can become an obsession. Especially when food concerns are presented in a dramatic, unbalanced way. There's even a medical term for this: *orthorexia nervosa*. It's when good eating habits actually become unhealthy and cause suffering and distress. People with orthorexia can have a high level of anxiety around food choices and experience social isolation due to not participating in activities over concerns about food options. Social media can contribute to this phenomenon by increasing the pressure to achieve unrealistically perfect diets or health status. The bottom line is that even as experts with influence can help educate about healthy eating habits, we should not be promoting unrealistic goals that cause harm. Yes, unless there is a specific medical reason why you can't, you can eat with your extended family on special occasions, even if Aunt Caroline has made those sweet potatoes with marshmallows again. And you can go out to dinner to catch up with old friends, even if they've chosen an eatery you wouldn't have. Yes, you can occasionally eat that conference food, or that intermittent birthday pizza or cake slice. Of course, we'll all do our best to limit those exposures to immune-harming foods and jump right back on plan once food is under our own control again. Trust your instincts and your ability to manage what you eat in a healthy way.

Your diet will be the bedrock of your immune health, so getting it tuned in will make a huge difference to your immune resilience. Next, we'll tackle how to supplement your diet to provide extra support where and when you might need it.

To view the references cited in this chapter, please visit
www.immuneresilienceplan.com/science.

CHAPTER 12

Immune-Boosting Supplements

Gems That Take Immune Support to the Next Level

Wander over to the supplement aisle in any supermarket or pharmacy and you'll find dozens, if not hundreds, of compounds that promise the world in terms of health. Many of these have centuries, even millennia of traditional use behind them. Now, with modern scientific techniques and research methods, we understand more and more about the mechanisms through which these compounds act against harmful pathogens and on our immune system. Just as their collective name implies, these compounds can help *supplement* the foods you eat, when you feel you need that extra safeguard, or when there are specific areas of your immune system you want to lend extra support. The only supplement I routinely recommend for most *everyone* is a quality multivitamin and mineral supplement. Beyond that, depending on what you determine to be the biggest holes in your immune resilience bucket, you'll find additional options for more specifically targeted support. But with so many options, which are the best to choose? This chapter presents a curated list of those that have the best science-backed effectiveness, broad range of immune-benefiting activity, and highest safety profiles.

A FOUNDATIONAL MULTIVITAMIN AND MINERAL

A multivitamin and mineral supplement is a valuable insurance policy for all of us. The only time I drop this recommendation is for someone who is consistently hitting nutrient intake targets from food sources. (I check this routinely with a diet nutrient calculator.) The multivitamin and mineral supplements I use in clinical practice contain the most biologically active forms of each nutrient and are rigorously tested for quality (you'll find my preferred brands listed, once again, in the Resources). As a summary, here are the basics to check for in your multi to support optimal immune function. Remember to follow any adjustments to this guidance that pertain to you from chapter 7.

WHAT TO LOOK FOR IN YOUR MULTI

- Vitamin A: a partial contribution to your Recommended Daily Allowance (RDA), ideally with a combination of preformed retinol (limited to 5,000 IU/1,500 mcg RAE per day) together with provitamin A carotenoids.
- Vitamins B_1, B_2, B_3, pantothenic acid (B_5), B_6, biotin (B_7), folate (B_9), and B_{12}: 100 percent of RDA. Note that many multivitamins exceed the RDA guidance for B vitamins by quite a bit. This is generally thought to be okay. However, in my experience not everyone does well with high-dose B vitamins. And there are data that suggest excessively high B vitamin intakes may not be as benign as has been thought. For those reasons it's best to seek out one nearest the RDA level.
- Vitamin C: 100 percent of RDA.
- Vitamin D: 100 percent of RDA (or more; see "Additional Vitamin and Mineral Support" below).
- Vitamin E: 80 percent to 100 percent of RDA.
- Copper: 100 percent of RDA.

- Iron: 100 percent of RDA for women in their reproductive years (with a menstrual cycle). Men and postmenopausal women should choose a multi without iron.
- Magnesium: At least 100 mg per day.
- Selenium: 100 percent of RDA.
- Zinc: 100 percent of RDA.

You can find your RDAs at the National Institutes of Health's Office of Dietary Supplements (https://ods.od.nih.gov/HealthInformation/Dietary _Reference_Intakes.aspx). It's best to check there directly since they vary by age and are periodically updated.

ADDITIONAL VITAMIN AND MINERAL SUPPORT

Provided in summary here and in more detail in chapter 7.

- Vitamin D: Add 1,500–2,000 IU for adults during winter months with reduced sunlight exposure or year-round for individuals with darker skin.
- EPA and DHA: Adding 250–500 mg per day supplemental EPA and DHA combined is a good idea for all, no matter the time of year. Vegan sources are available if you don't or can't eat fish.
- A note for individuals at risk for osteopenia and osteoporosis: Because calcium is, like magnesium, a very large nutrient, supplemental multivitamin and mineral products don't usually contain much of it. Just be aware that if you fall into this category, or even if you don't but your regular diet falls short on calcium, you'll likely need to source calcium, and possibly magnesium, in a separate supplement.

BOTANICALS AND MORE

Ashwagandha. *Antimicrobial. Antioxidant. Anti-inflammatory. Immune responsiveness. Anti-anxiety. Pain relieving. Blood sugar bal-*

Supplement Quality and Safety

Remember that just because a product is "natural," it doesn't automatically mean it's high quality or safe. Here's what to know when navigating dietary supplements:

- *Quality:* Since the supplement industry in the US is largely unregulated, we must all do our homework to find reputable sources. ConsumerLab.com, a company that performs independent testing of supplements and reports on quality issues routinely finds that some supplements available to purchase don't contain what they say they contain, or worse, contain something harmful such as toxins from contamination somewhere along the supply chain. There have also been several high-profile media reports of counterfeit supplements sold by third parties on marketplace sites such as Amazon.com. As a clinician, it's absolutely essential to me that I can trust the supplement brands that I recommend, as well as the resellers. In the Resources section, I've listed those companies whose quality processes I've vetted and I have most confidence in.

- *Safety:* Supplemental nutrients and herbs have real biochemical effects in your body and these can be quite potent. For that reason, and because we don't have safety data in certain populations, they are not suitable for everyone. Always check with a qualified and knowledgeable health care practitioner before using any supplement, and follow up again if you're using a supplement for a prolonged period of time. If you're pregnant, breastfeeding, or have any chronic health condition, you should be extra cautious. If you take any medication, it is important to check for potential supplement interactions using an up-to-date, comprehensive, and searchable database such as Medscape's Drug Interaction Checker available online.

ancing. Ashwagandha is a good choice for supporting immunity if you've identified stress resilience as a potential hole in your immune resilience bucket. Ashwagandha is an herb used in Ayurvedic medicine and is known as an *adaptogenic* herb because it helps to support resiliency against physiological and psychological stress. Several human clinical trials have demonstrated its potential to lower reported anxiety levels, thought to be due to its ability to modify neurotransmitter (dopamine, serotonin, and GABA) signaling and lower cortisol levels. Ashwagandha also seems to be able to mobilize macrophages and stimulate phagocytosis, as well as potentially restoring suppressed immune responses to healthier levels.

How to take: 400–800 mg per day encapsulated ashwagandha root extract, standardized to contain at least 2.5 percent withanolides. Can also be taken as a liquid extract.

Astragalus root. *Antibacterial. Antiviral. Antioxidant. Anti-inflammatory. Immune responsiveness. Healthy microbiota. Barrier stabilizing. Blood sugar balancing. Wound healing.* Astragalus, a Chinese medicine staple, has a broad-spectrum antimicrobial action and modulates the immune system by stimulating white blood cell production, as well as activating natural killer cells, macrophages, and B cells, and promoting the production of interferons. It has been long used for respiratory tract infections such as common colds. Also of interest are the specific prebiotic fibers found in astragalus, which have been shown to enhance beneficial microbial populations and reduce gut leakiness.

How to take: 1,000–2,000 mg per day astragalus root extract or 5–10 grams per day of the whole herb. Can also be taken as a liquid extract.

Caution: Since quite a significant portion of the scientific data we have on astragalus indicates immune-stimulating effects, there is a theoretical (though unproven) risk for individuals with autoimmune conditions. I have not seen this occur in practice, but it would be prudent to avoid astragalus if you have an autoimmune condition, or work with a practitioner who can help you monitor its potential effects.

Berberine. *Antimicrobial. Antibacterial. Antifungal. Antiparasitic. Antioxidant. Anti-inflammatory. Anti-diarrheal. Blood sugar balanc-*

ing. Berberine itself is not an herb, rather a phytonutrient constituent found in several herbal plants, including goldenseal (*Hydrastis canadensis*), goldthread (*Coptis chinensis*), Oregon grape root (*Mahonia aquifolium*), and barberry (*Berberis vulgaris*). Berberine is one of my go-to antimicrobials for addressing gut dysbiosis and digestive infections, especially in the context of insulin resistance and diabetes. Preliminary research suggests that an additional way that berberine may help with diarrhea is by blocking the secretion of water into the intestines that is triggered by some pathogens like *E. coli*. Berberine's blood sugar–lowering effects appear to be due to its ability to increase cellular insulin receptors, making it easier for blood glucose to be moved from the blood into cells.

How to take: 500 mg berberine two or three times per day with food. Start with a lower dose and gradually increase to this level.

Caution: Berberine can interact with a number of prescription medications so it's best to check with your health care practitioner if you are taking one or more.

Black elderberry. *Antiviral. Antioxidant. Anti-inflammatory. Immune responsiveness.* The berries of the black elder tree have a long history of traditional use for cold and flu symptoms. The active components of black elderberries have immune-boosting and antiviral activity, including to herpes simplex virus type 1 (the cause of cold sores), coronaviruses (the causes of respiratory tract infections including the common cold), and flu viruses. A recent meta-analysis of studies conducted to date concluded that, when used at the onset of cold and flu symptoms, it can substantially reduce the duration of symptoms. One additional study of black elderberry taken preventively against exposure to respiratory infections during air travel found that it reduced overall duration and severity of infections compared to individuals who didn't take black elderberry. Elderberry also has mucolytic (mucus-thinning) and anti-inflammatory properties helping to alleviate respiratory symptoms. Its anti-

How to Be Selective About Your Immune Supplements

The list of recommended immune supplements in this chapter isn't meant to suggest that you need to take *all* of these to support immune resilience. In fact, you may not feel the need to take any beyond your multivitamin! Myself, I take a pared-down short list that are most relevant to what I know about my immune system—that it does best with anti-allergy and detoxification support. For those reasons I routinely take N-acetyl cysteine (NAC) and quercetin alongside my multivitamin, fish oil (for EPA/DHA), and extra vitamin D. And I always have astragalus, black elderberry, garlic, and holy basil supplements on hand for additional support when I feel that I'm at greater risk of exposure or when my immune system is taking a hit from work stress, and for taking at the first sign of infection. (For more about what to do when you get sick, see chapter 15.)

If you would like to support your immune resilience by adding supplements from this chapter, here's how I recommend you prioritize, based on your own understanding of where you may need additional support:

- *All-around immune support:* Multivitamin and mineral, EPA/DHA, vitamin D, curcumin, ginger, NAC, probiotics, quercetin.
- *Blood sugar control:* Berberine, garlic, ginger, probiotics.
- *Cold and flu season:* Echinacea, black elderberry, NAC.
- *Detoxification support:* Garlic, glutathione, NAC, probiotics.
- *Immune aging:* Glutathione, melatonin, EPA/DHA.
- *Inflammation:* Curcumin, glutathione, probiotics.
- *Known dysbiosis or infections:* Berberine, black elderberry, echinacea, garlic, ginger.
- *Leaky gut (increased intestinal permeability)*:* Astragalus root, ginger, quercetin, EPA/DHA, probiotics.
- *Sleep support:* Melatonin.
- *Sluggish immune system:* Astragalus, echinacea.
- *Stress support:* Ashwagandha, holy basil, probiotics.
- *Wound healing:* Astragalus root, curcumin, garlic, holy basil, vitamin C.

*Note that even though they are not detailed in this chapter, other supplements including deglycyrrhizinated licorice (DGL), L-glutamine, marshmallow root, slippery elm, prebiotics, vitamin D, and zinc carnosine are routinely used to support gut integrity.

inflammatory properties are presumed to be due to its high flavonoid content, including quercetin and anthocyanins.

How to take: 500 mg black elderberry fruit extract capsules per day. Higher doses, up to 1,200 mg per day can be taken for up to two weeks at a time. Black elderberry is also available as a syrup.

Caution: Be cautious with homemade black elderberry preparations because they don't always apply the heat and evaporation that is necessary to denature the toxic, cyanide-like components present in raw elderberries. These have been known to cause gastric symptoms including nausea, vomiting, and diarrhea.

Curcumin. *Antimicrobial. Antibacterial. Antiviral. Antifungal. Antiparasitic. Anti-inflammatory. Immune responsiveness. Anti-allergy. Wound healing.* Curcumin is the active constituent of the spice turmeric and is responsible for its bright yellow color. Several viruses are known to be inhibited by curcumin in laboratory experiments—influenza virus, hepatitis C virus, HIV, Zika virus, human papilloma virus, and norovirus, as well as some bacteria including pathogenic strains of *Staphylococcus* (including *S. aureus*), *Streptococcus* (including *S. mutans* in the mouth), *Pseudomonas,* and *E. coli.* Antibiotic-resistant *S. aureus* appears to be vulnerable to curcumin's activity, too. Human studies have indicated that curcumin can be helpful against urinary tract infections and gingival infections—it is comparable to chlorhexidine in reducing gum inflammation and better at improving gum attachment and reducing plaque, according to clinical reports. Mechanistically, curcumin interacts with various components of our immune system including dendritic cells, macrophages, B cells, and T cells. In animal experiments, curcumin has been shown to increase antibody levels. It also improves the structure of tight junctions between the cells lining the digestive tract and offers anti-inflammatory protection against dietary insults that damage either the microbiota or the integrity of the gut lining. Last but absolutely not least, curcumin is a potent anti-inflammatory compound, modulating the release of immune cytokines to dampen down excess inflammation: In experimental animal models, curcumin reduces severity and improves survival in infections with a higher risk for hyperinflammation and sepsis, and offers some protection against lung injury during severe pneumonia.

How to take: 500 mg curcumin two or three times per day. Choose a phytosomal formulation (a preparation that helps make plant-based compounds more soluble) or one with piperine for enhanced absorption.

Echinacea. *Antimicrobial. Antibacterial. Antiviral. Antifungal. Antioxidant. Anti-inflammatory. Immune responsiveness. Healthy microbiota.* Most human studies that have put echinacea to the test agree that it can reduce the duration and severity of respiratory infections such as common cold viruses, as well as the risk for complications (like ear infections, sinusitis, or pneumonia) and antibiotic use. Results suggest it may also improve influenza vaccine responsiveness. Echinacea increases the activity of several immune components including macrophages, dendritic cells, natural killer cells, antiviral interferon production, and cytokine signaling. It also has direct antimicrobial activity against bacteria, viruses, and *Candida*. Among the many active components recognized in echinacea are a group called *fructans*. These fructans have nourishing effects on beneficial intestinal bacteria, act as immune-signaling molecules, and have antioxidant activity. Although it's often noted for its immune-stimulating effects, echinacea also has anti-inflammatory properties found to inhibit excess inflammation by suppressing excess NF-κB and other pro-inflammatory pathways.

How to take: 2,000–2,500 mg echinacea herb extract per day to support general resilience and 4,000 mg per day for up to one week during infections. *Echinacea purpurea* is the species most commonly used in scientific studies, although *Echinacea angustifolia* has also demonstrated positive outcomes.

Caution: Some scientists have pointed out that the variation in some of the research findings on echinacea may be due to the different products used, highlighting the importance of quality and efficacy in making product choices. Since, like astragalus, research on echinacea tends to focus on its immune-stimulating effects, there is a theoretical risk for those with autoimmune conditions. Once again, there are no scientific studies that confirm this, and I have yet to see this occur in practice, but err on the side of caution and avoid echinacea if you have an autoimmune condition or work with a practitioner who can help you monitor its effects.

Garlic extract. *Antimicrobial. Antibacterial. Antiviral. Antifungal. Antiparasitic. Antioxidant. Anti-inflammatory. Immune responsiveness. Detoxification. Healthy microbiota. Improves circulation. Blood sugar balancing. Wound healing.* Several well-designed human studies have examined the effects of one proprietary formulation of aged garlic extract. In one randomized, double-blinded, placebo-controlled clinical trial, aged garlic extract (2.56 grams per day for 90 days) improved T cell and natural killer cell activity, reduced the severity and duration of respiratory infections, and kept participants better able to continue with work or school activities. A slightly higher dose of 3.6 grams aged garlic extract used in a separate study of obese but otherwise healthy adults significantly reduced markers of inflammation. Natural killer cell activity also improved in a study of cancer patients given garlic (again aged garlic extract, but at a much lower dose of 500 mg per day) whose immune systems were declining.

How to take: 1,000–1,500 mg aged garlic extract twice per day. Unaged extracts as well as dehydrated garlic and garlic oils are also available and can be reasonable options. Look for enteric-coated capsules for dehydrated garlic so that its potential to develop active compounds is protected.

Caution: Garlic, especially when consumed in higher doses as found in supplements, has the potential to act as a blood thinner and to increase blood-clotting time. Avoid for two weeks prior to surgery and discuss with your doctor if you are also taking a blood-thinning medication.

Ginger extract. *Antimicrobial. Antibacterial. Antiviral. Antifungal. Antiparasitic. Antioxidant. Anti-inflammatory. Immune balancing. Barrier stabilizing. Digestive support. Healthy microbiota. Pain relieving. Blood sugar balancing. Anti-autoimmune. Anti-asthma.* Ginger has demonstrated immune balancing effects by helping to support the development of regulatory T cells. It also helps support healthy levels of beneficial *Lactobacillus* bacterial species in the digestive tract. It has been long used and well studied for digestive symptoms, especially nausea and vomiting; mechanistically, ginger increases the movement of food from the stomach to the small intestine and along the digestive tract. It also helps to protect the gut barrier and maintain its integrity.

How to take: For general immune support, 500–1,000 mg ginger root extract (standardized to 4 percent to 5 percent gingerols) two or three times per day.

Caution: Ginger in high doses has blood-thinning and glucose-lowering effects and so should be avoided for two weeks before surgery. Discuss with your doctor if you are taking a blood-thinning or anti-diabetic medication.

Glutathione. *Antibacterial. Antiviral. Antioxidant. Anti-inflammatory. Immune responsiveness. Detoxification.* Glutathione is produced naturally in your liver and is often considered your body's "master" antioxidant, helping to keep levels of inflammation under control. It also protects the health of your barriers and immune cells in the face of pro-oxidant and pro-inflammatory exposures and aids in detoxifying environmental chemicals. Glutathione itself also seems to have antimicrobial properties. In one study that first cultured antibiotic-resistant *S. aureus* (MRSA), *E. coli, K. pneumoniae,* and *P. aeruginosa,* glutathione completely inhibited the growth of these pathogenic bacteria. Early lab studies also suggest that glutathione fine-tunes the innate immune response and may be necessary for macrophage activation and function as well as antiviral responses.

How to take: 200–300 mg liposomal glutathione twice per day. Although there has been some controversy over whether supplemental glutathione is degraded by digestion and therefore no more useful than taking NAC (see box below), there is evidence that the liposomal form is quite effective, due to the particular delivery method whereby the active constituent is provided in tiny, fat-like particles that bypass digestion. I have certainly found it to be helpful clinically.

Additional Glutathione Support

Supplemental glutathione, while I do find it effective in liposomal form, can be quite expensive. Luckily, there are other ways to support natural glutathione production in your body. N-acetylcysteine (NAC), for example, is a compound that your body can use to make glutathione, and it is available and inexpensive in supplement form (more on NAC supplements below). Consuming foods high in the sulfur amino acids methionine and L-cysteine also supports glutathione production in the body: lean meats, fish, eggs, lentils, sunflower seeds, allium vegetables (such as garlic, onions, leeks, and shallots), and cruciferous vegetables (like broccoli, cabbage, kale, and rutabaga) are good sources. Whey protein, green tea, and fresh ginger also help support glutathione activity in the body.

Also good to know and avoid are those factors that contribute to a glutathione deficiency. These include a diet low in vegetables and fruits, cigarette smoke, and chronic conditions such as type 2 diabetes and obesity.

Melatonin. *Antibacterial. Antiparasitic. Antioxidant. Anti-inflammatory. Immune responsiveness. Barrier integrity. Pain relieving. Sleep support. Anti-stress.* As you know from chapter 9, melatonin is a hormone that your body naturally produces and that is involved in regulating your sleep. But it does more than just that. Melatonin is a key activator and regulator of immune function. It rivals glutathione in its protective antioxidant and anti-inflammatory capabilities, and it has demonstrated impressive immune recovery effects in those with decreased immune function due to cancer therapy or HIV/AIDS. It has also been described as "a molecule that can enhance the host's tolerance against pathogen invasions," and especially those that may otherwise produce severe effects, such as acute respiratory distress syndrome (ARDS) and sepsis. Research out of the Cleveland Clinic in 2020 found that melatonin supplementation use was associated with 28 percent reduced likelihood of contracting COVID-19, although prospective intervention studies are needed to confirm this association.

How to take: 1.5–3 mg daily 30 to 60 minutes before bedtime. Higher doses have been used for some specific conditions but should be appropriately supervised by a qualified health care professional.

Caution: Because of the potential for causing sleepiness, do not drive or use machinery for five hours after taking melatonin.

N-acetyl cysteine (NAC). *Antiviral. Antioxidant. Anti-inflammatory. Congestion relief. Detoxifying.* NAC is a cysteine-containing molecule that has a long history of use in hospital settings as an antidote to acetaminophen (paracetamol) overdose and as a mucolytic (mucus-degrading) intervention in conditions including cystic fibrosis and chronic obstructive pulmonary disorder (COPD). It also has numerous immune-related effects. NAC is used by your body to form glutathione. This is thought to be the mechanism behind its ability to dampen down excess inflammation and collateral damage during serious infections such as pneumonia, as has been demonstrated in human research. NAC has also been shown to have direct antiviral activity and, when taken for general immune support, studies suggest the potential to reduce the occurrence and severity of respiratory infections. Its ability to thin mucus secretions so they can be more easily cleared from the body is also useful in respiratory tract infections with mucus production.

How to take: 500–600 mg twice per day.

Probiotics. *Antimicrobial. Anti-inflammatory. Immune balance. Immune responsiveness. Barrier integrity. Healthy microbiota. Detoxifying. Anti-anxiety. Sleep support. Blood sugar balancing. Anti-allergy. Anti-asthma. Anti-autoimmune.* At this point, you are well aware of the benefits of beneficial microbes for a healthy, strong immune system—including antimicrobial activity against harmful species, reducing inflammation, supporting barrier health, and training your immune system to be vigilant and responsive, yet measured. Supplemental probiotics contain strains of bacteria and some fungi that are known to have health-promoting effects, including on the immune system. See the box (pages 252–254) on choosing probiotics that have activity against specific types of infections.

How to take: For general immune resilience, choose a multi-strain supplement with both *Lactobacillus* and *Bifidobacterium* species and between 2 billion and 50 billion CFUs.

Quercetin. *Antiviral. Antioxidant. Anti-inflammatory. Barrier integrity. Anti-allergy.* Quercetin is a natural, yellow-pigmented compound found in most plant foods. It truly is a workhorse intervention that I use in clinic for many different applications—from restoring gut integrity, to dampening environmental allergy responses, to its anti-inflammatory and antioxidant protection. Laboratory studies in cultured cells and animals demonstrate that quercetin and its metabolites are active against Zika virus, hepatitis virus, dengue virus, Ebola virus, Epstein-Barr virus, influenza viruses (H1N1 and H5N1), and common cold viruses. These effects may be due in part to its demonstrated ability to increase production of antiviral interferons by the innate immune system. Despite these promising findings, clinical science has as yet been slow to evolve all of these into human studies of infection. We are not entirely without human data, however: Supplemental quercetin dosed at 1,000 mg per day over 12 weeks reduced the number of sick days due to upper respiratory tract infection and decreased infection severity scores in people over forty years old, according to one study. In a separate

Choosing Probiotics Targeted Against Specific Situations

Probiotics That May Reduce the Risk of Infections of the Digestive Tract

Form to take: oral capsule
- *Bacillus coagulans*
- *Bifidobacterium animalis*
- *Bifidobacterium infantis*
- *Lactobacillus rhamnosus**
- *Lactobacillus reuteri*
- *Lactobacillus paracasei*
- *Lactobacillus casei*
- *Lactobacillus plantarum*
- *Lactobacillus acidophilus**
- *Saccharomyces boulardii**
- *Streptococcus thermophilus*

*These species are those with the most research supporting their use to reduce the risk of *Clostridioides difficile*-associated diarrhea. *Saccharomyces boulardii* is also one of the best studied for reducing the risk for antibiotic-associated diarrhea.

Probiotics That May Reduce the Risk of Infections of the Airways and Lungs

Form to take: chewable if possible, or oral capsule
- *Lactobacillus rhamnosus*
- *Lactobacillus casei*
- *Lactococcus lactis*
- *Lactobacillus bulgaricus*
- *Streptococcus thermophilus*
- *Streptococcus salivarius* (most studies have used the K12 strain)
- *Lactobacillus plantarum*
- *Bifidobacterium animalis*
- *Lactobacillus casei*
- *Lactobacillus bulgaricus*
- *Lactobacillus brevis*
- *Lactobacillus gasseri*

- *Bifidobacterium subtilis*
- *Lactobacillus paracasei*
- *Bifidobacterium bifidum*
- *Lactobacillus acidophilus*
- *Bifidobacterium longum*

Probiotics That May Reduce the Risk of Infections of the Gums

Form to take: chewable
- *Streptococcus salivarius* (most studies have used the K12 strain)
- *Lactobacillus rhamnosus*
- *Lactobacillus acidophilus*
- *Lactobacillus casei*
- *Bifidobacterium longum*
- *Bifidobacterium infantis*
- *Bifidobacterium lactis*
- *Bifidobacterium breve*
- *Bifidobacterium longum*
- *Bifidobacterium pseudolongum*
- *Bifidobacterium bifidum*

Probiotics That May Reduce the Risk of Urinary Tract Infections

Form to take: oral capsule
- *Lactobacillus rhamnosus*
- *Lactobacillus reuteri*

Probiotics That May Reduce the Risk of Vaginal Infections

Form to take: oral capsule, suppositories, or rinses
- *Lactobacillus acidophilus*
- *Lactobacillus rhamnosus*
- *Lactobacillus fermentum*

Probiotics That May Improve Skin Integrity

Form to take: oral capsule, although some are also available as topicals

- *Lactobacillus paracasei*

(cont.)

- *Bifidobacterium longum*
- *Lactobacillus rhamnosus*
- *Lactobacillus salivarius*
- *Bifidobacterium breve*
- *Lactobacillus plantarum*
- *Lactobacillus reuteri*

Probiotics That May Improve Vaccine Responsiveness

Form to take: oral capsule
- *Lactobacillus casei*
- *Lactobacillus fermentum*
- *Lactobacillus paracasei*
- *Lactobacillus rhamnosus**
- *Bifidobacterium longum*
- *Lactobacillus plantarum*
- *Lactobacillus acidophilus*
- *Lactobacillus lactis*
- *Lactobacillus salivarius*
- *Lactobacillus fermentum*
- *Bifidobacterium breve*
- *Bifidobacterium bifidum*
- *Streptococcus thermophilus*

**Lactobacillus rhamnosus* GG (Culturelle®) has been one of the most frequently studied with favorable impacts.

study of individuals with chronic hepatitis C virus infection, several experienced a "clinically meaningful" decrease in measured viral load using supplemental quercetin, and without any side effects. In exercise studies, while not all have shown benefit, it does appear that 1,000 mg of quercetin per day may reduce infections following intensive exercise.

How to take: 500–1,500 mg quercetin per day.

Resveratrol. *Antiviral. Antioxidant. Anti-inflammatory. Anti-immune aging. Immune balancing. Lowers blood sugar.* Resveratrol is a naturally occurring phytonutrient found in red grape skins, mulberries, and to a lesser extent in peanuts. When resveratrol was given to healthy human volunteers at a dose of 1 gram daily for 28 days, it significantly increased their levels of regulatory T cells and decreased markers of inflammation, suggesting that resveratrol is an effective immune balancer that can help dial down inflammation and unruly immune activity like allergies and autoimmunity. Other studies show similar results, especially of resveratrol's ability to lower inflammation. Resveratrol also appears to inhibit the growth of some viruses including cold and flu viruses, cytomegalovirus, and herpes simplex viruses. It may also promote natural killer cell activity. Resveratrol is additionally a long-used natural anti-aging remedy that is thought to mimic the beneficial effects of fasting on mechanisms of DNA repair and integrity. This anti-aging potential may protect against age-related declines in immune function.

How to take: 500 mg per day. Take with food containing fat to aid absorption.

Whey protein. *Antibacterial. Antioxidant. Anti inflammatory. Anti-allergy. Immune responsiveness. Detoxifying. Blood sugar lowering.* Laboratory and animal studies have shown that whey protein has antibacterial, anti-allergy, antioxidant, and anti-inflammatory effects. Whey is high in branched-chain amino acids, which are thought to provide a ready source of energy for immune cells that need to ramp up quickly in response to a harmful bug. It is also a source of gamma-glutamylcysteine, which is another compound your body can use to produce the antioxidant glutathione. Whey protein powders can be a good option to use in the smoothie recipes in part 4.

How to take: A serving containing 15–22 grams of protein per day.

What we consume through food, and support with supplements, is just half of the equation to immune resilience. You've read how our environment can also be a great threat to immune health, so let's now read how to double down with the right lifestyle choices.

To view the references cited in this chapter, please visit www.immuneresilienceplan.com/science.

CHAPTER 13

Your Lifestyle Plan

Practical Strategies for Exercise, Stress, Sleep, Nature, and Clean Living

A s you read in part 2, what we expose ourselves to in our everyday lives can affect our immune system just as much as our diet. So taking steps toward living the right kind of healthy lifestyle and mitigating the risks of dangerous pathogens that surround us is equally as important as changing the foods we eat. Hand in hand, diet and lifestyle changes can be that double act that ensures your immune system is as strong as it can be.

EXERCISE

I have an admission to make: I have never been a gym person. I know plenty of wonderful people who do like going to a gym and do so on a regular basis. Gyms are very convenient, of course—they come with equipment, trainers, classes, and . . . showers. All good stuff. Yet I can't seem to get myself there. On the other hand, put me outdoors (especially in the woods) and I can go for miles—up and down hills, on foot or on a bike, usually with our dog, Aslan. Water activities work great for me, too—swimming or paddleboarding in our local lake. I especially like to go with my husband and kids, or with other family and friends. I also like to do a lot of work in our yard and vegetable garden. The good news is, whether you are a gym lover or not, there are many different ways you can incorporate physical movement into your day.

Recall from chapter 9 that the best kind of exercise for immune resilience is regular, moderate-intensity exercise. That means exercising for 30 to 60 minutes, five days of the week, at between 60 percent and 80 percent of your maximum possible exertion level. Your maximum exertion level is unique to you and unique to you *in that moment of your life.* It's going to be different from your colleague's or neighbor's. It's going to change over time as you build fitness. If you have been more sedentary up until now, you'll need to build up slowly in both duration of exercise and intensity.

How to tell if you're exercising at 60 percent to 80 percent of intensity (target zone shaded gray):

Exercise Intensity	What it feels like
90%–100%	This is pushing yourself to your limits, only manageable for a minute or two before your body forces you to stop.
80%–90%	Breathless and hard to speak more than a few words. You're likely sweating hard now and couldn't sustain this for more than about 10 minutes.
70%–80% (target zone)	Breathing is a little labored, but you're able to speak a sentence. Singing is a challenge, though, and you feel ready to stop after about 30 minutes.
60%–70% (target zone)	Muscles feel warmed and your breathing has deepened. But you can easily hold a conversation or even burst into song. You could keep going in this zone for a while.
50%–60%	Easy movement that doesn't really feel like exercise at all.
0%–50%	Light daily activities or resting.

WHAT TYPE OF EXERCISE TO CHOOSE?

For immune resilience, you'll want to incorporate aerobic activity. Aerobic activities are the kind that get your heart rate going and your lungs breathing faster—brisk walking, hiking, jogging, swimming, cycling, dancing are all good examples. As are aerobic exercise classes, stationary bicycles, and treadmills. Housework such as active cleaning, yard work (like pushing a lawnmower or spreading mulch), or other home maintenance activities also count, as long as you're still getting your heart rate and breathing going.

The most vital thing is to choose a form of exercise that you like. And ideally that you *love*. Consider incorporating your exercise with time spent with family and friends or outdoors in nature. The companionship can help turn something otherwise monotonous into something you look forward to and is great for further reducing stress levels. Being outdoors can give you that additional vitamin D boost and harness those benefits of nature on your immune system. Recall from chapter 9 that "forest bathing," for instance, can improve immune cell function with effects that last a week or even more.

AVOID FALLING INTO THE SEDENTARISM TRAP IN BETWEEN EXERCISE SESSIONS

Have you heard that sitting is the new smoking? Being more sedentary, even if you do exercise at some point each day, is bad for your health and bad for your immune system. Yet many of us, myself included, have to spend several hours at a desk to do our jobs. To ward off the ill effects of too much sitting, get up and walk around for a few minutes, do a few stretches, or run on the spot, at least once every hour during the course of the day. There are also several desk accessories and configuration options that help you stay moving, including standing desks, treadmill desks, and under-desk bike pedals.

A NOTE FOR ATHLETES (OR ANYONE WHO EXPERIENCES REGULAR INTENSE, PHYSICAL STRESS)

One of the areas where exercise has been especially studied is in professional athletes, who are known to have increased susceptibility to common infections like colds and flu, or reactivation of certain latent viruses such as Epstein-Barr virus. The stakes for professional athletes are high, of course: getting sick can mean missing out on career-critical competitions. Immune suppression from the intense level of physical training may well be behind this connection, although other factors in an athlete's life—higher stress, sleep deprivation, jet lag, crowds, and being in travel hubs and in confined spaces with others, like on airplanes—may also contribute.

For competitive athletes and for anyone else who has to operate at a high level of intensity (I'm thinking of other professions with high physical demands like dancers, landscapers, construction workers, and firefighters), it's a good idea to work with a specialized nutritionist who can help you compensate for the stress on your body and immune system through resilience-building, anti-inflammatory, and antioxidant support, as well as mitigate the effects of ancillary factors such as stress and jet lag. The principles of the Immune Resilience Diet and lifestyle measures described in this book provide an excellent foundation. You'll also need to work out specific cycles of intensity and rest to balance negative effects. Specific supplemental nutraceuticals such as vitamin D, glutamine, bovine colostrum, phytonutrients, and mushroom-derived beta-glucans have also shown promise in countering the increased incidence of respiratory tract infections and boosting the numbers of white blood cells in athletes in regular training.

CATCHING ZZZ'S

Good sleep has become a luxury in our modern, light-filled, demanding, and distracting world. I am continually surprised by how many people, when I inquire, let out a long exhale and shake their head as they begin to tell me just how elusive a really good night's sleep is.

Our lives are set up so differently from those of our ancestors. Rather than rising on first light and retiring to bed once the sun has faded over the horizon, we live in environments where artificial light has become all-pervasive. For several hours a day, day and night, many of us are now fixated on our computer or other device screens, like televisions, smartphones, tablets, gaming systems, and computers. These are all sources of blue light, which is particularly potent at suppressing melatonin, your natural sleep hormone (and immune friend). And it's not just light that disrupts sleep. More than 15 percent of Americans are engaged in some form of shift work that impacts regular sleep timing. And many of us burn the candle at both ends during the week, with the goal of "catching up" on missed sleep over the weekends. All this takes its toll on your health and your immune system, as you know from chapter 9. Catch-up "recovery" sleep isn't a fail-safe either. Preliminary research data show that *some* biological immune function tests that are detrimentally affected by poor sleep can be normalized by recovery sleep. But not all.

When we sleep better, our immune system benefits. Extensive amounts of research put the ideal amounts of sleep at between seven and nine hours per night, but like most things, the right amount can be an individual thing. One reason for this is that it's not just quantity that's important. Quality is, too. Interestingly, in one research study, participants who slept less than seven hours per night but reported that they felt like they were getting adequate sleep did not have the same increased immune vulnerability (in this study, to pneumonia) as those who slept more but who didn't feel it was enough. Ask yourself this: Do I wake feeling rested and refreshed? Or do I still feel tired and have to drag myself out of bed? If you answered no and then yes, you still need to take a look at these sleep guidelines to help you get a more "productive" night's sleep.

GOOD SLEEP STRATEGIES FOR ALL OF US

SET UP YOUR BEDROOM

- Turn down the thermostat: You want to keep your bedroom cool. An ideal sleeping temperature is around 60 to 65 degrees Fahrenheit.
- Keep your bedroom completely dark for sleeping: turn off digital clock displays and get some blackout blinds if needed.
- Remove or turn off appliances in your bedroom that make noise (except for sound machines, which can help).

EVENING HABITS

- Keep a sleep routine: Try to go to bed at the same time each night to train your biological clock.
- Turn off screens at least two hours before bed: If you have to use a screen in the evening, use a light-filtering app or eyeglasses that reduce blue light emissions.
- Avoid anxiety-provoking activity before bed (anything from news, paying bills, checking your financial reports, to arguments and other difficult conversations).
- Do your aerobic exercise earlier in the day, preferably before 6:00 p.m.

FOOD AND DRINK

- Avoid eating large meals just before bed: aim to finish eating two to four hours before retiring.
- Avoid drinking more than 4 to 6 ounces before you go to bed.
- Stay away from caffeine-containing drinks and foods after 2:00 p.m.: if you're really sensitive you may need to limit yourself to just one drink in the morning, or none at all.
- Steer clear of alcohol: it may send you to sleep initially, but it tends to promote wakefulness during the second half of the night.

LAST BUT NOT LEAST
- Check your medications: some can have stimulating effects.
- Consider a sleep-tracking tool. There are several simple yet smart wearables that can measure how long you've slept as well as the kind of sleep you've had.

EXTRA SLEEP SUPPORT IF YOU NEED IT

If you've followed all the advice above and you're still struggling with good sleep, there is more you can do. First, make sure your diet is really dialed in—full of healthy and anti-inflammatory foods. The Immune Resilience Diet is your starting point for that. Second, look for any potential sources of inflammation beyond diet that could be disrupting your sleep—inflammation is known to interfere with sleep. This could be your microbiome, toxins in your everyday environment, or chronic infections of any kind. Following the guidance in this book, with particular attention to those areas, will help. Third, make sure you have your stress resilience well and truly nailed. Stress can disrupt sleep, and poor sleep can create stress. It's a self-reinforcing cycle that you'll want to break if you're in it. The next section of this chapter will give you some tools to work on stress resilience. Also consider some of these natural sleep aids that are my favorites and the ones I most regularly use in clinic:

- *L-theanine.* L-theanine helps to boost the levels of gamma-aminobutyric acid (GABA) in your brain, which counters the effects of excitatory signaling molecules. Research suggests that L-theanine works by helping your body fall asleep more readily and improving restorative sleep. 50–200 mg per day.

- *Melatonin.* Melatonin is highly effective for promoting healthy sleep, and I also find it useful to help counter the effects of jet lag and shift work. 1–3 mg per day, 30 to 60 minutes before bed.

- *Magnesium.* Magnesium is well known for its calming effect. It can actually get right in there at a biochemical level and block the activity of more stimulatory compounds that might be keeping you awake. 400–600 mg per day.

- *Tryptophan foods.* Tryptophan is the amino acid (a protein block) that your body uses to make serotonin, a feel-good hormone, as well as your sleep hormone melatonin. Foods high in tryptophan include chicken, turkey, oats, cheese, whole wheat, bananas, nuts, and seeds. Consuming these foods with some carbohydrate component (as is also found in wheat, bananas, nuts, and seeds) helps deliver that tryptophan into the brain, where it can get to work on your sleep mechanisms. Including these foods regularly can help give your body the materials it needs to induce sleep.

- *Omega-3 fats.* Getting more of these essential, anti-inflammatory fats appears to be key for sleep. Studies have shown that omega-3 fats can improve restorative sleep, increase sleep duration, and reduce night wakings. For extra sleep support, look for an omega-3 supplement that can provide a higher-than-normal DHA content of around 600 mg per day.

- *Herbal teas.* Valerian, chamomile, lavender, lemon balm, and passion-flower have all been researched for their sleep-promoting effects. In addition, the act of brewing tea and slowly sipping the warming liquid can be very relaxing and put you in the right mood for sleep.

STRESS

Destructive stress levels harm your immune resilience, no doubt about it. Not only that, but when we're stressed, it's almost impossible to keep other important immune resilience behaviors in line, too: our sleep can be disturbed, we might exercise less, skip important self-care habits, or binge on unhealthy food choices. Keeping your stress levels in check is essential.

Too often when we're talking about stress, we use the term *stress man-agement*. I really dislike the term. *Management* suggests that we need to introduce control. It's often taken to mean that we have to spend more time relaxing and try to avoid overly stressful situations. If we stay in a demand-ing job, then we're somehow failing at stress management. If we set our-selves overly ambitious goals, we're not doing right by ourselves. I do agree that we all need *some* downtime, but I can't get on board with the idea of trying to relinquish as much life stress as possible. It's not really feasible. And, in fact, just thinking about that is positively stressful!

I much prefer the term *stress resilience*. It's a theme I'm sure you're sensing. When we're stress *resilient*, we're not trying to overly control stressful situations that come our way. After all, life is unpredictable—we simply cannot control everything we must face on a daily basis. And life is not a walk in the park for most of us either. There are always bills to pay, dependents to care for, deadlines to meet, exams to pass, and curveballs that strike at some point, like job loss, divorce, or the death of a loved one. Stress resilience is about being able to successfully navigate—and even grow through—life's challenges. It's about finding your "eustress," or *you*-stress, level, that positive level of stress that fosters strength and wisdom even as it puts you outside your comfort zone. It's reflective of an attitude that doesn't shy away from emotions, that responds positively to chal-lenges and is open to growth.

One of my biggest ever aha! moments came when a wise educator in stress resilience explained that having some kind of regular mind-body practice (otherwise known as a stress management practice) wasn't just about relaxing in that moment, although that is a helpful piece of it. But, even more important, it's about training your mind so that it learns a dif-ferent response to stress. That way, even when you're not in the middle of your mind-training practice, your brain is still able to respond to stresses in a more resilient way. It helps you feel strong emotions when they come along without being debilitated by them. This training is about developing a skill, just like any other skill, which needs to be practiced in order for you to become comfortable with it. Patricia, whom you first met in part 2, faced unavoidable stresses on a daily basis, and was at first skeptical that this would work. But by using mind-body practices (the ones that best fit into her routine), she started to notice that she felt differently at other times of the day, too—less anxious and more relaxed. Many other individuals I've worked with have found the same.

One more related piece of the puzzle in my own journey came into place as I happily let go of "managing" my stressors. And that was that while we cannot control the events of each day, we *can* control how we respond to them. These mind shifts are much more powerful than simply asking a busy person to make space in their day to breathe deeply.

There are so many different kinds of mind-training practices. Once again, it's so important to find what speaks to you. My personal favorites are derived from the book *Peace Is Every Step* by Thich Nhat Hanh, a guide for incorporating mindfulness practices into everyday moments (perfect for those of us with busy lives!) and spending time in nature. There's something so humbling about being in the vast richness of the natural world that is incredibly grounding and resets your perspective on pretty much anything. Those activities, and talking with close friends and family, playing with our pooch, making a cup of tea, and simply watching our kids grow.

MIND-BODY PRACTICE OPTIONS

- *Meditation.* Meditation practices are about cultivating an awareness of ourselves, of our thoughts and emotions. Through meditation we can increase our mindfulness, our ability to be present and fully engaged in whatever we're doing in that moment. It helps minimize how much our thoughts dwell on what might have happened, or what's to come. It's about being nonjudgmental and non-fearful of ourselves, our thoughts, and our feelings. There are some great research studies out there showing how meditation can improve measures of immune function like reduced immune cell aging, improved antibody response, and reduced inflammation. There are also many books, apps, and in-person lessons to help you learn the techniques of meditation. You can find some of my favorites in the Resources section.

- *Tapping.* Tapping is more formally called "emotional freedom technique" (EFT). Similar to acupuncture, tapping focuses on certain energy points in the body (known as *energy meridians*), which are based on traditional Chinese medicine. But unlike acupuncture, tapping is something you can do easily at home on a regular basis. Studies have shown that tapping may significantly decrease measures of stress and anxiety.

- *Tai chi.* Tai chi is another technique that originates in China. It's sometimes known as "meditation in motion," which I often find is a great way for meditation newbies to start, since sitting still for long periods can initially be quite daunting and even difficult. But tai chi isn't just for newcomers. Regular tai chi practice has been shown to improve depression, anxiety, and general stress, as well as slow biological signs of aging.

- *Yoga.* Yoga doesn't just work on strength and flexibility; it is also a highly effective mind-body practice. Even in the scientific literature, yoga is recognized for its ability to retrain your outlook on stressful events, which researchers speculate may derive from the postures themselves as well as the increased mind and body awareness that is encouraged by the practice. The bottom line is that yoga can improve self-confidence, emotional resilience, and reduce anxiety.

- *Prayer.* Prayer is an important mind-body practice in large part because it is used so widely. The act of prayer elicits the relaxation response, reframes what is within our control and what is not, and can foster feelings of gratitude, compassion, and hope, all of which have positive effects on well-being and our response to stress.

- *Cognitive behavioral therapy (CBT).* CBT is an approach used by psychotherapists that looks at changing destructive thoughts, beliefs, attitudes, and behaviors and improving our ability to regulate emotions. Although I often recommend CBT when the techniques I've mentioned above aren't enough—for instance, when I'm working with someone who has experienced some form of trauma in their past or present—CBT is really an effective tool that anyone can use to help improve their resilience toward life's stressful situations.

OTHER HELPFUL THINGS FOR STRESS

- *Sleep*. When we're sleep deprived, our stress response (and immune) system becomes imbalanced. Research has shown that if we restrict sleep to four hours even on just one night, we tend to underproduce cortisol in the morning, when it should be helping us wake up. And we tend to overproduce cortisol later in the afternoon and evening. Once again, sleep quality plays an important role: poor-quality sleep, even without a reduced number of hours of sleep, can put our stress response system on hyperalert.

- *Exercise*. Exercise is a great stress buster! Exercise triggers your body's production of endorphins—natural "feel good" chemicals that help reduce feelings of anxiety and improve your mood. The net result is that exercise helps you feel calmer and more in control of your life.

- *Hobbies*. Doing something you love is a great way to unwind, maybe let your mind wander, and to spend time with others, if your hobby lends itself to that. Just try to choose something that doesn't involve screen time. If your hobby helps you stay healthy in other ways, too, all the better—for example, gardening, cooking, joining a walking club, dancing, owning a pet, or volunteering.

- *Life purpose*. A dramatic new increase in research into this subject has indicated that there are a host of potential benefits, including a more positive outlook and better stress resilience, waiting for those who commit to a purpose. You can find purpose in many ways—within your job, as a caregiver (yes, you parents and others who perform unpaid care for others!), as a hobby, as a mentor, or in charitable work.

- *A life edit*. Yes, I know I said that focusing on how you *respond* to stress is more important than reducing stressful situations. But there is a place for considering reducing your stress exposures when they *are* changeable and when they are pushing you beyond healthy levels. Do you really need to take on those extra commitments if your plate is already full? Or should you really keep up relationships you know are destructively stressful? Sometimes making those changes is essential to keep your stress resilience in balance.

NUTRITIONAL SUPPORT FOR STRESS RESILIENCE

Being a nutritionist, I have a ready tool set of nutritional interventions that can help promote a healthier stress response. Here are my favorites:

- *L-theanine.* L-theanine isn't just good for sleep. In fact, the mechanism by which it helps with sleep is by countering the stimulatory signals in your brain to bring better balance and calmness. 50–200 mg, one to three times per day. Green tea, mentioned just below, is also a source of L-theanine.

- *Magnesium.* As you read above, magnesium is a great de-stressor. Magnesium can be taken orally at up to 600 mg per day. I also like to recommend magnesium salt baths (such as Epsom salts or Dead Sea salts): the act of taking a bath is great for reducing feelings of stress and anxiety, and the magnesium is absorbed through the skin as you soak.

- *Ashwagandha (Withania somnifera).* Ashwagandha root is a long-used herb known for its helpful effects against emotional or mental strain. These effects have been studied in high-quality (randomized, double-blinded, placebo-controlled) human trials. See pages 240–242 for dosing.

- *Rhodiola (Rhodiola rosea).* Rhodiola is another wonderful anti-anxiety herb that helps bring balance to your stress response. Several clinical studies have reported on rhodiola's beneficial effects on mild forms of anxiety as well as its ability to help alleviate fatigue and improve mood and concentration. 200 mg twice per day. Note that some people experience difficulty sleeping if they take rhodiola in the afternoon or evening. If you notice this, stick to taking rhodiola only in the morning.

- *Herbal teas.* Valerian, chamomile, green tea, lavender, lemon balm, and passionflower have all demonstrated stress-reducing effects.

HOW TO TELL IF YOU'RE ACTUALLY IMPROVING YOUR STRESS RESILIENCE

In clinical practice, when I suspect an imbalanced stress response is a factor undermining someone's health and immune resilience, I often have them take a salivary cortisol test. While this can be a helpful snapshot, it's not something that individuals can use on a daily basis to tell how well they're doing in building good stress resilience. For that I turn to heart rate variability, something that can be easily measured at home and on the go, and that can provide the immediate feedback that is so useful in helping us all evolve our stress response.

Heart rate variability is a measure of the variation of time intervals between consecutive heartbeats. Surprisingly, perhaps, your heart isn't intended to tick as evenly as a metronome. Instead, a healthy heart has minute levels of variation in the time from one heartbeat to the next. These variations are a good thing, indicating that the subconscious part of your nervous system (known as the autonomic nervous system) is able to adjust continuously to its environment. In other words, it demonstrates its resilience. Sometimes you can really tell a difference—for example, when you take a few deep, slow breaths, and feel your heart rate slow. But most of the time the fluctuations are imperceptible to us. What is interesting in relation to stress is that having a higher resting heart rate variability is a good predictor of your ability to move through and recover from both mentally and physically stressful events.

Many wearable smart devices can track heart rate variability as well as sleep and other health parameters.

NATURE

As you learned from chapter 9, spending time outdoors and in nature can be highly beneficial for your immune system, increasing the capabilities of your special operations immune cells, boosting vitamin D, and supporting a healthier microbiota. Unfortunately, though, in our modern world the lack of nature is increasingly normalized—our living environments are ever more built up, we spend more time indoors, and even many of our plants are now plastic versions of their former selves. Children spend up to three times as many hours with computers and televisions as they do playing outside.

Having lived for some time in Switzerland, I got to see how one country's citizens, in love with the outdoors, make the absolute most of it. After work or on a weekend, Switzerland's natural environment is where it's at. Whether it's biking, hiking, horseback riding, sailing, lake swimming, rowing, paragliding (impressive), skiing, skating, or anything else you can think of—nearly everyone is doing something outside. And there's no age limit: I am ashamed to admit that I've been overtaken hiking up a Swiss mountainside by individuals who are in their seventies!

Here are some suggestions for embracing nature in your own way:

- *Start a garden.* Planting a garden, whether you have a backyard or a window ledge, immediately connects you with soil and plants. Studies have also shown that growing your own herbs, fruits, and vegetables is associated with *eating* more fruits and vegetables, which you know is a win for immune health.

- *Explore a local park.* Do you own "forest bathing" in your local park or green space. Go for a hike, have a picnic, or even just take a blanket to lie on and a book to read. You can also make it a social occasion with family and friends, or do your exercise while you're there, too.

- *Go camping.* Camping feels like the ultimate nature immersion. You are literally sleeping inches away from the dirt and undergrowth, and planting your feet in it from the moment you step out of your tent. Not only that, you're breathing in those beneficial volatile plant compounds all day and night.

- *Pick an outdoor hobby.* Gardening, hiking, fishing, or kayaking are just a few of the many options for outdoor hobbies. If those aren't your thing, consider collecting (flowers, fossils, stones, or shells, as long as the location allows for that), birdwatching, geocaching, or outdoor photography.

- *Integrate nature into what you're already doing.* Business meeting? How about making it a walking meeting outdoors? How about biking through the trails to work instead of driving? Meeting a friend for coffee? Make it a coffee-to-go and head to the woods together to hike.

CLEAN LIVING

Yes, hygiene has a special place in reducing our risk of catching a harmful germ, but recall that "clean" living in the context of immune resilience is all about reducing exposure to environmental chemicals that can get in the way of optimal immune function. We can do a lot to mitigate their effects on our body by supporting detoxification through good foods, exercise, and sleep. And, yes, it's impossible for us to avoid environmental toxins entirely. However, we're in an era of unprecedented levels of exposure to vast combinations of new, synthetic chemicals that affect our delicate hormonal, neurological, and immune systems in ways that are not yet well understood. And while the science is catching up, here (together with specific brand recommendations in the Resources section) are sensible ways you can reduce your risk levels and protect your health:

- *Foods:* Moving away from ultra-processed foods and getting to know your food supply chain gives you much more control over the environmental chemicals that you're exposed to. Shopping at farmers' markets, for example, is one of my favorite ways to find out more about where my food is coming from and is an incredibly gratifying, community-building way of sourcing food for dinner. In addition, choosing organic foods as much as possible is a good way to reduce your exposure to pesticides and herbicides. And careful fish selection reduces your exposure to mercury contamination. Hop back to pages 189–190 for more detailed guidance.

- *Food packaging:* Making conscious choices to avoid certain types of food packaging can make a big difference in your exposure to plastic-based chemicals like BPA, BPS, and phthalates. Choose unpackaged, fresh foods where possible and look for food storage alternatives made from more inert materials like glass and uncoated stainless steel.

- *Food utensils:* Avoid plastic food trays and wrapping, plastic drinks bottles, plastic-lined cans, cartons, and beverage cups, plastic plates and utensils, plastic straws, and plastic food storage containers. Especially avoid heating foods in plastic containers, or leaving plastic drinks containers out in the sun, since the higher temperature causes more chemical compounds to transfer into the food or drink inside.

- *Cookware:* Stainless steel, carbon steel, glass, properly glazed ceramic, enamel, stoneware, cast iron, and enamel-coated cast iron are good cookware choices. Ceramic cookware that is improperly glazed has been known to contain lead, so it's best to choose reputable brands that meet Proposition 65 standards (a California regulation that requires businesses to warn consumers about harmful chemical exposures). Newer nonstick cookware uses surfaces that are claimed to be free of some of the older perfluorochemicals. However, little is known about the new chemicals they use, so I prefer to stick to what I know is safest.

- *Water:* Use a good-quality water filter, at a minimum for cooking and drinking, or ideally for the whole-house water supply. A good choice is an activated carbon filtration system with a micron rating of 0.1 or less, since those are able to remove the most toxins, bacteria, and even some viruses, as well as metals and chlorine. Reverse osmosis filters are even more effective, filtering down to particle sizes of 0.001 microns, which catches more of the tinier particles like viruses, pesticides, and pharmaceutical contaminants. However, since they additionally remove nutrient minerals like calcium and magnesium, you'll need to be extra careful to source these fully through diet or supplementation. Using a combination of carbon filtration and reverse osmosis is most effective at minimizing contaminants. If you want to test your water (also something I highly recommend, especially if you're not sure about investing in a home filtration system), there are good options through National Testing Laboratories (watercheck.com) and Tap Score (mytapscore.com).

- *Indoor air:* Choose a HEPA filter in your vacuum cleaner and an air purification system that can remove most small particles and microbes from the air. Look for a system that is designed to handle the space you have—some handle smaller areas only. Avoid ionic air purifiers, since those generate ozone, which comes with its own health concerns. Support air purification with regular wet-mop and wet-

Hygiene Practices

While shoring up your immune defenses through food and lifestyle, don't forget that simple hygiene practices still protect you, especially when you know a particularly high-risk bug is circulating in your vicinity or if your immune system is compromised due to illness or medications. During the COVID-19 pandemic, social distancing, limiting group interactions, good indoor ventilation, hand washing, and sanitizing, as well as using face masks, were all demonstrated to be effective at reducing the risk of catching SARS-CoV-2. Basic hygiene practices also protect us from many other germs.

cloth cleaning (using a nontoxic cleaning solution, of course) to wipe up surface toxins.

- *Personal care products:* One of the best places to start to look for healthier personal care alternatives is the Environmental Working Group's Skin Deep database (available at ewg.org). It's a fantastic resource for learning about chemicals in personal care products as well as for finding products that do the job without harming your immune resilience.

- *Cleaning products:* Choose natural cleaning products that are free of chemicals such as phthalates. I use diluted household vinegar for many cleaning purposes like floors, windows, and counters. It removes grime and germs, helps prevent mold growth, and is odorless after it dries. One of the most challenging cleaning products to replace, I found, was my stainless-steel appliance cleaner. That is, until I discovered that a diluted vinegar solution to clean the grease off, followed by a polish with olive oil (other oils would work, too), was just the thing to get that satisfying, high-shine polished finish.

- *Scents and candles:* Scented candles and room fresheners can be a source of phthalates and other chemicals. Naturally fragranced or unscented beeswax or vegetable wax candles are a better choice.

- *Home décor:* There are good sources for toxin-free furniture, carpeting, decorating, and building materials that you can seek out over time.

- *Lead in older homes:* Any home built in the US before 1978 may still have lead paint on walls, trim, and other surfaces. If you live in an older house, it's a good idea to perform at least a basic evaluation. Home assessment kits for lead are available in hardware and building supply stores, or online. You can use these on old painted surfaces or even on ceramic serve ware. There are also more robust laboratory testing options available via the EPA's National Lead Laboratory Accreditation Program (NLLAP) and you can find an NLLAP-recognized laboratory through their directory. Licensed lead risk assessors, authorized by local health departments, can also perform the most thorough analysis, including evaluating whether the lead is an increased risk because the paint is chipping or spreading through house dust.

- *Lead in newer homes:* Even if you own a home built after 1978, you aren't necessarily guaranteed that it is lead free. Lead is still found in many brass plumbing fixtures and can also enter your house through municipal water than has been run through lead pipes.

- *Leave toxins at the door:* A simple but effective practice to reduce the toxins that are picked up and tracked into your home is to remove your outdoor shoes when you come inside.

- *Yard care:* Organic alternatives to pesticides and weed killers are increasingly available and work for many purposes by using a combination of natural ingredients like essential oils, lemon juice, or vinegar. Mulch and corn gluten meal also act as effective barriers to control weed growth. Much more information about natural solutions, including simple homemade preparations, can be found online.

- *Vegetable garden soil:* Many of my clients have found harmful levels of toxic metals including lead and arsenic when they test the soil they're using for homegrown veggies. These contaminating metals can come from vehicle exhaust, industrial waste, runoff from other properties, old fertilizers and pesticides (especially in old orchards), railroad ties and other treated lumber, old paint chips, or past floods. A soil test is the best way to determine if any toxic metals are contaminating your garden soil. Many universities offer excellent and affordable soil-testing services. Since it can be very difficult to remove toxic metals from soil, the best remediation is often to use a raised planter with clean topsoil.

We've covered a lot of ground in this chapter. Depending on where you're starting from, all these "to dos" may seem a little overwhelming. If that's what you're feeling, don't worry. Pick just two to three things that you want to start working on first. Then you can circle back to working on another batch when those feel like they are comfortably ingrained into your routine.

_____

To view the references cited in this chapter, please visit www.immuneresilienceplan.com/science.

CHAPTER 14

Underlying Conditions That Can Derail Immune Resilience

And What to Do About Them

What does diabetes have to do with immune resilience against infections? What about constipation or heartburn? Depression or low thyroid function? It turns out, they can sometimes hamper your immune system quite a bit.

You read earlier about how a compromised immune system can be a significant contributor to most chronic diseases. Now in this chapter, we'll look at the unfortunate reciprocal situation in which some chronic conditions can negatively affect your immune system. The good news is that all these underlying conditions are in large part lifestyle diseases, meaning that they can be worsened or improved by how we live and how we eat. They are perfect targets for naturally shoring up our immune function, as well as improving overall health. You'll also be pleased to know that the Immune Resilience Diet is still *the* foundational diet to follow for each and every one of these underlying conditions. Simply make the adjustments recommended in this chapter to tailor your diet, lifestyle, and supplements if you have any one of the following: prediabetes or diabetes, weight issues, low thyroid function, depression or grief, chronic constipation, dry mouth, heartburn, or low stomach acid, or if you are simply interested in addressing immune changes that relate to aging. If you have none of these, you can skip ahead to the next chapter. As always, if you do have any medical condition, speak with your physician before making any changes.

PREDIABETES AND TYPE 2 DIABETES

Poorly regulated blood sugar that characterizes prediabetes and type 2 diabetes is associated with defects in all three pillars of the immune system: barriers, immune cells, and microbiota. Too much circulating blood sugar damages cells, blood vessels, and organs throughout the body. We looked at some of the ways it does this in chapter 6, when we discussed about how barrier cells, from your skin to your gut, to even the corneas of your eyes, start to lose their integrity and ability to heal in a high-sugar environment. Excess sugars may also damage salivary glands, undermining another important first line of defense and protector of oral health. Researchers have also observed sluggish responses from patrolling white blood cells in individuals with type 2 diabetes: defective respiratory bursts, weakened phagocytosis, impaired use of those biochemical "weapons," and weaker communication signals between cells. Sugars also nourish bad bugs at the expense of good ones, so disturbances in the microbial ecosystems of the gut as well as other sites around the body is another characteristic of type 2 diabetes.

At the same time that immune protection falters, inflammation gets ramped up—turned on by the inflammatory effects of higher blood sugar as well as the bad bugs in your microbiota that start to make more "noise." This effect has been observed and reported in top-tier journals such as *The Lancet,* in which scientists have also connected diabetes with deadlier COVID-19 and H1N1 influenza infections. Other scientists have observed that higher levels of insulin, which can be seen years before blood glucose even starts to trend higher, can promote inflammation by "potentiating" the effects of lipopolysaccharides (LPS) coming from bad bacteria in the gut on immune cells, essentially giving them a megaphone that then startles those immune cells into a higher level of distress and inflammation signaling.

Using a Continuous Glucose Monitor (CGM) to Better Understand Your Blood Sugar

Science has recently discovered that your glycemic response to food (the degree to which a particular food raises your blood sugar) differs from the next person's. Sometimes quite substantially. A continuous glucose monitor, which tracks your blood sugar levels throughout the day and night, helps you identify what works for you and what doesn't. I find it much more illuminating than intermittent finger prick tests, which miss the fluctuations. Some of the useful things my clients have discovered (or confirmed) through using a continuous glucose monitor are:

- Once you have prediabetes or diabetes, you can't always eat a generic healthy diet (such as one that includes whole grains, legumes, and fruits) and expect to turn the tide of blood sugar dysregulation. Your body is at this point responding in a dramatically different way to these foods than that of someone without insulin resistance.

- Whole grains (like whole-wheat bread or pasta) often drive up blood sugar nearly as much as their "white" counterparts. Oatmeal, often recommended as a breakfast option for diabetes eating plans, can do the same.

- Large increases in blood sugar triggered by the wrong foods set off a pattern of imbalance (high and low blood sugar readings) that can last several days before it normalizes, even if you immediately go back to eating the right way. That's why it's important to stick strictly to avoiding high-carbohydrate foods.

- Low blood sugar dives (that most often follow the highs) are often associated with intense cravings that drive a vicious cycle of poor food choices. Another reason why control can be hard to regain if you eat off plan.

- Blood sugar can go up when you *don't* eat. Your body has built-in mechanisms to release glucose from stored locations and provide short-term glucose supplies to critical organs during the early stages of fasting. Sometimes this "rebound" effect can push your blood sugar higher than if you stick to regular eating patterns. If you find this is happening, try sticking to regular eating times and counter any spikes you notice with a low-carbohydrate, high-fiber snack or meal.

- Pay attention to stress. Sometimes it's not just food that's driving up your blood sugar. Spikes can be seen after stressful events or even a poor night's sleep.

The downsides to CGMs are that they are expensive, insurance coverage varies, and (at the time of this writing) they aren't easily available without a prescription. You can find more information about the latest CGM options in the Resources section and at the companion website for this book: www.ImmuneResiliencePlan.com.

All this helps explain why those with type 2 diabetes have a higher risk for many types of infections and almost universally suffer more when they do get sick. Osteomyelitis, pneumonia, cellulitis, peritonitis, urinary tract infections, foot infections, wound or surgical site infections, periodontal disease, and worsened COVID-19 are all more common in those with type 2 diabetes. And the risk for hospitalization for these illnesses is much higher. Hospitalization rates for COVID-19, for example, are up to six times higher in those with type 2 diabetes than in those without.

TWEAKS TO YOUR IMMUNE RESILIENCE DIET

Diet is your biggest lever when it comes to lowering your blood sugar. And the most impactful way you can change your diet is to lower your carbohydrate intake. The reason is that once your body has lost its tolerance for carbohydrates, it cannot manage them in the same way as the body of someone who is metabolically healthy. That's why simply eating a healthy version of a higher-carbohydrate diet is not usually enough to bring blood sugar back under control. I've witnessed reams of absolute transformations in the metabolic health and blood sugar control of individuals who have followed a lower-carb approach, especially when used alongside support for other potential blood sugar influencers—your microbiota (yes, having the wrong kinds of bugs living in your gut spells bad news for blood sugar), environmental toxins, exercise, stress, and sleep—together with targeted supplemental support. For those of us carrying excess weight, this approach drops pounds, too. Here's how to do this to get those same benefits:

- Strictly avoid all sources of sugars and other refined carbohydrates including candy, sweetened drinks, juices, white pasta, white rice, pizza, and ice cream. In other words, shift from an 80 percent "flexible" approach to as close to 100 percent avoidance as you can while your metabolism is under this kind of stress; it can't appropriately deal with excursions.
- Steer clear of all foods containing starchy potatoes (white and sweet potatoes), grains, legumes, and fruits with the exception of the following low-glycemic fruits: avocados, berries, lemons, limes, and olives.
- Make a solid effort to shift from conventionally reared animal foods to organic ones, since the type of saturated fats that are higher in conventionally reared animals are linked with insulin resistance.
- Add good blood sugar regulators to your diet: fibrous vegetables, sea vegetables such as kelp or wakame, fermented foods, cinnamon, and green tea are good choices.
- Practice intermittent fasting (see page 226).
- If you have dry mouth, consider the strategies on page 291.
- Use a continuous glucose monitor (CGM) to learn how your body's blood sugar responds to different foods (highly recommended).

TWEAKS TO YOUR LIFESTYLE

Following the lifestyle recommendations in this book is another key component of regulating your blood sugar. Cortisol, a major stress hormone, is a potent stimulator of increased blood sugar. Remember: this happens because your body thinks it needs to run away from a predator and therefore makes its primary energy source (glucose) more readily available to be used by your muscles and brain. The best way to counter this is through daily downtime and stress-response training, as well as good sleep practices and regular exercise. Flip back to chapter 13 for ideas.

Many endocrine-disrupting toxins are also well known to interfere with your metabolism and promote higher blood sugar and weight gain. These are even known scientifically as *obesogens*. Some of the biggest culprits you'll already now know from chapter 8—BPA, PCBs, phthalates, and flame retardants, which are collectively pervasive in food packaging, cosmetics and personal care products, and home furnishings. High fructose corn syrup also falls into this category.

SUPPLEMENT CONSIDERATIONS

- Choose a multivitamin that contains chromium (as chromium picolinate, 100–200 mcg per day for up to six months at a time), since this trace mineral is needed for cells to use glucose.
- Berberine improves insulin sensitivity and microbial balance in the gut; it also counters inflammation. 500 mg three times per day with food (start with once per day and gradually increase to three times to avoid nausea and abdominal discomfort).
- Garlic extract. 1,000–1,500 mg twice per day.
- Ginger root extract. 500–1,000 mg (standardized to 4–5 percent gingerols) two to three times per day.
- Probiotics. 10–50 billion CFUs in a multi-strain product.

WEIGHT ISSUES

We know from the science that being underweight or overweight is associated with a greater chance of getting infections.

Being underweight (having a body mass index, or BMI, of less than 18.5) can result from inadequate food intake as well as conditions that either impair nutrient absorption, metabolism, or utilization, or excessively use nutrients so as to drain body reserves. This malnutrition affects all the body's essential functions, including the immune system, due to the insufficient availability of calories, protein, and other nutrients needed for it to work well. Studies have shown that low weight–associated malnutrition leads to reduced cytokine production, barrier breakdown, and reduced phagocyte function. Acquired immunity is impaired, too, since T cells are diminished, as is sIgA production and B cell activity.

In several large studies, obesity (having a body mass index of 30 or greater) has been associated with increased risk of acquiring any kind of infection. In a study of nearly 1,500 individuals in Germany, obese participants consistently reported a higher frequency of both upper and lower respiratory tract infections. In a study of more than 39,000 Swedish adults, obesity was linked with increased infection risk in both women and men. It has been shown that overweight and obese individuals produce fewer B cells in response to vaccines, making immunizations less effective. Being overweight also tends to increase overall inflammation throughout the body.

Weight Associations with Specific Infections, by Age Group in Developed Countries

	Children and Adolescents	Adults
Underweight	Respiratory tract infections Surgical site infections	Community-acquired infections Community-acquired pneumonia Influenza-associated pneumonia
Obese	Acute bronchitis Urinary tract infections	Community-acquired infections Community-acquired pneumonia Influenza-associated pneumonia Hospital-based infections Skin infections Urinary tract infections Surgical site infections Sepsis

The reasons for underweight issues can be diverse and complicated. It's best to work with a qualified practitioner who can help determine whether that underweight status is an issue and help address it if needed. If you're struggling at the other end of the weight spectrum, with being overweight or obese, the ideal first step is to follow the recommendations above for prediabetes and diabetes, since those also effectively address the excess weight that is harming your metabolism and immune system. Also review the next section on low thyroid function (and get your thyroid hormone levels checked), since this can also promote excess weight gain.

LOW THYROID FUNCTION

Thyroid hormone affects the level of activity in every single cell you have. It's like the "master key" that turns on metabolic activity in every cell that it touches. Normally, circulating levels of thyroid hormone are kept in balance, keeping cell operations running smoothly. However, when we have too much or too little thyroid hormone circulating, things can start to go wrong. According to the American Thyroid Association, an estimated 20 million Americans have some form of thyroid disease, but up to 60 percent are unaware of it.

Thyroid conditions that result in low hormone output are most relevant for immune resilience. In some parts of the world where iodine deficiency is prevalent, the lack of this nutrient is the most common cause of low thyroid hormone. However, in the US, the most common cause is a process of autoimmunity where the immune system mistakenly attacks and slowly destroys the thyroid gland, the site of thyroid hormone production. This condition is called Hashimoto's thyroiditis. Over time, this process causes the levels of circulating thyroid hormone to go down, which can lead to the classic low thyroid symptoms: fatigue, weight gain, constipation, depression, dry skin, cold sensitivity, and thinning hair.

Although there has been very little research into the effects of low thyroid function on the risk for infection, what science has uncovered suggests that there are potential associations with impaired immune activity. Immune cells, such as natural killer cells, dendritic cells, and macrophages, are all under the master regulatory control of thyroid hormone, just like other cells; in general, low thyroid hormone leads to a less activated immune system. Individuals with diagnosed low thyroid function, for instance, don't mount a fever against an infection as readily as those with normal thyroid function. However, inflammatory pathways can be turned on, perpetuating that state of chronic inflammation. Not least, the very nature of the destructive and inappropriate immune behavior that is the process of autoimmunity is a sign of an immune system that is unhappy.

Identifying and managing low thyroid function through your primary care physician and endocrinologist is essential to keep the effects of low thyroid function to a minimum. In addition, there are dietary and lifestyle tools that you can use to address some of the newly understood underlying reasons why your immune system became so distressed and erratic in the first place. When I work with someone who has Hashimoto's thyroiditis, we look at all areas of their diet and lifestyle. We remove pro-inflammatory foods and, at first, gluten-containing foods, since gluten is known to stimulate this particular autoimmune process in some individuals. We look at other factors that can disturb immune balance like the microbiota, intestinal permeability, environmental toxins, stress, and sleep.

If you have Hashimoto's thyroiditis, here are steps you can try at home:

TWEAKS TO YOUR IMMUNE RESILIENCE DIET

- Strictly remove all sources of sugars and other refined carbohydrates including candy, sweetened drinks, white pasta, white rice, pizza, and ice cream.
- Avoid all sources of gluten for a period of at least eight weeks, ideally while tracking the effects of this change on the levels of thyroid antibodies your body is producing. (This is a blood test that your physician can help you with or that is also available through some direct-to-consumer labs noted in the Resources section.) After eight weeks,

slowly bring gluten back into your diet, tracking how you feel and seeing how it affects your next blood test reading.

SUPPLEMENT CONSIDERATIONS

- Probiotics. 10–50 billion or more CFUs in a multi-strain supplement.
- EPA/DHA. 2–4 grams per day.
- Curcumin. 500 mg three times per day.

For anyone with Hashimoto's thyroiditis, I strongly recommend also being evaluated for celiac disease, since the prevalence is higher than in the general population. If celiac disease is confirmed, then the recommendation to avoid gluten should become permanent. If you feel that you need additional support, work with a qualified practitioner in functional medicine or personalized nutrition to explore and address any other underlying contributors to the autoimmune process.

Gluten-Containing Foods

The following grains contain gluten: barley, bulgur, kamut, oats (unless specified gluten free), rye, semolina, spelt, triticale, wheat, and wheat germ. Gluten can often appear in prepared foods that you might not expect, including beer, bouillon and broths, candy, chewing gum, cold cut meats, chips and other snacks, condiments, flavored teas, fish sticks, gravies, hot dogs, instant drink mixes, and sauces. More detail can be found at websites catering to those with celiac disease (the most recognized gluten-related disorder) such as celiac.org.

DEPRESSION AND GRIEF

If you've recently suffered a significant loss—like losing a loved one, going through a divorce, or losing your job—your immune system can be affected.

A recent scientific review paper that looked at all the studies on bereavement over the last forty-five years found that there was significant evidence for detrimental immune changes happening after a major loss. These included higher levels of systemic inflammation, altered immune cell behavior, and lower antibody responsiveness.

Even without significant grief, ongoing subclinical mild depression (levels too low for an official diagnosis) is a form of stress that can undermine your immune resilience and weaken immunity. According to the American Psychological Association, duration of depression has the biggest impact on your immune system—more so than its severity. The same goes for social isolation and feelings of loneliness, which have both become more prominent as a result of social contact restrictions during the COVID-19 pandemic.

Some kinds of emotionally challenging and stressful situations just can't be avoided. Focusing on shoring up other factors that support healthy immunity becomes ever more important to compensate for this particular challenge. This means utilizing the healthy, immune-supportive eating habits in the Immune Resilience Diet. It means weeding out anything that feeds inflammation, like processed foods and sugars, an uncared-for microbiota, and environmental toxins. It means incorporating some moderate exercise, good sleep, and time out in nature. In addition, focusing on stress resilience skills that help your mind (and body) reset their responses to those real stressors makes a measurable difference to immune function.

TWEAKS TO YOUR IMMUNE RESILIENCE DIET

- Understand that depression and grief are risk factors for poor food choices and insufficient nutrient intake. Seek support if you are unable to maintain a healthy weight and food intake during this time.
- Focus on stocking your pantry and freezer with real food: healthy go-to meals and snacks that you can grab quickly when you're not feeling in the mood to cook.
- Avoid caffeine, alcohol, sugary drinks, and refined carbohydrates; these are going to make you feel worse rather than better. Keep them

out of your house and avoid situations where you'll be overly tempted to indulge.

- Drink herbal tea. Herbal teas are not only great for your immune system, but the routine of making a warm tea, inhaling the aromas, and slowly sipping it is a great way to bring relaxation, nourishment, and immune support into your day. Passionflower, chamomile, rooibos, and echinacea teas are good choices for both relaxation and immune support.

TWEAKS TO YOUR LIFESTYLE

- Adopt a stress resilience technique that you can practice daily. See page 264 for ideas.
- Find a way to exercise regularly, ideally with a friend. One easy way is to meet outside for a walk, preferably in nature.
- Find something you're interested in—a hobby or passion—and let it provide a positive focal point to help bring some lightness to your day.
- Find ways to help others. We can derive a great deal of positive feeling from helping others improve their situation.

SUPPLEMENT CONSIDERATIONS

- Rhodiola (*Rhodiola rosea*) can be particularly helpful. 200 mg twice per day. Note that some people experience difficulty sleeping if they take rhodiola in the afternoon or evening. If you notice this, stick to taking rhodiola only in the morning.

Did You Know? Inflammation Feeds Depression

Even as feelings of grief and depression feed inflammation, so too does inflammation feed a low mood. This has been shown in many research studies. This only makes it ever more important to interrupt that cycle by clearing up sources of inflammation in the body wherever you can—through your diet, your gut microbes, toxins, and lifestyle.

• See additional supplement recommendations on page 244 for stress resilience.

CHRONIC CONSTIPATION

Movement keeps ecosystems healthy. When the movement of our bowels is blocked, we get more stagnation, and the removal of potential pathogens and toxins is compromised. It's no surprise then that scientists find higher levels of pathogenic bacteria and fungi in the digestive tracts of constipated individuals compared with those without constipation. They also find lower concentrations of beneficial bacterial species and increased gut leakiness. They see immune changes as well, including reduced phagocytosis and elevated antibody levels to pathogenic *E. coli* and *Staphylococcus aureus* species.

Constipation can also promote urinary tract infections, since a backup of contents in the rectum and colon can put pressure on the bladder and urethra, preventing them from emptying completely. This promotes bacterial retention and growth in the urinary tract that can lead to infection. In one study of 209 children with chronic UTIs, 65 percent showed improvement after an intervention targeted at reducing constipation that included higher-fiber foods and more exercise. Nutrition and lifestyle solutions to chronic constipation are often effective and relatively easy.

TWEAKS TO YOUR IMMUNE RESILIENCE DIET

Increased insoluble fiber and fermented foods are best for chronic constipation, both of which you'll be getting plenty of on the Immune Resilience Diet. Just be sure to pay extra attention to these foods, as well as your fluid intake.

• Insoluble fiber foods: whole grains, nuts, seeds (flaxseeds and chia seeds are good choices), beans, legumes, cauliflower, green peas, prunes, dark leafy greens, berries, apples (with skins).
• 2 tablespoons of flaxseed oil or olive oil first thing in the morning.

- Fermented foods: see pages 183–184 for ideas.
- Good hydration: an easy rule of thumb is to aim to drink half your body weight (in pounds) in fluid ounces of water or unsweetened, uncaffeinated drinks per day.

TWEAKS TO YOUR LIFESTYLE

- Focus on the exercise portion of your Immune Resilience lifestyle plan, since the movement of physical activity helps stimulate movement within your digestive tract.
- Sing and gargle: both stimulate your vagus nerve, which runs from your brain to all the key organs of your digestive tract. Stimulating this nerve can help support healthy digestive movements.

SUPPLEMENT CONSIDERATIONS

- Magnesium citrate: 400–800 mg per day.
- Vitamin C: up to 2 grams per day (start low and increase the dose gradually up to this amount or until you can "go" regularly).
- Laxative herbs for occasional use only: rhubarb, senna, aloe vera (juice or edible gel).
- Laxative herbs suitable for regular use: burdock root, triphala.

DRY MOUTH

As you now know, saliva is one of your body's first-line immune defenses: a guardian of resistance against mouth and airway infections as well as a protector of overall oral health. And you know that if oral health declines, the knock-on effects can impact other important organs and systems, such as your heart, joints, and immune system. Saliva washes billions of microbial cells from your mouth every day. It contains important biological chemicals that lubricate and break down foods to help you extract the nutrients they contain, that keep your teeth and gums healthy, and that inhibit the growth of bad bacteria.

Signs that you may have low saliva production include a dry or sticky feeling in your mouth, thickened saliva, bad breath, difficulty chewing and swallowing, a dry throat, and a dry or grooved tongue. Hundreds of medications can have the side effect of dry mouth, in particular antidepressants, blood pressure medications, pain medications, antihistamines, decongestants, and muscle relaxants. Sjögren's syndrome and diabetes are associated with increased risk for dry mouth. Stress decreases saliva production. Saliva production also declines as we age, making it even more common in older adults.

When I'm working with an individual who is experiencing dry mouth, there are several strategies we can use to help improve saliva production:

TWEAKS TO YOUR IMMUNE RESILIENCE DIET

- Get into the habit of cooking your meals rather than buying them or letting someone else cook for you, since the sights and smells of cooking will stimulate saliva production.
- Chew food thoroughly—up to thirty times per bite! This also stimulates saliva production.
- Drink herbal teas: ginger tea is a good choice, since ginger is known for its saliva-stimulating properties. Frequent sipping on unsweetened teas or water can alleviate dry mouth symptoms.
- Avoid caffeine, alcohol, carbonated drinks, smoking, and all sugars.

TWEAKS TO YOUR LIFESTYLE

- Adopt a favorite mind-body practice.
- Avoid peroxide- or alcohol-containing mouthwashes.

SUPPLEMENT CONSIDERATIONS

- Sugar-free lozenges (ginger, zinc, or xylitol).
- Marshmallow root slurry, a mixture of marshmallow root powder and water, swished for 20 seconds. Can be spat out or swallowed.

HEARTBURN
(GASTROESOPHAGEAL REFLUX, OR GERD)

It's important to talk about heartburn in relation to immune health because medications used to suppress acid production go against this important component of your body's natural barriers (as you learned in chapter 3). As a practitioner interested in getting to the root cause of health concerns rather than simply patching symptoms to mask an underlying issue, I prefer to look to solve heartburn naturally where possible. This can both alleviate the potential problems of heartburn medications and keep the function of stomach acid intact for immune health.

Low stomach acidity due to long-term use of certain acid-suppressing medications, especially proton pump inhibitors such as omeprazole, increases the risk for many different digestive infections such as bacterial infections and *Candida*, including those caused by drug-resistant strains. It also increases the risk for chest infections, thought to be because the lack of acid in the stomach promotes dysbiosis in both the stomach and esophageal tract, which can then contaminate the microbiota of the airways, especially when reflux occurs. Long-term use of acid-suppressive medications also increases the risk for nutrient deficiencies, including those that are used by our immune system since an acidic stomach environment is essential for the digestion and release of many nutrients, including protein, iron, and vitamin B_{12}.

Now I'm not suggesting you just discontinue a prescribed medication. Any changes you make to your prescriptions should be done in concert with your physician. However, there may be less risky pharmaceutical options for managing heartburn, such as bedtime H2 blocker medications, which predominantly suppress only nighttime acid production and carry less risk of dependence. In addition, heartburn is often driven by dietary and lifestyle factors and many instances can be alleviated by following these practices:

TWEAKS TO YOUR IMMUNE RESILIENCE DIET

- Identify and avoid trigger foods such as caffeine, alcohol, fried and fatty foods, chocolate, and carbonated beverages. Sometimes it may also be necessary to avoid spicy foods, tomato-based foods, citrus fruit, mint, garlic, and onion.
- Avoid overeating; instead, eat smaller, more frequent meals.
- Do not eat for two to three hours before going to bed.
- Eat slowly, deliberately, and chew your food completely.

TWEAKS TO YOUR LIFESTYLE

- Offer a few words of gratitude before a meal to allow your "rest and digest" response to kick in.
- Don't smoke.
- Address constipation, if this is a problem (see above).

Note that lack of sleep, chronic stress, and inadequate exercise have all been shown to play a role in some manifestations of heartburn, so be sure to pay attention to those components of your Immune Resilience Plan. In addition, read the following section on low stomach acid, which can also (surprisingly) be a cause of heartburn.

LOW STOMACH ACID

Having too little stomach acid independently of acid-suppressing medications can create the same immune problems that acid suppressants do. Common symptoms of low stomach acid include immediate bloating and indigestion after a regular meal, as well as burping and flatulence. Heartburn can also result from the stagnation of food in the stomach and from the stomach's increased mechanical action (churning) to try to compensate for too little acid. Longer-term effects relate to impaired nutrient digestion and can include iron deficiency, brittle fingernails, and fatigue, as well as immune impairments.

Identifying low stomach acid can be difficult and should be done by a qualified practitioner. However, you can try this at-home test to see if you are *likely* to have low stomach acid:

- Mix ⅛ teaspoon sodium bicarbonate into ⅓ cup room temperature water.
- Drink the mixture on an empty stomach (it will have a slightly salty taste).
- If you experience burping within five minutes of drinking the mixture, this may indicate low levels of stomach acid.

TWEAKS TO YOUR IMMUNE RESILIENCE DIET
- Avoid caffeine and alcohol.
- Avoid drinking excess fluids right before a meal.
- Eat slowly, deliberately, and chew food completely.
- Add fermented foods to your daily diet.

TWEAKS TO YOUR LIFESTYLE
- Good sleep, regular exercise, and having a healthy stress response can help improve stomach acid production, so don't skip any of those in your Immune Resilience Plan.
- Say or think some words of gratitude before a meal to allow your "rest and digest" response to kick in.

SUPPLEMENT CONSIDERATIONS
- Herbal bitters: gentian root, artichoke leaf, milk thistle, dandelion root.
- Peppermint oil (only if heartburn is *not* a symptom).
- Digestive enzymes, especially peptidases and proteases, which help break down protein.
- Betaine HCl (only under the guidance of a qualified practitioner).

OBSTRUCTIVE SLEEP APNEA

Obstructive sleep apnea (OSA) is a condition where your breathing is intermittently blocked during sleep by the over-relaxation of your throat muscles. When this happens, breathing typically resumes with a gasp, snort, or body jerk. You may not notice this, but it increases sleep restlessness and reduces the amount of oxygen your body receives while you're sleeping. Common signs of OSA include unexplained daytime tiredness, snoring, sudden nighttime wakings, irritability, anxiety, memory and concentration issues, and headaches.

There are several potential consequences of untreated OSA, including high blood pressure, heart problems, type 2 diabetes, mood disorders, and—according to the American Sleep Association—a weakened immune system that leaves you more vulnerable to infections and illness.

OSA is treated with a breathing-aid known as a CPAP machine, which provides a constant air pressure in the airways at nighttime to prevent their closure. Dentists can help address sleep apnea with nighttime oral appliances that help to promote unrestricted air flow. There are other things to consider, however, that can help address the complex underlying causes of OSA. Happily, eating an anti-inflammatory diet, getting enough exercise and sleep, and cultivating stress resilience are all important for improving OSA, and all of these are core components of your Immune Resilience Plan. In addition, the following can be helpful:

TWEAKS TO YOUR IMMUNE RESILIENCE PLAN

- Tackle other underlying conditions such as blood sugar dysregulation, GERD, and overweight/obesity, since all of these can contribute to OSA.
- Consider testing for nutrient deficits, microbiome dysregulation, food sensitivities, hormonal and neurotransmitter imbalances, as well as for sources of inflammation through the advanced laboratory testing options I've listed in the Resources section. All of these can play a role in OSA.

TWEAKS TO YOUR IMMUNE RESILIENCE DIET

- Avoid alcohol, since it can overly relax airway muscles.
- Consider an elimination diet to identify food sensitivities.
- Focus even harder on including anti-inflammatory foods—colorful plant foods, herbs, spices, and sources of omega-3 fats—as well as removing pro-inflammatory foods, like ultra-processed foods, sugars, and other refined carbohydrates.

SUPPLEMENT CONSIDERATIONS

- Vitamin D at a dose to achieve 40–60 ng/mL 25-OH-D on your blood test.
- Magnesium: 400 mg daily.
- EPA/DHA: 1.5 grams daily.
- Curcumin: 500 mg twice daily.

AGING

Okay, so aging isn't exactly a disease. However, aging is associated with a number of physiological changes that can undermine our immune resilience and increase the risk for infection, autoimmunity, and cancer—all immune-related conditions. While signs of age-related immune deterioration can appear from around age fifty onward, they tend to be most pronounced as we reach and surpass our seventy-year mark. This is why older adults can be more vulnerable to catching whatever's going around, like the flu, and to suffering more from it. And why vaccines become less effective in older individuals.

Some of the age-related changes affect our immune cells, particularly T and B cells involved in germ-specific immune responses and immunological memory. Other immune responses, like antiviral interferon gamma production, weaken, too. It is also well understood that, as we age, levels of inflammation gradually increase. There's even a word for this: *inflammaging*. This level of inflammation isn't always enough to be identified as any particular disease or even always manifest in apparent symptoms (although sometimes it is: many of the diseases of aging involve an inflammatory component). However, it can cause hidden changes in physiology including within the immune system.

While we can't avoid its inevitable end point, aging is a progression that is to a certain extent alterable. Scientists today are studying what makes some people age faster than others, and—perhaps no surprise—how we eat and live makes a big difference.

TWEAKS TO YOUR IMMUNE RESILIENCE DIET

- For those aged sixty-five years and older, increase protein intake to 1.2 grams per kilogram (2.2 pounds) of body weight daily.
- Practice intermittent fasting, as long as you are not underweight or have any other contraindication (see page 226).
- Increase vitamin E foods: nuts, nut oils, nut butters, seeds, seed oils, seed butters, avocados, or consider adding supplemental vitamin E (below).
- Add resveratrol foods: bilberries, blueberries, cranberries, peanuts. (Although red wine is a source of resveratrol, I don't recommend relying on it as an anti-inflammatory food since it can simultaneously promote inflammation. If you do already drink wine, it is okay to enjoy it occasionally, in moderation and alongside other foods.)

SUPPLEMENT CONSIDERATIONS

For those aged fifty years and older:

- Vitamin E: 200–400 IU per day (ideally, mixed natural tocopherols and tocotrienols).
- Curcumin: 500 mg twice daily.
- EPA/DHA: 1.5 grams daily.
- Vitamin C: 400–600 mg daily.
- Zinc: 15 mg daily.
- Probiotic: 2 billion CFUs or more in a multi-strain probiotic. While probiotics are generally considered to be extremely safe, for the very

aged or immunocompromised, consider using heat-killed probiotic species to avoid the very rare but potential risk for probiotic-related complications such as sepsis.

To view the references cited in this chapter, please visit
www.immuneresilienceplan.com/science.

CHAPTER 15

What to Do When You Get Sick

Short of living in complete, sanitized isolation, you are going to encounter germs. Many of them. And occasionally one is going to come along that makes you sick. Even if you follow the Immune Resilience Diet and lifestyle plan to a T! In this chapter, you'll find everything you need to know to help naturally address the mild symptoms you'll feel as your body mounts its immune response (something you'll have prepared it for well) to common infectious attacks and help your body defend itself quickly and powerfully so that you can bounce back to your usual self in no time. These are tried-and-true tools that can help manage minor symptoms at home and help give your immune system a leg up against the invading germ. Just remember: if your symptoms become severe or prolonged, you should always seek appropriate medical care.

FIRST, THE BASICS: FOR ALL KINDS OF MALADIES

Mom's advice bears repeating: proper rest can give your immune system the space and energy it needs to get you feeling better sooner. Especially when you're feeling achy or chilled, and certainly if you have a fever, all of which mean you're likely contagious. Sleep is what your body naturally craves when it's sick, anyway. And if you give yourself the space to do so when you notice that first sign of a congested nose or tickle in your throat, you can help your immune system fight back more effectively.

Second to sleep is how you eat and drink. All of the recommendations in this chapter assume you're using the Immune Resilience Diet principles as your baseline, even though there are adjustments noted under each illness type. Drinking plenty of fluids is even more important when you're ill, since you can be more prone to becoming dehydrated due to a fever, diarrhea, or vomiting. Keeping on track with healthy, immune-boosting foods will also go a long way. For example, chicken soup, a traditional home remedy for many ailments, actually has good scientific backing: The glutamine-rich bone broth provides an important energy source for your immune cells. The vegetables nourish your microbiome and, together with the easily digestible (long-cooked) chicken, provide quality nutrients for your immune system. And the steamy aromas gently moisten your mucous membranes, helping to ease congestion. I think that's pretty neat.

In addition to foods, we are fortunate to have good scientific evidence for the use of many nutrient and botanical supplements to ease symptoms and shorten the duration of several types of infections. You'll find all those here, too. Important to know is that early interventions tend to produce the best outcomes. So learn to tune in to your body and pay attention to those first signs and symptoms that tell you something is "off."

Now on to what to do for those everyday infectious illnesses. The list of options in each of the tables in this chapter is intended to provide considerations rather than a prescriptive list of interventions to follow all at once. You can be selective and choose either what you have on hand or what best fits each circumstance.

RESPIRATORY TRACT INFECTIONS

Infections of the respiratory tract include coughs, colds, flu, and sinusitis. They tend to be characterized by congestion in the nasal passages, throat, and/or lungs and can be caused by several different kinds of viruses.

Foods for all respiratory symptoms	• Chicken soup (see recipe on page 327). • Herbal teas: chamomile, echinacea, ginger, green tea, peppermint, sage, tulsi. Inhale the steam from the tea, too. • Fire cider (see recipe on page 358). • Raw, dark honey: a good congestion buster, sore throat and cough soother, and antimicrobial. Can be added to teas. • Fresh ginger. • Citrus fruits.
Supplements (taken orally) for all respiratory symptoms	• Vitamin C: 1,000–2,000 mg daily for up to 1 week; decrease dose if it causes diarrhea. • Vitamin D: 10,000 IU for 3 days. • Echinacea: 4,000 mg daily of a standardized extract for up to 1 week. Can continue with 2,000–2,500 mg daily for up to 8 weeks. • Black elderberry: 1,200 mg daily for up to 2 weeks. • Umckaloabo (*Pelargonium sidoides*) liquid herbal extract (Eps 7630): 30 drops three times daily for up to 3 weeks.
For congestion	• N-acetyl cysteine (oral): 600–800 mg twice per day for up to 2 weeks. • Humidifier in the bedroom. • Saline or xylitol nose spray. • Steam inhalation (see instructions below). • Steamy bath or shower. • Essential oil diffuser with eucalyptus, rosemary, lavender, frankincense, and/or tea tree oil.

For a sore throat	• Soothing herbs: chamomile, marshmallow root, slippery elm (as teas or lozenges). • Zinc lozenge (oral): up to 75 mg per day for a maximum of 10 days; gives additional immune support and is directly antimicrobial. • Chewable probiotic containing *S. salivarius* (also works against strep throat).* • Herbal throat spray (such as Biocidin; see Resources). • Salt water gargles: mix 1 teaspoon salt into ⅓ cup warm water and stir to dissolve. Gargle for 15 seconds up to six times per day.
For a dry cough	• Soothing herbs: chamomile, marshmallow root, slippery elm, thyme (as teas or lozenges).
For a wet cough	• N-acetyl cysteine (oral): 600–800 mg twice daily for up to 2 weeks. • Ivy leaf syrup (oral; see Resources).

See a doctor if you think you may have strep throat.

TECHNIQUE: HOW TO USE A STEAM INHALER

This simple technique is something any of us can do at home with very little equipment.

- Equipment and ingredients: Water that has just been boiled, a medium or large kitchen mixing bowl, essential oils (optional), a kitchen towel or hand towel.
- Add the steamy water to the bowl along with 2 to 3 drops of essential oil.
- Place the towel over your head and lean over the bowl. Hold the towel out to trap the steam vapors around your face. Breathe in deeply.
- Intermittently clear congestion by blowing your nose and then return to the steam.

TECHNIQUE: HOW TO MAKE
A MEDICINAL-STRENGTH HERBAL TEA

There is a whole treasure trove of natural remedies hiding in your kitchen spice cabinet and tea cupboard. To turn everyday herbs and spices into therapeutic teas with medicinal qualities, you just need to know two simple techniques. Both produce a tea that can be enjoyed warm or cold.

Infusion method: An herbal infusion is best for extracting the beneficial properties of leaves and flowers like green tea, peppermint, or chamomile. Make your infusion by pouring just-boiled water over the herbs and letting it all sit, covered, for 10 to 15 minutes. Then strain the tea (or remove the tea bag).

Decoction method: An herbal decoction is best for spices made from the seeds, bark, or root of a plant, or for medicinal mushrooms. In these plants, the beneficial compounds are a little more tightly locked up and need a little more effort to extract them. Make your decoction by simmering the herbs in water in a pot with the lid on for 20 to 30 minutes, then strain.

What if I'm making a blended tea where some ingredients need the decoction method and some the infusion method? Simply make the decoction first, and then add your herbs to be infused and let them steep off the heat.

Using a Humidifier

When the air is cold in wintertime, it can't hold as much moisture. Indoor heated air and airplane cabins are also very drying. These conditions dry up mucus and prevent it from effectively expelling debris and germs. Scientists at Yale University have proven that dry air prevents efficient removal of germs, prevents airway barrier cells from repairing infection-induced damage, impedes the strength of our immune system alert signals, and reduces antiviral interferon gamma production. I highly recommend an air humidifier if your environment is dry, and especially if you're suffering with mucus congestion, with a goal to keep air humidity in the range of 40 percent to 50 percent. (Don't go above 55 percent because that can lead to mold growth.) Intriguingly, experiments have shown that when we are in that optimal range of humidity, our heart rate variability goes up, a sign of reduced stress. And less stress has beneficial effects on our immune resilience: a win-win!

INFECTIONS OF THE DIGESTIVE TRACT

Acute infections of the digestive tract can be characterized by pain, nausea, vomiting, and/or diarrhea.

Foods for all infections of the digestive tract	• Electrolyte-replenishing drink options: • Bone broth • Coconut water • Homemade electrolyte support formula (see below)
Supplements (taken orally) for all infections of the digestive tract	• Multi-strain probiotic with at least 5 billion live CFUs daily for up to 4 weeks. Take at least 2 hours away from berberine, if using. • Berberine: 500 mg three times per day while symptoms last. • Bovine colostrum: 1,000–2,000 mg three times per day while symptoms last. • Over-the-counter electrolyte formula: look for sugar- and additive-free versions.

For diarrhea	• Increase fiber intake with soft-cooked whole grains, legumes, vegetables, and fruits. • Stay well hydrated. • Probiotic (oral) with *Lactobacillus rhamnosus* GG: This species has some of the best science to support its use for diarrhea. Take at least 2 hours away from berberine, if using. • Curcumin (oral): 500 mg three times per day; blocks the activity of many diarrhea-causing microbes.
For nausea and vomiting	• Pay attention to hydration if vomiting. • ¼ teaspoon ground dried ginger mixed into 2 teaspoons manuka (or other raw) honey, taken orally every hour for up to 3 hours while symptoms last. Or: • Ginger extract (oral): 1,000 mg three times per day while symptoms last. • Cinnamon (oral, in capsule form): 1,000 mg twice per day while symptoms last.

HOMEMADE ELECTROLYTE SUPPORT FORMULA

Combine:

¼ teaspoon of sodium chloride (table salt)

½ teaspoon sodium bicarbonate (baking soda)

½ teaspoon potassium chloride (e.g., Morton's lite salt)

4½ cups water

Stir until dissolved. Drink this amount slowly throughout the day, making a new batch each day, while diarrhea symptoms last. You can add freshly squeezed lemon or lime juice, mint leaves, and/or raw honey for flavor and additional immune support (optional).

This formula provides (per day): 1.75 grams sodium and 0.7 grams potassium, suitable for mild diarrhea and dehydration only. For severe diarrhea and dehydration, consult a physician for medical rehydration.

URINARY TRACT INFECTIONS

Urinary tract infections (UTIs) are associated with a persistent urge to urinate, a burning sensation during urination, cloudy urine, and/or pelvic pain. They can sometimes become chronic and, when treated with repeated rounds of antibiotics, increase the risk for antibiotic resistance. These natural alternatives for mild UTIs help restore balance without the risk of antibiotic resistance.

For all infections of the urinary system	• Unsweetened cranberry juice: 8 fluid ounces up to three times per day while symptoms last. • Parsley tea (recipe and instructions on page 308). • Increase potassium foods: avocado, beans, butternut squash, cantaloupe melon, coconut water, cucumber, broccoli, spinach, sweet potatoes. • Avoid caffeine and alcohol. • Phytoestrogen plant foods for post-menopausal women: soybean (organic, fermented), flaxseed. (Estrogen balance helps counter UTIs.) • Address constipation, which can block urinary flow (see page 290).
At first sign of an infection and while symptoms last (taken orally, in capsule form)	• Uva ursi: 200 mg daily. • Berberine: 500 mg three times per day. • Cranberry concentrate or extract: 400–600 mg twice per day.

For chronic UTIs	*One or more of the following can be taken regularly (orally) to reduce recurrence:* • Cranberry concentrate or extract (capsules): 400–600 mg twice per day. • Hibiscus tea: two to three times per day. • D-mannose (capsules or powder): 250–500 mg three times per day. • Multi-strain probiotic: at least 5 billion CFUs per day. For women, look for one that is designed to support vaginal health (which has knock-on effects on urinary tract health) such as Azo Complete Feminine Balance or Jarrow Formulas Fem-Dophilus. • Vitamin D: 2,000 IU daily and get your levels checked (see page 116 for more about getting your vitamin D levels right). • Marshmallow root (capsules or powder): 100–400 mg daily. *Additionally, prioritize regular, moderate exercise.*

PARSLEY TEA

Bring 5 cups of water to a boil in a large saucepan. Add one medium bunch of parsley, washed but not destemmed or chopped. Simmer for 8 minutes and then strain, reserving the liquid as the tea. Consume over the course of the day, warm or cold.

ORAL INFECTIONS

Most commercial oral care products contain chemical agents, many synthetic, that can disrupt the important balance of healthy microbes in the mouth, even as they combat harmful species. These include alcohols, detergents, and triclosan (the compound now banned in the US in soaps for personal use). In addition, many oral microbes are developing resistance to antibiotics and synthetic chemicals. Natural alternatives can help keep harmful microbes at bay, while still supporting a healthy oral microbiota and providing additional benefits such as antioxidants and gum healing.

For all oral infections	• Herbal tea made with rosemary, thyme, ginger (see recipe on page 304). • Prioritize fermented foods, shiitake mushrooms, fish, and garlic.
For gingivitis and dental caries	• Homemade oral rinse (see page 360). • Chewable, sugar-free probiotic ideally containing *S. salivarius.* • Sugar-free xylitol chewing gum. • 2.5 grams EPA plus 1.5 grams DHA omega-3 fatty acids: for up to 3 months (see page 128 for cautions). • Coenzyme Q$_{10}$: 100–150 mg daily in oral capsule form or, even better, choose a liquid liposomal formula and swish it around your mouth before swallowing. • Choose a natural toothpaste without harsh chemical ingredients and with gentle antimicrobials such as aloe, tea tree, or manuka honey. For dental caries, include a remineralization toothpaste with calcium hydroxyapatite. • Consider using a traditional "oil pulling" technique using unrefined, virgin coconut oil (see below). • Follow a regular oral hygiene routine including gentle brushing over gums as well as teeth, flossing, and rinsing.

For canker sores (aphthous ulcer)	• Wet black or green tea bags applied to the sore for a few minutes at a time are a time-honored remedy for canker sores (the tannins have astringent and analgesic properties). • Black elderberry extract (oral): 1,200 mg daily for up to 2 weeks. • B vitamins in your multivitamin can help counter canker sores. • Improve stress resilience. • Consider sensitivities to foods (most common possibilities include gluten, dairy, soy, egg, corn, nuts, and foods that cross-react with pollen allergies, i.e., oral allergy syndrome). For a list of food-pollen cross-reactions, visit aaaai.org and search "oral allergy syndrome."
For cold sores (herpes simplex)	• Reishi mushroom extract (oral): 500–1,000 mg twice per day for up to 4 weeks. • Black elderberry extract (oral): 1,200 mg daily for up to 2 weeks. • Topical lemon balm or tea tree essential oil*, diluted in a carrier oil or salve (see salve recipe on page 361). • Lysine (oral): 2,000–3,000 mg daily for up to 6 months (or longer under the guidance of a qualified practitioner). • Mint or parsley tea: brewed to medicinal strength (see page 308 for instructions). • Zinc (oral): 75 mg daily for up to 10 days.
For thrush	• Strict avoidance of all sugars and refined carbohydrates. • Abundant, colorful plant foods. • Mouth rinse made with 1 tablespoon coconut oil plus 2 drops food-grade tea tree oil, swish for 20 seconds, then spit, three times per day until symptoms subside. *If these home remedies don't work quickly for thrush, it's best to see your physician.*

Note that a small but significant proportion of people have allergic contact sensitivity to tea tree oil. If this is the first time you are using tea tree oil, and especially if you have sensitive skin, it's best to apply a small, diluted amount to the arm first to be sure you won't react to it.

RECIPE: TEA FOR ORAL INFECTIONS

Bring 4 cups of water to a boil in a saucepan. Add 1 tablespoon dried rosemary, 1 tablespoon dried thyme, and 1 inch ginger, peeled and sliced. Simmer for 20 minutes and then strain. Sip over the course of the day, swishing a little before swallowing to coat the gums.

TECHNIQUE: OIL PULLING

Oil pulling is a traditional practice that has been used in Ayurveda for thousands of years. It involves holding around 2 teaspoons of oil in the mouth for several minutes, while swishing it over the gums and teeth. Recently, oil pulling with virgin coconut oil (10 mL, equivalent to 2 teaspoons, held for 10 minutes) has been evaluated in modern clinical studies and found to be as effective as chlorhexidine, the commonly used pharmaceutical ingredient in prescription mouthwashes for some infections.

EYE INFECTIONS

Eye infections such as conjunctivitis or a stye can be caused by viruses or bacteria. They are usually highly contagious and can spread quickly. In addition to the herbal compress recommendation below, follow basic hygiene practices such as gentle cleansing with a wet cotton pad, avoiding eye makeup, and washing your hands before you touch your eye.

Eye infections	• Make a warm (not hot) herbal compress by using just a teabag of eyebright and/or chamomile. Most infections of the eyelid or conjunctiva are very responsive to warmth.

EAR INFECTIONS

Ear infections can be caused by bacteria, viruses, or fungi. The following options can be used for mild ear infections lasting one to two days. However, if there is any possibility of a ruptured ear drum, do not introduce any drops into the ear and seek immediate medical attention.

Foods	• Reishi mushrooms.
Supplements	• Black elderberry extract (oral): 1,200 mg daily. • 5 billion to 10 billion CFUs multi-strain probiotic, ideally chewable and containing *S. salivarius*. • Garlic and mullein oil ear drops: 2 to 3 drops in the ear, three times per day.
Other	• For recurrent ear infections, consider sensitivities to foods (common possibilities include gluten, dairy, soy, egg, corn, and nuts).

VAGINAL INFECTIONS

Vaginal infections are most commonly bacterial or fungal. While antibiotics work for most bacterial infections, they don't work for fungal infections and can even make them worse by creating more dysbiosis. Plant antimicrobials and other natural immune supportive interventions have the benefit of working simultaneously against both bacterial and fungal pathogens.

Foods	• Fermented foods such as live yogurt. • Strictly avoid sugar and alcohol.
Supplements	• Multi-strain probiotics taken orally that include *Lactobacillus* species (*L. acidophilus*, *L. plantarum*, *L. rhamnosus*, and *L. fermentum* are good species to look for). As mentioned above, several probiotic products are specifically designed to support vaginal health, such as Azo Complete Feminine Balance or Jarrow Formulas Fem-Dophilus. • Garlic extract capsules taken orally: 1,000–1,500 mg twice daily while symptoms last.
Other	• Avoid scented personal care products and douches. • Choose breathable, cotton underwear and sanitary pads. • Choose chemical-free sanitary pads and tampons and change them several times per day during your period. • Homemade coconut oil and tea tree (or probiotic) suppositories (see recipe below). • Prioritize moderate exercise and avoid long periods of sitting.

ANTIMICROBIAL VAGINAL SUPPOSITORIES

For this recipe, you'll need a suppository mold tray available at some pharmacies and online. To make 25 2mL suppositories, use 50 mL melted coconut oil combined with 8 drops tea tree oil. Stir well and distribute into the molds. Refrigerate until hardened. Use with a sanitary pad.

Variation: Add the contents of 5 probiotic capsules containing one or more of the species listed under "Supplements" above instead of the tea tree oil.

WOUNDS AND SKIN INFECTIONS

An open wound is an invitation to infection, so it's important to care for any damage to your skin.

Wound care	• Topical salve: see recipe on page 361. • Tea tree oil, diluted in carrier oil and applied topically. • Raw, dark honey applied topically. Manuka honey is a good option. • Zinc (oral): 75 mg daily for up to 10 days. • Vitamin C (oral): 1,000–6,000 mg daily for up to 1 week; decrease dose if it causes diarrhea. • Additional dietary protein is required for extensive wounds and surgery.
Mild skin infection	• Topical salve: see recipe on page 361. • Tea tree oil, diluted in carrier oil and applied topically. • Manuka honey, applied topically.
Athlete's foot (ringworm)	• Oral echinacea: 4,000 mg per day for 1 week followed by 2,000–2,500 mg per day for up to 7 weeks if needed. • Tea tree foot soak: Prepare a warm water foot bath and add 4–6 drops tea tree essential oil. Soak feet for 20 minutes. • Leave feet barefoot as much as possible. • Dust feet with cornstarch powder (a safer talc alternative) to keep them dry.

CHRONIC INFECTIONS

Oftentimes in clinic we work with individuals who have chronic symptoms associated with an infectious disease whose acute stage has long passed, yet who are dealing with lingering, associated issues. Lyme disease, Epstein-Barr virus, and now SARS-CoV-2 (the so-called long COVID) are known to cause all kinds of problems in susceptible individuals. These might include prolonged fatigue, joint pain, muscle aches, immunosuppression (recurrent infections of any kind), autoimmune disease, and anxiety.

What makes an individual susceptible isn't yet fully understood, yet it's likely to be a combination of genetic vulnerability, the health of their immune system, and the other stresses that their body is dealing with. Certainly, my clinical experience is that working on restoring immune resilience and removing as many of the additional physiological (and psychological) stressors as we can is by far the most effective way to make meaningful improvements in health and quality of life. Some specific considerations for chronic infections are listed below, which I highly recommend. Beyond that, there are specific herbal and nutraceutical interventions that can be used to jump-start the process and to help manage symptom flares. However, they are best used under the guidance of an experienced practitioner and are beyond the scope of this book.

The supplements listed below are intended to be taken orally.

Essential nutrients	• Vitamin D: 2,000 IU daily and more if a deficiency is identified. • Vitamin C: 1,000–2,000 mg daily. • 100% of your RDA for zinc and selenium.
Anti-inflammatory supplements	• EPA/DHA: 2–4 grams per day. • Curcumin: 500 mg three times per day. • Boswellia: 350–500 mg twice per day. *Boswellia, also known as Indian frankincense, is a resin that comes from the* Boswellia serrata *tree. I find it especially useful in the context of chronic infections to help combat unruly inflammation.*

Cellular energy support (mitochondrial health)	• B vitamins (B_1, B_2, B_3, B_5, B_6, folate, and B_{12}) as part of your multivitamin. • Coenzyme Q_{10}: 100 mg per day. • American ginseng root extract: 500 mg twice per day (if fatigue is present). *American ginseng, also known by its Latin name* Panax quinquefolius, *is a natural energy booster that can sometimes help improve the tiredness that is often present alongside chronic infections.*
Digestive tract support	• L-glutamine: 2,500–5,000 mg per day (see box below). • Slippery elm: 100–400 mg per day. • Marshmallow root: 100–400 mg per day. • Zinc carnosine: providing 15 mg zinc per day.
Stress resilience	Reining in chronic stress feelings is key, especially since chronic infections tend to disturb the autonomic nervous system (which can lead to elevated levels of anxiety) and, in my experience, our bodies find it very difficult to heal when in a high stress-response state. I highly recommend a heart rate variability monitor and the stress resilience practices in chapter 13.

Caution: L-Glutamine and Cancer

There is some controversy over the use of *supplemental* L-glutamine if there is known cancer in the body or a history of prior cancer, since some cancer cells preferentially use L-glutamine for energy. Conversely, L-glutamine supplementation has a long history and evidence base as a safe and effective support for the digestive tract. It has also been shown to be useful in reducing the effects of cancer cachexia and chemotherapy side effects, and may even inhibit other cancer types. If you have, or have a history of, cancer, it's best to discuss L-glutamine supplementation with your oncologist or other qualified health care provider.

To view the references cited in this chapter, please visit
www.immuneresilienceplan.com/science.

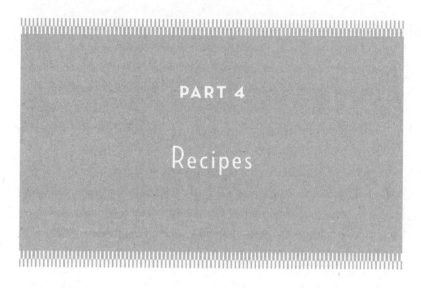

PART 4

Recipes

By now, you have read all about the good foods to eat and bad foods to avoid to build up your immune resilience. The following recipes I hope will help inspire you to incorporate those foods in your diet in a delicious way. Rich in fiber, vitamins and minerals, antioxidants, and phytonutrients, these are meals that can be enjoyed by your entire family.

BREAKFAST

BIRCHER MUESLI

I got into making this deliciously satisfying muesli while in Switzerland. A European staple, muesli was first developed by Swiss physician Maximilian Bircher-Benner around 1900 for his hospital patients. Its main ingredient, oats, contains high amounts of beta-glucans, fibrous prebiotic foods that feed those good bacteria that help keep our barriers strong and our immune cells behaving appropriately. I like to add flaxseeds and walnuts, high in immune-building omega-3 fats, as well as the optional orange zest—it lends a brightness to the flavor and adds in those beneficial citrus phytonutrients.

The great thing about muesli is that you can make a large batch of the dry mixture in advance and then just set your individual portion to soak overnight when you want it to be ready for you in the morning.

SERVINGS: 6

ACTIVE TIME: 20 MINUTES

INACTIVE TIME: 8 TO 12 HOURS,
OR MORE IF DRYING YOUR OWN ORANGE ZEST

FOR THE DRY MIX:

1½ cups whole-grain rolled oats

2/3 cup walnuts, finely chopped or pulsed in food processor

½ cup pumpkin seeds, finely chopped or pulsed in food processor

½ cup ground flaxseeds

½ teaspoon salt

dried zest of 1 orange (see Note), optional

TO SERVE:

½ cup dry mix

½ cup dairy milk *or* unsweetened nondairy milk

1 scoop unsweetened plain thick yogurt

1 apple

Combine the oats, walnuts, pumpkin seeds, flaxseeds, salt, and dried zest (if using) and store in an airtight container until ready to use. The mixture will keep for up to 2 months in a dark, cool place.

When ready to use, scoop a single serving (½ cup) of dry mix into your serving bowl the night before you want to serve it. Add the milk and stir to combine. Leave overnight in the refrigerator.

In the morning, add a scoop of yogurt, grate the apple over your muesli, and stir to combine. Enjoy!

Note: Drying your own orange zest is super simple, but it requires a little advanced planning. Zest the orange using a citrus zester, then spread out the zest on a piece of waxed paper on a small plate and leave it in a cool, dry place for 8 to 12 hours.

Tip: You can use the remaining orange for juice or as a healthy immune-boosting snack!

SUPERIMMUNITY OMELET

Start your day with this hearty and satisfying recipe and you'll have hit 100 percent of the daily value targets for vitamin A, vitamin C, and zinc. Plus you'll get a great jump-start on other important nutrients with daily selenium, copper, vitamin E, iron, magnesium, and vitamin D, if you source vitamin D–enriched eggs. It also delivers on essential fatty acids with 2 grams of omega-3 fats and 3 grams of omega-6.

Oh, and trust the addition of oysters: they lend a salty, umami flavor to the dish and are what allows you to get all that great zinc. If you prefer to leave them out, that's okay—just look for other sources of zinc throughout your day, such as meats, poultry, beans, nuts, seeds, and whole grains.

SERVINGS: MAKES 1 OMELET

ACTIVE TIME: 20 MINUTES

1 tablespoon olive oil or ghee

½ small red bell pepper, diced

4 medium mushrooms, diced

¾ cup fresh spinach, chopped

1½ tablespoons canned unsmoked oysters, chopped

2 medium eggs, vitamin D-enriched if possible

salt and pepper, to taste

Gently heat the olive oil or ghee in a medium sauté pan over medium heat. Add the bell pepper and mushrooms and cook for 7 to 10 minutes until softened. Add the spinach and oysters and cook until the spinach is fully wilted.

In a separate dish, whisk the eggs together and season with salt and pepper. Add the whisked eggs to the pan with the other ingredients and gently stir together just until everything is evenly distributed and the egg has a chance to coat the bottom of the pan.

Let cook, undisturbed, for 2 to 3 minutes, checking the underside for doneness. If it's starting to look golden brown, it's time to fold the omelet in half. Cover and let it cook for another 2 to 3 minutes or until fully cooked through. Serve.

PARSLEY POWER SMOOTHIE

This bright-green smoothie has a fresh flavor, thanks to the power combo of lemon, parsley, and celery. The apple and banana (if using) cut through the tartness and give you just the right balance of sweetness. If this is your breakfast, you may want to add a good-quality protein powder (organic protein powder, if you can, without unwanted additives).

SERVINGS: 2

ACTIVE TIME: 7 MINUTES

½ cup packed parsley

½ cup chopped celery (about 1 stalk)

1 apple, cored and quartered

juice of 1 lemon

½ banana (optional, if needed for sweetness)

protein powder of choice (optional)

milk of your choice

Mix all the ingredients in a blender with enough milk to blend to a smoothie consistency. I like to start with a half cup of milk and then add more if needed, slowly.

BERRY BLEND SMOOTHIE

This smoothie combination, deeply flavored with berries, brightened with lemon, is made extra creamy by the addition of cashews. Once again, I recommend adding a protein powder if you are making this a meal; I've listed some of my favorites in the Resources section.

SERVINGS: 2

ACTIVE TIME: 5 MINUTES

½ cup raspberries, fresh or frozen

½ cup blueberries, fresh or frozen

1 handful of cashews (about ⅓ cup)

1 small apple, peeled and cored

juice of 1 lemon

1 cup unsweetened milk of your choice (such as dairy, almond, or coconut)

1 teaspoon raw, dark honey (optional)

Place the raspberries, blueberries, cashews, apple, lemon juice, and honey (if using) in a blender with enough milk to blend to a smoothie consistency.

ORANGE-CINNAMON SWEET POTATO BREAD

This bread is so much more than just "bread." It is a meal in itself—made with sweet potatoes, almonds, apples, and orange, baked together with aromatic spices. You won't miss the added sugar, since the sweet potato and applesauce lend a natural sweetness that tastes just right.

I like to make this recipe using sweet potato I've cooked and then saved from dinner the night before. To cook the sweet potato, I bake it whole, unpeeled, and pricked several times with a fork, in a 400°F oven. A medium sweet potato takes about an hour to cook through using this method. Once cooled, you can slice it in half and scoop out the cooked flesh. Alternatively, you can pick up frozen ready-to-cook sweet potato that can be steamed or oven roasted more quickly.

SERVINGS: 6

ACTIVE TIME: 20 MINUTES
(NOT INCLUDING SWEET POTATO COOKING TIME)

INACTIVE TIME: 60 MINUTES

DRY INGREDIENTS:

1½ cup whole wheat or spelt flour

½ cup ground almonds

1 teaspoon baking soda

¾ teaspoon baking powder

1½ teaspoons ground cinnamon

½ teaspoon ground ginger

¼ teaspoon ground allspice

¾ teaspoon salt

WET INGREDIENTS:

2 large eggs

1 cup cooked sweet potato, mashed

⅓ cup unsweetened applesauce

zest and juice of 1 medium orange

¼ cup olive oil plus more for oiling the loaf pan

1 teaspoon vanilla extract

Preheat your oven to 375°F. Lightly oil an 8- or 9-inch loaf pan and line it with parchment paper.

Whisk the flour, ground almonds, baking soda, baking powder, cinnamon, ginger, allspice, and salt together in a large mixing bowl. In a separate bowl, whisk the eggs, sweet potato, applesauce, orange zest and juice, olive oil, and vanilla extract until combined. Pour the wet mixture into the dry and stir the mixture with a spatula until you have no remaining bits of dry ingredients visible. Do not overmix.

Pour the mixture into the loaf pan and bake for 45 minutes or until a cake tester inserted into the center comes out clean. Allow to cool in the pan for 10 minutes and then turn out onto a wire rack to finish cooling.

SIMPLE OAT-FLAX BREAD ROLLS

This single-rise roll recipe comes together in a flash, making you feel positively superhero-ish. I love using olive oil here (and generally in my baking), but if you prefer a more subtle taste, use sunflower oil instead. If you don't have a dish exactly the right size, you can also bake these rolls on a baking sheet.

MAKES 8 ROLLS

ACTIVE TIME: 25 MINUTES

INACTIVE TIME: 30 MINUTES

1½ cups whole-grain spelt flour, plus more for dusting the baking dish and making any adjustments during mixing

½ cup oat flour

⅓ cup flaxseed meal

2 teaspoons active dry yeast

½ teaspoon salt

¼ cup olive oil, plus more for the baking dish

1 cup warm water (110–115°F), plus more for any adjustments during mixing

Grease an 8-inch-by-12-inch Pyrex or other oven-proof glass, earthenware, or enameled cast-iron casserole dish with olive oil. Dust with a fine coating of flour. Set aside.

Add the spelt flour, oat flour, flaxseed meal, yeast, and salt to a large mixing bowl or a stand mixer. Whisk to combine. Combine the oil with the water and add to the dry mix. With your hands or using a mixer with the paddle attachment, bring the dough together until the wet and dry ingredients are fully incorporated. Adjust with more water or flour to reach a bread dough consistency. (I like to use a wetter dough as I find it yields softer rolls, but it also makes kneading a little more challenging.)

Knead the dough (on a floured surface if necessary) for about 10 minutes or until you can stretch it without it breaking.

Separate the dough into 8 pieces using kitchen scissors or a bench scraper for ease, since the dough will otherwise become stringy when pulled apart. Roll each piece into a ball, dust with flour, and place in two evenly spaced rows of four in your prepared baking dish.

Set two racks in your oven, one on the lowest rack and one on the middle rack, but don't turn the oven on. Instead, fill a loaf or cake pan with 3 cups of boiling water and place it on the bottom rack. Place your rolls on the top rack, close the oven door, and let the dough rise for 30 minutes.

Remove the water pan from the oven but leave the rolls inside. Set the oven temperature to 350°F and your timer for 23 minutes. The rolls will continue to rise and cook as the temperature heats up.

Remove from the oven and let cool for 10 to 15 minutes before serving.

SOUPS

MAMA'S CHICKEN SOUP

This soup has been known to cure a broken heart (just saying!). And of course, it's also a staple immune-resilience dish that is both warming and comforting, while also helping to ease congestion and feed immune cells. It works well as leftovers, too. Just remember to taste before adding salt because some store-bought versions of chicken stock are already well salted.

SERVINGS: 4

ACTIVE TIME: 45 MINUTES

INACTIVE TIME: 30 MINUTES

2 tablespoons ghee or olive oil

4 large chicken thighs, bone in, skinless

2 tablespoons flour or cornstarch

4 cups bone broth (see recipe on page 353 or use a good-quality store-bought version)

2 medium onions, peeled and diced

2 medium carrots, peeled and diced

3 celery ribs, diced

1 medium white potato, peeled and diced

6 cloves garlic, peeled and minced

½ inch ginger, peeled and pressed or minced

2 bay leaves

salt and pepper, to taste

In a large saucepan over medium heat, melt the ghee or olive oil. Dust the chicken thighs with the flour or cornstarch and add to the pan, cooking until the chicken is slightly browned. Add the chicken stock, onion, carrots, celery, potato, garlic, ginger, and bay leaves, bring to a boil, and simmer gently for 30 minutes. Remove the bay leaves and discard. Remove the chicken thighs onto a cutting board and carefully separate the meat from the bone and return the meat to the soup. Bring back to a boil and simmer for 5 minutes, season with salt and pepper to taste, and serve.

MINESTRONE SOUP

Minestrone, from the blue-zone region of Sardinia, Italy, is considered to be an important contributor to the local population's impressive longevity. Feel free to substitute seasonal vegetables for the zucchini and green beans—yellow squash, winter squash, and peas work well, too.

SERVINGS: 4

ACTIVE TIME: 25 MINUTES

INACTIVE TIME: 35 MINUTES

2 tablespoons ghee or extra-virgin olive oil

1 small onion, peeled and diced

1 carrot, peeled and diced

2 celery ribs, diced

1 small zucchini, diced

½ cup chopped green beans

1 can (16 ounces) diced tomatoes, with their liquid

3 cups bone or vegetable broth (recipe for bone broth on page 353 or store-bought options in the Resources section)

3 tablespoons tomato paste

4 cloves garlic, peeled and pressed or minced

1 sprig fresh thyme or ½ teaspoon dried

2 sprigs fresh oregano or ½ teaspoon dried

pinch of red pepper flakes

½ cup dried whole-grain orzo pasta

½ cup canned cannellini beans, rinsed

juice of half a lemon

salt and pepper to taste

In a large saucepan, sauté the onion, carrots, and celery in ghee or oil to soften, stirring intermittently, for 7 to 10 minutes. Add the zucchini, green beans, tomatoes, broth, tomato paste, garlic, thyme, oregano, red pepper flakes, orzo, cannellini beans, lemon juice, salt, and pepper, and bring to a gentle boil. Cover with a lid and simmer for 25 minutes, stirring frequently to prevent the orzo sticking to the bottom. Remove the fresh herb sprigs if using. Adjust the seasoning as necessary before serving.

CURRIED BUTTERNUT SQUASH SOUP

This is a silky smooth, vibrant orange soup with just a hint of sweetness. Butternut squash is a rich source of provitamin A carotenoids that play an important role in gut and immune health. Time-saver tip: If you use pre-cubed squash instead of cooking whole squash, you can put the raw squash cubes into the soup pot and cook along with the other ingredients.

SERVINGS: 4

ACTIVE TIME: 20 MINUTES

INACTIVE TIME: 1 HOUR 45 MINUTES

1 large (3 to 4 pounds) butternut squash

4 cups bone or vegetable broth (recipe for bone broth on page 353 or store-bought options in the Resources section)

2 teaspoons garlic powder

2 teaspoons onion powder

1 tablespoon ground cumin

1 teaspoon ground turmeric

zest and juice of 1 lemon

salt and pepper to taste

FOR TOPPING:

½ cup fresh cilantro, chopped

Yogurt or sour cream, unsweetened and with live cultures

To bake the butternut squash: Heat the oven to 180°F. Make two deep piercings in your squash, rub it with oil, and place it on a medium baking sheet or in a casserole dish. Bake for 1 hour 15 minutes or until it is completely cooked though (soft when tested with a knife).

Let the squash stand until cool enough to handle (about 30 minutes). Cut it in half lengthwise, then scoop out and discard the seeds. Scoop out the cooked squash and place it in a large saucepan and cover. Add the broth, garlic powder, onion powder, cumin, and turmeric. Bring to a simmer and cook for 15 minutes, stirring intermittently to break up the squash. If the squash isn't fully broken up after 15 minutes, puree the soup using an immersion blender.

Add the lemon zest and juice and then season to taste. Serve into four bowls and top each with fresh cilantro and either yogurt or sour cream.

CHICKEN NOODLE SOUP WITH SPINACH AND FRESH PESTO

This is a super-quick recipe, especially if you already have cooked chicken and/or pesto on hand. Speaking of pesto, it's a great addition to any recipe for a quick flavor and immune boost.

SERVINGS: 4

ACTIVE TIME: 20 MINUTES

INACTIVE TIME: 30 MINUTES

8 ounces chicken breast, diced

2 tablespoons flour

2 tablespoons ghee *or* olive oil

4 cups bone *or* vegetable broth (recipe for bone broth on page 353 or store-bought options in the Resources section)

1 large onion, peeled and diced

4 ounces brown rice noodles (such as pad thai noodles)

4 cups tightly packed baby spinach leaves, washed

6 tablespoons Immune-Boosting Pesto (recipe on page 350)

salt and pepper to taste

Dust the chicken pieces with the flour. Using a large saucepan, melt the ghee or heat the olive oil. Then add the chicken. Cook until the chicken is slightly browned (it doesn't have to be fully cooked through at this point).

Slowly add the stock, stirring. Add the onion and cover with a lid. Simmer for 30 minutes until the onion is completely translucent and the chicken cooked through. Add the noodles for the last 5 minutes of the cooking time, stirring so they don't stick together.

Remove from the heat. Mix in the spinach leaves to wilt. Stir in the pesto and season to taste.

PHYTONUTRIENT-LOADED SALAD

There's one simple rule for creating a salad that is bursting with beneficial phytonutrients—color! In this salad, you'll find a full spectrum of phytonutrients and harmony of flavor that I hope will become a regular in your lunch routine and will inspire you to create your own versions.

SERVINGS: 1

ACTIVE TIME: 5 MINUTES

1 small red onion, diced

8 cherry tomatoes, quartered

½ medium yellow bell pepper, halved and diced

½ avocado, diced

1 small orange, peeled and diced, omitting the center pith and seeds

⅓ cup blueberries

1 packed cup arugula leaves

¼ cup pumpkin seeds

Toss all ingredients together and place on your plate or bowl. Serve as is or with Uber-Simple Tahini Dressing (recipe on page 351).

IMMUNE-BOOSTING TABBOULEH

Tabbouleh is an easy, flavor-packed recipe that stars some of my favorite culinary herbs: parsley and mint. The flavors are fresh and punchy, yet balanced and satisfying. It makes a great light lunch, either alone or alongside some cooked chicken. I like to cook the bulgur wheat in advance, usually the night before. You can easily use quinoa as a substitute for the bulgur if you are gluten sensitive.

SERVINGS: 2

ACTIVE TIME: 20 MINUTES,
PLUS TIME TO COOK AND COOL THE BULGUR

- 2 teaspoons apple cider vinegar
- 1 tablespoon flaxseed oil
- 2 cloves garlic, minced
- 1 cup flat-leaf parsley leaves, chopped (about 1 bunch)
- ¼ cup mint leaves, chopped
- 2 cups whole-grain bulgur wheat, cooked and allowed to cool (see headnote above)
- 2 cups cherry tomatoes, quartered
- ¼ red onion, finely chopped
- Salt and pepper, to taste

Combine the apple cider vinegar and flaxseed oil and add the minced garlic in a small bowl. Let it sit a few minutes to marinate (minimum 15 minutes and up to 2 hours) while you prepare the other ingredients.

In a medium bowl, combine the parsley, mint, bulgur wheat, tomatoes, onion, salt, and pepper and toss gently.

When you're ready to serve, add the garlic mixture and continue to toss until evenly distributed. Divide into two servings and enjoy!

JEWELED COLESLAW WITH REAL MAYO

The combination of purple and green cabbage, flecked with orange carrot and deep green parsley, makes for an attractive dish. Remember, the longer the cabbage and onion marinate, the more sulforaphane and allicin they'll give off. This recipe also adds a good quantity of vitamins and quercetin, as well as fiber. Be sure to use a good-quality mayonnaise like the homemade one I use here, or a store-bought one that passes your ultra-processed food screening.

FOR THE COLESLAW

SERVINGS: 4

ACTIVE: 15 MINUTES

INACTIVE TIME: 30 MINUTES

½ small purple cabbage, thinly sliced (see Note)

½ small green cabbage, thinly sliced

1 medium onion, finely diced

2 medium carrots, peeled and grated

2 teaspoons salt

¼ cup mayonnaise (recipe below)

¼ cup chopped fresh parsley

Place the cabbages, onion, and carrots in a large mixing bowl. Rub the salt into the vegetables by hand. Let sit, covered, for 30 minutes.

Drain any liquid, stir in the mayonnaise and parsley, and serve immediately.

Note: For the best texture, you'll want to slice your cabbage as thinly as possible. I prefer to do this in a food processor with the slicing disc attachment, but you could also use a mandolin or a sharp chef's knife. You could also use the shredder disc attachment for the onions and carrots.

FOR THE MAYONNAISE

MAKES ABOUT 1 CUP

ACTIVE TIME: 15 MINUTES

1 medium pasteurized egg*

1 tablespoon Dijon mustard

1 tablespoon apple cider vinegar

½ teaspoon salt

⅓ cup avocado oil

½ cup expeller-pressed, non-GMO organic canola oil *or* a mild-tasting flaxseed oil

*Pasteurized eggs are those that have been heat treated to reduce the slight risk of food-borne illness. They are a better choice in recipes that call for consuming raw or lightly cooked egg.

Crack the egg into a blender and blitz just for a few seconds until the white and yolk are combined. Add the mustard, vinegar, and salt, and process for another few seconds until combined. With the blender on low, slowly add the avocado oil, just a drop at a time to allow an emulsion to form. Add the canola oil slowly, in a very thin stream.

This mayo keeps well in a sealed jar in the refrigerator for up to 1 week.

Note: If, despite achieving inhuman levels of patience, your mayo separates, don't panic. You can usually fix the problem by adding either another teaspoon of Dijon mustard or an extra egg yolk and slowly blending it in.

EASY SAUERKRAUT

This is such a simple recipe for fermenting cabbage. If you want to get more fancy you can add 1 to 2 teaspoons of a spice, such as juniper berries, caraway seeds, or celery seeds. But I like it just as much plain. You'll need a large

mixing bowl, a couple of mason jars, and a fermentation weight. A fermentation weight will keep your cabbage submerged in the brine during fermentation, which is what protects it from rotting. You can pick up a fermentation weight in your local kitchen supply store or online. I like to use glass fermentation weights, sized specifically for mason jars. You can also find stainless steel spring fermentation weights as an alternative to glass.

Make sure all your equipment is super clean and sterilized—including your large mixing bowl, mason jar(s), and fermentation weights. The high-heat sterilization setting on your dishwasher is a convenient way to do this.

SERVINGS: APPROXIMATELY 40

ACTIVE TIME: 30 MINUTES

INACTIVE TIME: 1 TO 3 WEEKS

1 medium head of cabbage, weighed and shredded (1½ pounds of cabbage fills about a 1-quart wide-mouth canning jar)

1 tablespoon salt for every pound of cabbage, and more for the covering liquid

water

In a large bowl, mix the chopped cabbage and salt. Massage it well with clean hands to distribute all the salt. Let it rest for an hour.

Pack the cabbage tightly into one or two jars using a spoon or by hand, depending on the size of the jars. Mason jars work well for this. Really press down as you go. Leave at least 2 inches of space at the top. Pour any juice that has released from the salted cabbage into the jar(s) and loosely screw on the jar lid(s).

Let the cabbage sit in a cool place, outside of direct sunlight, for 24 hours. Then open up the jar(s) and press down again. You should see that the cabbage will have released quite a bit of juice by this point. Top up the liquid level with water mixed with additional salt (1¼ teaspoons salt per 1 cup water) to cover the cabbage by about 1 inch.

Weigh the cabbage down in each jar using a fermentation weight. Put on the lid(s) and set out of direct sunlight at a cool room temperature for at least 1 week and up to 3 weeks. You'll need to open the jar(s) daily to release the carbon dioxide formed by the microbes busy at work (otherwise known as "burping"). Taste the sauerkraut now and again to see how it's doing. Once it's reached your preferred "doneness," transfer it to the refrigerator, where it can stay for up to 3 months.

Add 1 to 2 tablespoons to a meal to boost your probiotic and phytonutrient intake.

GARLICKY RICED CAULIFLOWER WITH PARMESAN CHEESE

Cauliflower, like its cruciferous cousin broccoli, contains the means to make sulforaphane, a powerful phytonutrient that can dial down inflammation and reduce the effects of aging on your immune cells. But it does that only when the enzyme it uses to make sulforaphane is activated—and that is done by chewing or chopping. Chopping cauliflower into small pieces, letting it rest, then cooking it just briefly, helps it develop the most of its sulforaphane. Garlic also benefits from chopping and letting its antimicrobial and immune-boosting compounds develop before you use it. Just a touch of ghee and Parmesan (from a good-quality pastured and antibiotic-free source, of course) rounds out the flavor and fat profile beautifully.

SERVINGS: 2

ACTIVE TIME: 25 MINUTES

INACTIVE TIME: 30 TO 90 MINUTES

1 small cauliflower head, cut into florets *or* one 16-ounce bag of frozen riced cauliflower

4 cloves garlic, minced

1 tablespoon ghee

1/8 cup water

2 tablespoons grated Parmesan cheese

salt and pepper, to taste

First, "rice" the cauliflower in a food processor. (If you don't have a processor, you can do this by hand by chopping the cauliflower into a small dice.) Let the cauliflower pieces and minced garlic sit separately for 30 minutes (or up to 90 minutes if you have time) to allow the sulforaphane and allicin content to develop.

Place a large sauté pan over a medium-high heat source for 3 to 4 minutes to bring it to temperature. Melt the ghee to coat the bottom of the pan. Add the cauliflower and stir as it starts to sauté for 2 minutes. Add the garlic and stir through. Continue to sauté for 1 to 2 minutes.

Drizzle the water over the cauliflower and garlic. It should start to sizzle and immediately develop steam. Cover with a lid to capture the steam and leave for 30 seconds. Then remove the lid and cook for another minute until the water evaporates.

Remove from heat and stir in the Parmesan cheese. Season with salt and pepper and serve immediately.

MAIN COURSES

PESTO PASTA PRIMAVERA

Pasta dishes don't need to be pasta heavy. Or cheese heavy, for that matter. There are ways to incorporate pasta without overloading on carbs and dairy, and without forgoing fiber and phytonutrients. Once you make the switch, you'll find lots more ways to fit your favorite pasta dishes into the Immune Resilience Diet. I sometimes like to use a spelt pasta or gluten-free pasta (like Trader Joe's quinoa pasta) in place of wheat pasta to mix it up a bit and make sure that I am not getting stuck into using too much gluten. This recipe is also great served cold and makes an excellent dish to bring to a picnic or potluck.

SERVINGS: 2

ACTIVE TIME: 25 MINUTES

1 cup dry bite-sized pasta such as penne, rigatoni, or fusilli

¼ cup pesto (see recipe on page 350)

1 medium red onion, thinly sliced

⅔ cup fresh or frozen peas

8 to 10 asparagus spears, trimmed and chopped into bite-size pieces

1 red or yellow bell pepper, stalk and seeds removed, cut into 1½-inch strips

1 cup broccoli, cut into florets

8 cherry tomatoes, halved

2 scallion stalks (green and white parts), trimmed and diced

salt and pepper, to taste

TO SERVE:

extra-virgin olive oil

2 tablespoons Parmesan shavings (optional)

Fill a large, lidded saucepan with water and bring to a boil over medium heat. Once boiling, reduce the heat to a simmer and add the pasta. Cook according to the directions on the packet and then drain. Toss with the pesto and set aside, still in the saucepan.

Meanwhile, place the onion, peas, asparagus, bell pepper, and broccoli into a steamer and cook for 7 to 12 minutes, until the vegetables are just tender but retain their bright color.

Add the vegetables to the pasta, along with the cherry tomatoes and scallions. Season to taste and toss gently until everything is evenly distributed.

Divide the pasta into two bowls or onto plates. Drizzle with olive oil and sprinkle with Parmesan if using. Serve immediately.

PORK AND LENTIL CASSOULET

Meat is great for adding flavor and nutrients, but it doesn't always have to be the star on your plate (by volume). When you use meat in a smaller, supporting role, you leave room for those all-important plant foods, high in fiber and phytonutrients, and create a meal that is anti-inflammatory while still being highly nutritious and absolutely delicious.

White button mushrooms, cremini, or portobello mushrooms will work well in this recipe, but if you can find medicinal mushrooms, like shiitake or maitake, which have extra anti-inflammatory and immune-enhancing properties, all the better. One last note: I like to choose jarred rather than canned tomato sauce to reduce any potential contamination with BPA and BPS.

SERVINGS: 4

ACTIVE TIME: 15 MINUTES

INACTIVE TIME: 1 HOUR 30 MINUTES

½ cup lentils (green, brown, or black)

½ pound boneless pork shoulder, cut into ¾-inch cubes

2 cups onions, diced

2 cups mushrooms, diced

2 medium carrots, peeled and diced

6 garlic cloves, minced

1½ cups bone broth (recipe on page 353 or store-bought options in the
    Resources section)

2 teaspoons dried thyme *or* 2 sprigs fresh

1 teaspoon dried rosemary *or* 1 sprig fresh

2 tablespoons tomato paste

one 15-ounce jar tomato sauce

1½ teaspoons salt

¼ teaspoon black pepper

Preheat the oven to 375°F. Into a medium-size (4- to 6-quart) casserole dish or Dutch oven, place the lentils, pork, onions, mushrooms, carrots, garlic, bone broth, thyme, and rosemary. Stir gently to combine, making sure that the lentils all end up submerged in the liquid portion.

Cover and cook for 1 hour, then remove from the oven to add the tomato paste, tomato sauce, salt, and pepper. Stir to combine. Return to the oven and cook for another 30 minutes.

This recipe pairs well with the Garlicky Riced Cauliflower with Parmesan Cheese (page 337) and a couple of tablespoons of sauerkraut (page 335).

Note: This recipe also works very well in a slow cooker or Instant Pot. For a slow cooker, the first phase of cooking can be set for 8 hours at low heat. Then add the tomato paste and sauce, along with the seasonings, before cooking on high for a further 45 minutes. If using an Instant Pot, the first phase of the cooking time can be reduced to just 20 minutes.

HERBED MUSHROOM AND SPINACH RAGOUT

Mushrooms of all stripes have immune-enhancing properties. From the humble white button mushroom to the well-known medicinal varieties like shiitake, mushrooms increase secretory IgA antibody production, activate certain immune cells, and dial down inflammation. But being good for you doesn't mean having to sacrifice flavor. This dish is bursting with taste and pairs very well with wild rice.

SERVINGS: 4

ACTIVE TIME: 30 TO 40 MINUTES

2 tablespoons ghee or extra-virgin olive oil

4 cups white, cremini, or portobello mushrooms, sliced

4 cups wild mushrooms (such as shiitake*, oyster, porcini, maitake, chanterelle, or trumpet), sliced

4 cloves garlic, minced

2 tablespoons flour

1 cup bone broth (recipe on page 353 or store-bought options in the Resources section)

6 cups baby spinach, washed

2 teaspoons dried thyme or 2 sprigs fresh

1 teaspoon dried rosemary or 1 sprig fresh

1 teaspoon dried oregano or 1 sprig fresh

⅓ cup flat-leaf parsley, finely chopped

juice of half a lemon

salt and pepper, to taste

*Larger shiitake mushrooms tend to have tough stems. Remove these before slicing.

TO SERVE:

4 servings wild rice, cooked according to the packet directions

sauerkraut, 2 tablespoons per serving (recipe on page 335)

Heat a large sauté pan over medium heat. Add the oil and allow it to warm for a minute. Add half the mushrooms and stir until they begin to shrink down in size (about 5 minutes). Add the rest of the mushrooms and continue to cook until all the mushrooms are tender, about 15 to 20 minutes. (If there is a lot of liquid released from the mushrooms, turn up the heat and continue stirring until the liquid is nearly all gone.)

Add the garlic and stir through. Sprinkle the flour over the mushrooms and stir in until the flour has disappeared. Slowly add the bone broth, spinach, thyme, rosemary, and oregano, gently stirring intermittently for 10 to 15 minutes. Add up to ⅓ cup of water if needed, to thin the sauce.

To serve, remove from the heat and stir in the parsley and lemon juice. Season to taste and add wild rice and sauerkraut to each plate.

ONE-PAN WILD SALMON WITH ASPARAGUS AND LEMON

This supremely bright and tasty dish will make you feel like a star in the kitchen. If this is your first experience with one-pan baking, I know you'll find lots more opportunities to stretch your legs with this technique. It's quick and easy, and cleanup is a breeze.

SERVINGS: 2

ACTIVE TIME: 10 MINUTES

INACTIVE TIME: 20 TO 25 MINUTES

2 salmon fillets, around 3 to 4 ounces each

4 tablespoons ghee or extra-virgin olive oil

4 garlic cloves, minced

1 teaspoon red pepper flakes

2 tablespoons bone broth (recipe on page 353 or store-bought options in the Resources section) or water

1 pound asparagus spears, woody ends trimmed

1 medium red onion, thinly sliced

1 small lemon, sliced into rounds

salt and pepper, to taste

¼ cup flat-leaf parsley, finely chopped

Preheat the oven to 375°F. Grease the bottom and sides of a wide oven dish or baking sheet (with raised sides) with 2 tablespoons of the ghee or extra-virgin olive oil.

In a small bowl, mix the remaining ghee or olive oil with the garlic and red pepper flakes. Set aside.

Place the salmon fillets on one-half of your oven dish. On the other half, place the asparagus spears, evenly distributed and topped with the red onion slices. Drizzle the bone broth or water over the asparagus.

Rub the vegetables and salmon with the garlic and red pepper flake mixture. Layer the lemon rounds over the top, sprinkle with salt and pepper, and bake for 20 to 25 minutes until everything is just cooked through. Serve topped with the chopped parsley.

CHICKPEA CURRY WITH SWEET POTATO AND KALE

This is another easy dish that comes together effortlessly in a casserole or Dutch oven. If you don't like things too spicy, you can easily omit the chili pepper and still retain the overall mellow spice flavor (not to mention the immune benefits). Be sure to include the toppings, which provide additional probiotics in the yogurt as well as the benefits and brightness of the fresh herbs and lime.

SERVINGS: 4

ACTIVE TIME: 20 MINUTES

INACTIVE TIME: 45 MINUTES

1 medium onion, diced

1 medium sweet potato, peeled and diced

2 cups cooked chickpeas (garbanzo beans)

6 leaves of kale, stems removed and roughly chopped into bite-size
pieces

1 to 2 fresh red chili peppers, deseeded and minced, *or* ¼ to ½ teaspoon
red pepper flakes

6 cloves garlic, minced

1 inch fresh ginger, peeled and minced, *or* ¾ teaspoon ground ginger

1 tablespoon ground cumin

1 teaspoon ground turmeric

⅛ teaspoon ground cinnamon

¾ cup bone broth (recipe on page 353 or store-bought options in the
Resources section) *or* water

4 tablespoons tomato paste

TO SERVE:

cooked whole-grain rice or millet (cook according to the packet directions)

plain thick yogurt, such as Greek or Skyr, with live cultures

¼ cup chopped cilantro

lime wedges

Preheat the oven to 375°F. Place the onion, sweet potato, chickpeas, kale, peppers, garlic, ginger, cumin, turmeric, cinnamon, bone broth or water, and tomato paste into a medium (4- to 6-quart) casserole dish or Dutch oven. Stir to combine. Cover and bake for 45 minutes. Check the sweet potato for doneness before serving.

Serve alongside a whole grain like rice or millet, with a dollop of live yogurt, chopped cilantro, and a squeeze of lime.

SNACKS

LOADED PESTO HUMMUS

In my opinion, there's nothing better than a luscious, creamy hummus dip. And it's very hard to find that in a store-bought version. This homemade gem, with immune-boosting additions, takes classic hummus to a whole new level. It's also an excellent way to use some of that powerful pesto you made on page 350.

It's nutritionally best to soak, sprout, and cook your own chickpeas (see how to do this on page 188). However, this recipe uses the store-bought, pre-cooked variety that will work when you haven't had time to plan for that. Try to find precooked chickpeas that come in glass jars rather than cans (which inevitably have a plastic lining). They are out there; Eden Foods and Jovial Foods are two brands that use glass jars.

SERVINGS: 4

PREPARATION TIME: 15 MINUTES

1½ cups cooked chickpeas (about one 15-ounce store-bought can or jar), drained and rinsed

¼ cup tahini (pureed sesame seeds)

4 tablespoons flaxseed oil

juice and zest of 1 small lemon

salt and pepper, to taste

¼ cup lemon basil pesto (page 350)

Place the chickpeas, tahini, flaxseed oil, lemon juice and zest, salt, and pepper in a food processor and blend until completely smooth. You may need to pause and scrape down the sides intermittently to make sure everything gets incorporated.

Scrape out the hummus into a serving dish. Drizzle the pesto over the top and serve immediately with cut-up vegetable sticks like bell peppers, celery, jicama, carrot, or zucchini.

NO-BAKE ENERGY BITES

If you recall, I mentioned earlier in the book that in my twenties and thirties, when I didn't know any better, I'd reach for something easy and sugary to pick me up from that midafternoon energy crash. Well, I have since found something better to reach for: these little balls of yum! I've especially crafted these to give you a little of all the kinds of fats we need—omega-3s, omega-6s, in the perfect 1:3 ratio, and a roughly equal distribution of good-quality whole-plant-based polyunsaturated, monounsaturated, and saturated fats. Plus, some prebiotic oats and honey. And I've snuck in some tasty cacao nibs—they are packed with phytonutrients, but without the sugar you get from most chocolate chips.

MAKES APPROXIMATELY 24 1-INCH OR 16 1½-INCH BALLS

ACTIVE TIME: 20 MINUTES

¾ cup rolled oats

⅓ cup walnut halves

¼ cup ground flaxseeds

¼ cup unsweetened, shredded coconut

¼ cup almond butter

¼ cup coconut butter, melted

⅓ cup raw honey

¼ cup cacao nibs

½ teaspoon vanilla

pinch of salt

Place the oats, walnuts, flaxseeds, and coconut in a food processor and pulse until the nuts and oats are finely chopped. Add the almond butter, coconut butter, honey, cacao nibs, vanilla, and salt and then pulse some more, until everything is evenly combined.

Form the mixture into bite-size balls. Enjoy right away or store in the refrigerator for up to 2 weeks. For storing, it works best to place each ball in a mini-muffin paper cup to keep them separated.

PUMPKIN SPICE TRAIL MIX

This trail mix is loaded with high omega-3 and other unsaturated fats and makes a perfect snack on the go or topping for a good-quality, unsweetened yogurt. The coconut and spices add antimicrobial and anti-inflammatory benefits.

SERVINGS: 8

ACTIVE TIME: 15 MINUTES

INACTIVE TIME: 15 MINUTES

1 cup walnuts

1 cup pumpkin seeds (pepitas)

½ cup flaxseeds

½ cup unsweetened coconut flakes

1 teaspoon ground cinnamon

¼ teaspoon ground ginger

¼ teaspoon ground allspice

½ teaspoon salt

¼ cup pureed cooked pumpkin

2 tablespoons apple juice (one with no added sugar)

1 tablespoon olive oil, plus more for greasing the baking sheet

Preheat the oven to 350°F. Grease a large baking sheet, preferably one with sides.

Combine the walnuts, seeds, and coconut flakes in a large mixing bowl. Separately, mix the spices, salt, pureed pumpkin, apple juice, and olive oil, and then add to the dry mixture and stir to coat evenly.

Spread the mixture evenly onto the baking sheet and bake for 12 to 15 minutes until starting to crisp. Remove from the oven and allow to cool completely. Transfer to an airtight container to store for up to 1 week.

IMMUNE-BOOSTING PESTO + VARIATIONS

Pesto always makes a meal feel fancy, yet it's incredibly simple to make. Plus, it's just bursting with flavor that elevates any food pairing. These pesto variations provide research-based immune support using the ingredients you've learned about. They are great stirred into pastas, lentils, beans, or vegetables, as a topping for hot or cold meats and vegetarian dishes, or simply as a dip or spread.

MAKES ¾ CUP OF PESTO

ACTIVE TIME: 10 MINUTES

4 cloves of garlic

⅓ cup nuts: pine nuts (traditional), cashews, almonds, pistachios, or walnuts

¾ cup basil leaves

¼ cup grated Parmesan cheese

⅓ cup good-quality olive oil

1 teaspoon salt

¼ teaspoon black pepper

Combine garlic, nuts, herbs, cheese, olive oil, salt, and pepper in a food processor and pulse until you reach your desired consistency, scraping the sides occasionally. Use immediately or store in an airtight container with an extra covering of olive oil (1 to 2 tablespoons) to keep the basil from darkening. These pestos can be frozen, too, for up to 3 months—divided into mini freezer bags or portioned into ice cube trays.

VARIATIONS

Walnut and thyme. Use walnuts as your nut choice, then add ⅓ cup thyme leaves and ¼ cup parsley leaves instead of the basil.

Holy basil (tulsi). Use pine nuts or cashews as your nut choice, then add ¼ cup holy basil leaves and ½ cup regular basil instead of the full amount of basil.

Lemon basil. Use either pine nuts, cashews, or almonds and add the juice and zest of one lemon.

UBER-SIMPLE TAHINI DRESSING

If you're not familiar with tahini, it's a Middle Eastern condiment made from ground sesame seeds. A little magic happens when you mix tahini with a little bit of cold water: first it gets thicker, then it gets whiter, and then it gradually smooths out into a luscious dressing that seems far too indulgent to be healthy. I also highly recommend adding the lemon juice—it really takes it up a notch. This dressing is super simple and quick to make.

MAKES 1 SERVING
(BUT EASILY DOUBLES, TRIPLES, QUADRUPLES . . .)
ACTIVE TIME: 5 MINUTES

1 heaped (drippy) tablespoon of tahini
3 tablespoons cold water
juice of half a lemon (optional)
½ teaspoon salt

Place the tahini into a small bowl. Slowly add the water and the lemon juice, if using, 1 tablespoon at a time, mixing each one in thoroughly. Adjust the water quantity as needed to get to your desired consistency. Stir in the salt and serve.

OMEGA-3 HONEY MUSTARD DRESSING

Flax oil adds a boost of those important omega-3 fats to this dressing and to any salad or cooked vegetables, for that matter. I also use a small amount of manuka honey, which has amazing antimicrobial properties, as do garlic and mustard. Raw apple cider vinegar contains beneficial probiotic organisms that support a healthy microbiota and happy digestion.

SERVINGS: 2

ACTIVE TIME: 10 MINUTES

¼ cup flaxseed oil

1 clove garlic, pressed or minced

½ teaspoon Dijon mustard

2 tablespoons raw apple cider vinegar

1 teaspoon manuka or other good-quality raw honey

½ teaspoon salt

Combine the flaxseed oil, garlic, mustard, vinegar, honey, and salt in a blender until emulsified and smooth. Serve either straightaway or keep in the refrigerator for 2 to 3 days.

Note: This dressing can be made easily by hand, if you prefer, by whisking the minced garlic with the Dijon mustard, apple cider vinegar, and manuka honey in a medium mixing bowl. Slowly add the flaxseed oil while continuing to whisk to a creamy emulsion. Stir in the salt and serve.

IMMUNE BONE BROTH

This recipe is one part Mama's home cooking, one part centuries-old remedy, one part modern science. Bone broth by itself is high in glutamine and for that reason is often used for healing the gut as well as nourishing you when you're feeling under the weather. In this recipe, I up the ante with the additional use of therapeutic mushrooms, astragalus root, garlic, and ginger (check Resources for sourcing tips). You'll need at least a 6-quart stockpot or slow cooker for this.

> 4 pounds organic bones (chicken or beef)
>
> 1 cup dried mushrooms (chaga, reishi, shiitake, or turkey tail, optional)
>
> 3 pieces of astragalus root (optional)
>
> 1 medium onion, skin removed and halved
>
> 5 cloves garlic, skin removed and crushed
>
> 2 inches fresh ginger root, peeled and cut into slices
>
> 1 tablespoon apple cider vinegar
>
> salt and pepper to season

Place bones, dried mushrooms, astragalus root (if using), onion, garlic, ginger, and vinegar into a large pot. Add water to cover by an inch or so. Bring to a simmer and cook on low for 8 to 12 hours for chicken bones, 24 to 32 hours for beef bones, keeping an eye on the water level and adding more water as needed. When it's done cooking, strain the stock liquid into a heat-resistant container, discard the solids, and season the liquid to taste. Serve as a hot drink or use in soups and casseroles.

HOMEMADE CLARIFIED BUTTER (GHEE)

Ghee is rendered butter fat. By heating butter, you boil off its water content and separate out the solids, leaving just the fat behind. Ghee is a rich natural source of butyrate that can supplement the butyrate produced in your gut. You can use ghee anywhere you would normally use regular butter—as a healthy cooking fat, melted over steamed vegetables, or in baking.

MAKES JUST UNDER 1 POUND

ACTIVE TIME: 45 MINUTES

1 pound good-quality organic butter from grass-fed cows

Place the butter in a medium saucepan over medium heat. Without stirring, allow the butter to melt and then begin to boil slightly. Reduce the heat to a simmer, letting the butter bubble gently. Stir intermittently.

As the water boils off, the butter should start to separate and foam. Continue to simmer for another 25 to 30 minutes until the foam is nearly all gone. The mixture will be a little more golden and slightly darker. You should be left with a clear layer on the top, and a more solid layer on the bottom. Stir only to prevent the bottom from sticking too much. Monitor the saucepan and adjust the temperature as needed so that the bottom doesn't burn.

Remove from the heat and skim any remaining foam off the top, and then pass the mixture through a cheesecloth-lined strainer to catch (and discard) the solid parts.

Carefully pour the clear oil into sterilized, airtight containers. Store in the refrigerator for up to 6 months. It will harden at cold temperatures.

BEVERAGES

A PAIR OF IMMUNE-BOOSTING TEAS

Drinking tea can be a surprisingly powerful way to add immune-supportive superfoods. The aromas teas release also work on our sinuses and airways as well as our digestive tract. Not least, the ritual of drinking tea is a perfect antidote to our modern, stressful lifestyles.

The recipes that follow are two of my favorite hot teas. One is a warming chai-inspired version, perfect for sipping on a cold day in a cozy pair of slippers and an oversized sweater. The other is light and refreshing, ideal for bright spring or summer days, or anytime you want to feel refreshed and energized.

SERVINGS: 2 LARGE MUGS
(ONE FOR NOW . . . ONE FOR LATER, OR TO SHARE)

PREPARATION TIME: 15 MINUTES

OPTION 1: WARMING

1 rooibos tea bag

1-inch piece of turmeric root, peeled and sliced, *or* ½ teaspoon ground turmeric

1 cinnamon stick, *or* ½ teaspoon ground cinnamon

½-inch piece of fresh ginger root, peeled and sliced, *or* ¼ teaspoon ground ginger

5 black peppercorns

4 cardamom pods (optional)

1 teaspoon manuka honey or ¼ teaspoon stevia (optional)

OPTION 2: REFRESHING

1 green tea bag

1 sprig fresh rosemary or ¼ teaspoon dried

1 sprig fresh thyme or ¼ teaspoon dried

½ inch fresh ginger root, peeled, or ¼ teaspoon ground ginger

rind (use a peeler to remove 3 to 4 strips) and juice of 1 small lemon

1 teaspoon manuka honey or ¼ teaspoon stevia (optional)

Measure 2 large mugs of water into a medium saucepan. Bring the water to a simmer over medium heat. Add all the ingredients of your tea to the pan, cover, and turn off the heat. Let everything steep for 10 minutes.

To serve, pour the liquid through a sieve to remove the herb and spice pieces, as well as the teabag. Then divide into two mugs and enjoy warm. The Refreshing tea also works very well as an iced tea.

GOLDEN TURMERIC MILK WITH GHEE

Golden milk is a traditional Indian drink with origins in Ayurvedic medicine. With the addition of ghee, it is a perfect anti-inflammatory, immune-regulating, and gut-nourishing combination. Plus, it's comforting and just delicious.

SERVINGS: 2

ACTIVE TIME: 10 MINUTES

2 tablespoons ghee (see recipe on page 354)

1 tablespoon honey

1 tablespoon ground turmeric

½ teaspoon ground ginger

½ teaspoon ground cinnamon

⅛ teaspoon ground black pepper

⅛ teaspoon allspice

pinch of salt

2½ cups unsweetened milk of your choice (such as dairy, almond, or coconut)

In a medium saucepan, heat the ghee until melted. Whisk in the honey, turmeric, ginger, cinnamon, pepper, allspice, salt, and milk, and continue to heat until almost boiling. Remove from the heat and strain if preferred. If you want to make your drink frothy, blend with a manual frother (as you would a cappuccino) or an immersion blender before serving.

GARDEN SPRITZER

If golden turmeric milk was made for cold, wintry days and cool evenings, this spritzer is ideal for hot days when you want to feel refreshed but still keep an eye on your immune health. Perfect to enjoy with your family and friends.

SERVINGS: 6

ACTIVE TIME: 5 MINUTES

2 lemons, sliced into rounds

2-inch stick of cucumber, sliced into rounds

1 cup mint leaves

2 cups ice

1 liter sparkling water

Mix the lemon, cucumber, mint, ice, and sparkling water in a large pitcher. Serve cold.

NO-WAIT FIRE CIDER

Fire cider is a generations-old herbal remedy that packs a huge punch of immune-boosting goodies and a good cold remedy. The trouble is that it usually takes quite some advanced planning . . . in fact, weeks of planning. This recipe delivers on potency but within just a tiny fraction of the time. Around 5 minutes, to be exact.

SERVINGS: 18

ACTIVE TIME: 5 MINUTES

1 teaspoon ground ginger

1 teaspoon onion powder

1 teaspoon garlic powder

1 teaspoon ground turmeric

1 teaspoon ground cinnamon

1 teaspoon ground cayenne pepper or horseradish powder

½ teaspoon ground black pepper

zest and juice of 1 organic lemon

1 cup raw apple cider vinegar

1 tablespoon raw, dark honey

Place the ginger, onion powder, garlic powder, turmeric, cinnamon, cayenne pepper or horseradish powder, black pepper, lemon juice and zest, vinegar, and honey in a glass jar and shake well. To use, add 1 tablespoon of the Fire Cider mixture to 5 ounces of just-boiled water. Inhale the aromas and, once it has cooled a bit, sip slowly. Take three times per day while symptoms last or to ward off winter bugs.

OATMEAL BATH SOAK

This recipe delivers on a combination of goodies for the skin microbiota, which will in turn promote skin health:

- *Glucomannan and beta-glucans, present in oats, have been identified as an important prebiotic for healthy skin microbes.*

- *Raw, unprocessed honey contains oligosaccharides, which feed healthy bacteria, as well as phytonutrient compounds such as rosmarinic acid and quercetin, which support microbial balance and skin integrity. Honey has been used in wound healing due to its ability to both stimulate immune activity and suppress excess inflammation.*

- *Lavender is a mild antimicrobial that has been found to block the activity of potentially harmful skin microbes. It also stimulates collagen renewal, wound healing, and immune activity.*

Honey and lavender oil give this recipe extra umph for sure, but if you haven't got them on hand, you can even go it alone with oats—you'll still derive all their stellar prebiotic benefits.

MAKES ENOUGH FOR 3 BATHS

3 cups rolled oats
6 tablespoons raw, dark honey (optional)
6 drops lavender essential oil (optional)

In a food processor, combine the oats, honey (if using), and lavender (if using) and pulse until the oats are coarsely ground and everything is evenly distributed. You may need to scrape down the sides intermittently. Store in the refrigerator until ready to use.

When ready to use, take 1 cup of the mixture and place it in a fine-mesh bag, tie a knot in the top, and add the whole "bag" to your bath. Soak for at least 20 minutes and then simply rinse off with fresh water as you leave the bath. Discard the used oatmeal baggie.

The mixture keeps well in the refrigerator for up to 2 weeks. Just remember to label it!

HOMEMADE ORAL RINSE

This comes together surprisingly easily and can be tweaked to meet your current oral health needs. You'll need an empty glass bottle with a screw cap (a quart jar is perfect) or other beverage container that can hold 2 cups of water and that you can run through the dishwasher on the high-heat, sterilization setting. See the Resources section for food-grade essential oils and herb powders.

2 cups boiling water

2 teaspoons baking soda

2 teaspoons granulated xylitol

10 drops peppermint essential oil *or* spearmint essential oil

OPTIONAL, FOR ADDITIONAL HEALING PROPERTIES:

For mouth sores, add 2 teaspoons marshmallow root *or* calendula flower powder.

For visibly coated tongue, add 6 to 8 dried cloves *or* 3 drops clove essential oil.

For gingivitis, add 6 to 8 drops tea tree essential oil.

For anti-plaque action, add 6 to 8 drops rosemary essential oil.

Combine the water, baking soda, xylitol, peppermint oil, and any additional optional ingredients in a heat-proof jar. Let stand for 10 minutes, stirring intermittently. Using a funnel, pour into your empty glass bottle, and allow to cool completely. That's it!

Store in the refrigerator and use within 1 to 2 weeks.

SIMPLE SKIN SALVES

Skin salves are useful for all kinds of minor skin problems. I use this one on dry skin, chapped lips, cuts and scrapes, eczema, and even on diaper rash. Essentially, the process is to infuse your oil with the herbs and let it solidify again—simple! Some recipes also call for beeswax or other kinds of cosmetics, but I only use that if I particularly want to use a more liquid oil like olive or almond.

There are so many variations of salves, but I've included my favorite base essential oil choices here. Beta-carophyllene, a cannabinoid compound in lavender and rosemary oils, has recently been shown to improve wound healing and, along with the coconut, has antimicrobial properties. Frankincense oil has a long history of use for skin rejuvenation and has anti-melanoma properties.

BASE INGREDIENTS:

4 ounces base oil (about 8 tablespoons or ½ cup, measured in liquid form)

½ ounce beeswax (about 1 tablespoon), optional, only if you live in warmer climates where the base oil you choose won't stay solid at room temperature

OPTION 1: GENERAL WOUND HEALING, MILD INFECTION, OR INSECT BITES
Choose coconut oil as your base oil.

ADDITIONAL INGREDIENTS:

3 drops rosemary essential oil

3 drops lavender essential oil

OPTION 2: ANTI-AGING

Choose shea or cacao butter as your base oil.

ADDITIONAL INGREDIENTS:

3 drops frankincense essential oil

½ teaspoon matcha green tea powder

Heat the oil in a double boiler. Add the remaining ingredients and stir well. Once the beeswax has fully melted, pour into a small, sterilized container and let cool to room temperature. Keeps for up to 1 year.

I'm guessing that you picked up this book because you were interested in doing more for your immune health, perhaps more for your health in general, and because (like me) you think there is a place for natural interventions in our health care system. I feel extraordinarily lucky to be surrounded professionally by brilliant, highly educated scientists, practitioners, and patients who also believe the same. While I fully recognize the vital role of modern medicine (and I use it without hesitation when I need it), I also know that, to have the best health (and health care) we can, we must give due weight to nutrition and lifestyle. *An exigent volume of scientific evidence, together with a health care system buckling under the burden of ever-increasing (diet- and lifestyle-driven) chronic disease, demands that we do.*

Although the seed of this book, and the material gathered for it, was planted and growing well before the COVID-19 pandemic, it was propelled forward by what felt like a real need to share this information in a timely way. My family has been touched both directly and indirectly by the spread of this virus, as have the families of just about everyone I know. It has been a stark reminder of just how important our immune defenses are in the face of new germs, especially those that take modern medicine by surprise.

But immune resilience was never just about COVID-19. Since the time infectious microbes were first recognized as disease-causing agents, we humans have had a fragile relationship with them. We know that even medical breakthroughs like vaccines and antibiotics, while they have been game changers in many ways, ultimately aren't panaceas. On top of that, most of us (myself included) have at some point or other taken our immune system for granted. We haven't appreciated just how sophisticated and complex it really is. How it affects our resilience and our ability to resist the threat of infections. The role it plays in so many chronic diseases. And, importantly, how much it is responsive to the inputs that we choose to give it.

My goal was that this book could both broaden and focus our collective thinking about what it means to support immune resilience. I am honored that you have taken the time to read it, and I also hope, as you turn these last pages, that you feel inspired, encouraged, and ultimately empowered to make good food and lifestyle choices with an understanding of how they connect with immune health.

After all, you can't predict the future, but you can be prepared for it.

The Use of Animal Research in Science

Several studies that I've cited in this book are animal-based research, and I want to fully acknowledge and address the reality that animal research generates controversy among animal rights proponents. While I don't claim to be able to live as virtuously as many amazing activists, I do consider myself a compassionate human being toward all creatures, furry or otherwise. And I have dearly loved all the animals I've known over the years—dogs, cats, horses, guinea pigs, rabbits, hamsters, birds, and others. That said, being immersed in the scientific world does give you a different perspective and understanding of the need for tests on animals to be conducted. That young child whose leg was just crushed in a car accident, that college football star with a dislocated hip, that COVID patient who needs help to keep breathing, that dog whose bowel needs urgent surgery due to a lodged piece of Lego he swallowed. Not to mention vaccines. Virtually anything a physician, paramedic, pharmacist, *or veterinarian* can use to treat their patients was only made possible by animal research. (Yes, even animals are helped by animal research.)

Animal research is essential to help scientists and practitioners understand the effectiveness and safety of any new interventions, as well as the mechanisms of both diseases and the interventions themselves. Animal research is usually a requirement of any scientific review committee (there's one of these overseeing every clinical research facility) before human studies can begin. And animal research can be the *only* research option for certain situations, such as when it comes to studying harmful agents like infectious diseases or toxins.

The bottom line is that animal research, performed as humanely as possible, is an unfortunate necessity for us to be able to help many more individuals and animals as a result.

ACKNOWLEDGMENTS

||||||||||||||||||||||||||||||||||||||||||||||||||||||||||||||

I am indebted to so many individuals who helped shape my understanding of the inner workings of our immune systems, food, and lifestyle, and made this book possible:

Thank you to the University of Bridgeport Human Nutrition Institute, the Institute for Functional Medicine, the American Nutrition Association, and the Academy of Nutrition and Dietetics for your excellent teaching and ongoing programs.

Thank you to colleagues, mentors, and educators in this field who I have learned so much from, including Sidney Baker, MD; Victoria Behm, MS, CNS; Elizabeth Bird, MD; Jeffrey Bland, PhD, CNS; Corinne Bush, MS, CNS; Stacey Cantor Adkins, MD; Kara Fitzgerald, ND; Leo Galland, MD; Sezelle Gereau, MD; Patrick Hanaway, MD; Kristi Hughes, ND; Datis Kharrazian, PhD; Liz Lipski, PhD; Kenneth Litwin, MD; Richard Lord, PhD; Robert Luby, MD; Dan Lukaczer, ND; Helen Messier, PhD; Deanna Minich, PhD; Dana Reed, MS, CNS; Robert Rountree, MD; Thomas Sult, MD; Terry Wahls, MD; Samuel Yanuck, DC; Lara Zakaria, PharmD; and Heather Zwickey, PhD.

In particular, thank you to my friend, colleague, and mentor, Kara Fitzgerald, ND, for expanding my thinking across the many facets of immune health and for encouraging me to push boundaries and step out of my comfort zone. And for always radiating a can-do, do-what-you-love attitude.

Thank you to Robert Rountree, MD, for your scientific expertise and review of this manuscript.

Thank you to Lara Zakaria, PharmD, CNS, Karen Herb, CNS, and the rest of my clinic team for holding the fort in so many ways as I took time to write.

Thank you to my agent Stephanie Tade for taking my humble book proposal and helping create this amazing opportunity for me to write and publish this book.

Thank you to Kathy Huck for your kind and patient guidance and brilliant editing. I hope to write many more books with you!

Thank you to the amazing team at Penguin Random House: Megan Newman, Lucia Watson, Suzy Swartz, Leah Marsh, Ryan Richardson, Lisa D'Agostino, Laura Corless, Tom Whatley, Alex Casement, Anne Kosmoski, Casey Maloney, and Sara Johnson, and my copyeditor and proofreader, Patricia Romanowski Bashe and Kim Lewis.

Thank you to Paul Girard for your perfect illustrations.

Thank you to my invaluable recipe tester, Karin Michalk, and to my support testers Iona Hodges, Anne Powell, Zoe Powell, and Sophie Seaman.

Thank you to Lindley Wells, CNS, for your help organizing and formatting all my (700+) references for this book.

Thank you to my husband, David Hodges, for your love, patience, and support. Thank you to Henry Hodges for your excellent analogy ideas. And thank you to our dog Aslan, who kept me company and slept on my feet throughout nearly the entire writing journey.

And thank you to all the individuals who've trusted me to walk with them on their health journey—I've learned the most from you.

RESOURCES

||||||||||||||||||||||||||||||||||||||||||

I get it. We all have busy lives, and one of the biggest obstacles that will stand in your way to becoming more resilient is feeling that you don't have the time or resources to help keep on top of things. Hopefully, this book will help with the bulk of that, but in addition, below is a curated list of products, brands, and apps that can help keep your immune system ready for anything.

NUTRITION TOOLS

- Calorie Calculator, calculator.net/calorie-calculator.html (daily calorie needs estimator)
- ConsumerLab.com, consumerlab.com (independent testing and reviews of brand name supplements)
- Cronometer, cronometer.com (nutrient intake tracking)
- Dietary Supplement Fact Sheets, ods.od.nih.gov (includes Recommended Dietary Intakes and Tolerable Upper Intake Levels for vitamins and minerals)
- Drug Interaction Checker, reference.medscape.com/drug-interactionchecker
- Drug-Nutrient Depletion Checker, mytavin.com

FOOD RESOURCES

- American Grassfed Association, americangrassfed.org (search for grassfed animal products)
- Brodo, brodo.com (organic bone broth)

- Eat Wild, eatwild.com (search for pastured meat, eggs, and dairy products)
- EPA Fish and Shellfish Advisories, epa.gov/fish-tech (provides information about fish and shellfish contamination including mercury and PCBs by region)
- Frontier Natural Products Co-op, frontiercoop.com (organic herbs and spices)
- Green Chef, greenchef.com (meal kits made with organic, whole foods)
- Local Harvest, localharvest.org (search for local farms and community-supported agriculture [CSA] programs)
- Lundberg Family Farms, lundberg.com (organic rice products tested to be free of arsenic contamination)
- Melissa's/World Variety Produce, melissas.com (organic fresh fruit and vegetable delivery)
- Numi, numitea.com (organic herbal teas)
- Pacific Botanicals, pacificbotanicals.com (organic herbs and spices, sea vegetables)
- Pete's Paleo, petespaleo.com (meal delivery service using fresh, whole foods)
- Sunbasket, sunbasket.com (meal kits made with organic, whole foods)
- The Osso Good Co., ossogood.life (organic bone broth)
- Thrive Market, thrivemarket.com (organic food brands at lower prices, including good options for dark chocolate and bone and vegetable broths)
- Traditional Medicinals, traditionalmedicinals.com (organic herbal teas)
- US Wellness Meats, grasslandbeef.com (grass-fed and pasture-raised meats and poultry, and wild-caught seafood)
- Vital Choice, vitalchoice.com (wild-caught fish, shellfish, and more)
- Wild Alaskan Company, wildalaskancompany.com (sustainable wild-caught fish)

DIETARY SUPPLEMENT SUPPLIERS

The following are available through many retail health stores and online:

- Banyan Botanicals, banyanbotanicals.com (great for quality bulk-buy turmeric, teas, and more)
- Carlson Products, carlsonlabs.com (especially good for fish oils and plant-based DHA)
- Culturelle, culturelle.com (widely available, researched probiotics)
- Feel Good Organics, fgorganics.com (teas, herbs, and spices)
- Gaia Herbs, gaiaherbs.com (I especially like their black elderberry, echinacea, and astragalus products)
- Garden of Life, gardenoflife.com (good, easily available, and with a wide product line)
- Mountain Rose Herbs, mountainroseherbs.com (good for bulk herbs, like astragalus root, and cosmetic ingredients)
- Mushroom Harvest, mushroomharvest.com (source for medicinal mushrooms)
- Naked Nutrition, nakednutrition.com (for their organic brown rice protein powder)
- Natural Vitality Calm, naturalvitality.com (especially their Natural Vitality Calm® Sleep)
- Nature's Way, naturesway.com (especially for their Bronchial Soothe Ivy Leaf Extract)
- New Chapter, newchapter.com (good-quality multivitamins and more)
- Nordic Naturals, nordicnaturals.com (especially good for omega-3s)
- Now Foods, nowfoods.com (a solid all-around supplement company that's widely available)
- Omega Nutrition, omeganutrition.com (for their organic pumpkin seed protein powder)
- Salus Haus, salus-haus.com (excellent herbal tonic combinations)

The following are available through practitioners only, whom you can ask for these brands specifically. Each stocks a wide range of useful products from multivitamins, vitamins, and minerals to herbs and protein powders.

- Bio-Botanical Research, biocidin.com (I regularly use their herbal antimicrobial Biocidin products which come in capsules, drops, toothpaste, and throat spray)
- Biotics Research, bioticsresearch.com
- Designs for Health, designsforhealth.com
- Douglas Labs, douglaslabs.com
- Innate Response Formulas, innateresponse.com
- Integrative Therapeutics, integrativepro.com
- Klaire Labs, klaire.com (especially good for probiotics)
- Metagenics, metagenics.com
- Pure Encapsulations, pureencapsulations.com
- Thorne, thorne.com
- Xymogen, xymogen.com

ESSENTIAL OIL SUPPLIERS
- DoTerra, doterra.com
- Mountain Rose Herbs, mountainroseherbs.com
- Young Living, youngliving.com (I especially like their antimicrobial blend "Thieves")

FASTING RESOURCES
- ProLon®, prolonfast.com (Fasting Mimicking Diet®)

ADVANCED MEDICAL AND NUTRITION LABORATORY TESTING
The following sites are good resources for a list of advanced testing available to determine immune health, nutrient status, toxin load, metabolic activity, and more. They also offer "find a practitioner" services. It is important to work with a qualified practitioner to help you interpret test results.

- Diagnostic Solutions Laboratory, diagnosticsolutionslab.com
- Doctor's Data, doctorsdata.com
- Genova Diagnostics, gdx.net
- Great Plains Laboratory, greatplainslaboratory.com
- KBMO Diagnostics, kbmodiagnostics.com
- Precision Analytical, dutchtest.com
- Precision Point Diagnostics, precisionpointdiagnostics.com
- Thorne HealthTech, thorne.com
- US Biotek, usbiotek.com
- Vibrant Wellness, vibrant-wellness.com

NONPRESCRIPTION SOURCES OF CONTINUOUS GLUCOSE MONITORS (CGMs)

At the time of this writing, CGMs are mostly only available with a prescription. The following services, though on the expensive side, offer a nonprescription route where CGM testing is combined with nutritional counseling. These may still be valuable for some individuals.

- January, january.ai
- Levels, levelshealth.com
- NutriSense, nutrisense.io
- Signos, signos.com

FIND A NATURAL HEALTH PROFESSIONAL TO WORK WITH

These websites have useful "Find a Practitioner" sections:

- The American Nutrition Association, theana.org (for personalized nutrition practitioners)
- The Institute for Functional Medicine, ifm.org (for functional medicine practitioners)

RESOURCES FOR PERSONAL CARE AND BEAUTY

- Lotion Crafter, lotioncrafter.com (for their ceramide complex)
- Making Cosmetics, makingcosmetics.com (ingredients for homemade personal care products)

- Mountain Rose Herbs (for their beeswax and more)
- Skin Deep, ewg.org/skindeep (independent analysis of the safety of personal care product ingredients)
- Whole Foods Market, wholefoodsmarket.com Beauty and Body Care Department

RESOURCES FOR A HEALTHIER HOME ENVIRONMENT

- 3M Lead Check Swabs, available at hardware stores and online (instant lead tests)
- Aizome, aizomebedding.com (zero synthetic chemicals, organic bedding)
- Aquasana, aquasana.com (water filtration with activated carbon)
- Austin Air, austinair.com (air purifiers)
- Blue Air, blueair.com (air purifiers)
- Charlie's Soap, charliesoap.com (nontoxic laundry and household cleaner)
- Cora Ball, coraball.com (a laundry ball that catches plastic microfibers so they can be disposed of properly)
- Greenguard Certified, ul.com/resources/ul-greenguard-certification-program (building materials, furniture, furnishings, and equipment that meets determined toxin emissions limits)
- H_2O at Home, us.h2oathome.com (natural cleaning products, including those that work with just water)
- IQ Air, iqair.com (air purifiers)
- Molekule, molekule.com (air purifiers)
- Multipure, multipure.com (water filtration with activated carbon)
- My Chemical-Free House, mychemicalfreehouse.net (resource for nontoxic interiors)
- National Testing Laboratories, watercheck.com (water testing)
- Organic and Healthy Inc., organicandhealthy.com (resource for nontoxic interiors)
- Slo Active, sloactive.com (plastic-free swimwear)
- Tap Score, mytapscore.com (water testing)

- The National Lead Laboratory Accreditation Program (NLLAP), https://www.epa.gov/lead/national-lead-laboratory-accreditation-program-nllap (source for finding accredited lead-testing laboratories)
- University Soil Testing Programs, various (many colleges and universities offer low-cost soil-testing programs including for toxic metals like arsenic and lead)

RESOURCES FOR EXERCISE, STRESS, AND SLEEP MANAGEMENT
- Apple Watch, apple.com/watch (exercise, stress, and sleep tracker)
- Calm, for iOS and Android devices (sleep and meditation app)
- Fitbit, fitbit.com (exercise, stress, and sleep tracking)
- Flux, justgetflux.com (software that reduces blue light emissions from personal computing devices)
- Headspace, for iOS and Android devices (meditation app)
- HeartMath, heartmath.com (heart rate variability monitor)
- Oura Ring, ouraring.com (wearable health tracker that measures heart rate variability, sleep, physical activity, and more)
- The Tapping Solution, for iOS and Android devices (app for guided Tapping meditations)
- Thich Nhat Hanh, Buddhist monk and author (books such as *Peace Is Every Breath*, published by HarperOne, reprinted 2011).

More resources can also be found at immuneresilienceplan.com.